Self-Assessment Color Review
Small Animal Clinical Oncology

Self-Assessment Color Review

Small Animal Clinical Oncology

Joyce E. Obradovich
DVM, DACVIM (Oncology)
Animal Center and Imaging Center
Canton, MI, USA

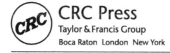

CRC Press
Taylor & Francis Group
Boca Raton London New York

CRC Press is an imprint of the
Taylor & Francis Group, an **informa** business

Dedication

This book is dedicated to the memory of my father, David Obradovich, and to my mother, Eileen Obradovich, and my daughter, Diana Obradovich, whose love and endless support throughout my lifetime allowed me to pursue my passion.

CRC Press
Taylor & Francis Group
6000 Broken Sound Parkway NW, Suite 300
Boca Raton, FL 33487-2742

© 2017 by Taylor & Francis Group, LLC
CRC Press is an imprint of Taylor & Francis Group, an Informa business

No claim to original U.S. Government works

Printed on acid-free paper
Version Date: 20160607

International Standard Book Number-13: 978-1-4822-2539-6 (Paperback)

Visit the Taylor & Francis Web site at
http://www.taylorandfrancis.com

and the CRC Press Web site at
http://www.crcpress.com

Contents

Preface

Cancer is a leading natural cause of death in dogs and cats. Despite the fear and emotions that the word cancer invokes, it is not always an automatic death sentence. Cancer is not just one disease, as it is often perceived, but hundreds of diseases with different treatments and entirely different outcomes. Many forms of cancers can be cured and many can be effectively treated, resulting in extension of a good quality of life. For those patients whose cancers are too advanced or aggressive to treat, palliative therapies can be very beneficial. Maintaining quality of life should always be our principal focus in the practice of veterinary oncology.

This book is a compilation of a wide variety of clinical oncology cases that challenge the reader to make decisions regarding diagnosis, staging, and treatment. There are also cases presented that explore palliative therapeutic options or more conservative alternatives for pet owners not able to pursue definitive or curative–intent treatments. Veterinary oncology is a rapidly expanding field of medicine in which information is constantly changing and evolving. While every attempt has been made to provide the most up to date information, the reader needs to be aware that a new study or clinical trial conducted subsequent to the publication of this text could dramatically change the standard of care for a particular type of cancer. For this reason, I would encourage the practitioner to use the information presented here as a guideline, but to keep current on the latest information available for a particular cancer type through reviewing recent journals and publications. It is also important to realize that each tumor type and clinical situation may not be represented in the literature, and therefore consultation with specialists in the field to explore their clinical experience can be very rewarding. I have tried to present information in the most objective manner possible supported by peer-reviewed publications, but invariably there are biases in the approach to case management that are based in the oncologists' training and personal experiences.

I hope that the veterinary practitioner finds this book a resource for their medical practice and that the veterinary student, intern, or resident find it a useful study tool.

Joyce E. Obradovich

Acknowledgments

The author would like to thank Dr. Richard Walshaw, DACVS, and Dr. Marta Agrodnia, DACVS, for performing the surgical procedures pictured in this book; Dr. Michael Wolf, DACVIM (Neurology), for providing the MRI studies and neurologic assessments; and Dr. Matti Kiupel, PhD, DACVP, and the Michigan State University Diagnostic Center for Population and Animal Health for the photomicrographs of biopsy specimens and for performing and interpreting all immunohistochemistry. The limb salvage procedure in Case 113 was performed by Dr. Stephen Withrow, DACVS, DACVIM (Oncology), at the Colorado State University Flint Animal Cancer Center.

Abbreviations

ABC	aneurysmal bone cyst
ASGAC	anal sac gland adenocarcinoma
ALP	alkaline phosphatase
ALT	alanine aminotransferase
BCC	basal cell carcinoma
BCT	basal cell tumor
BTA	bladder tumor antigen
BUN	blood urea nitrogen
CBC	complete blood count
CEOT	calcifying epithelial odontogenic tumor
CLL	chronic lymphocytic leukemia
CNS	central nervous system
CHOP	cyclophosphamide, doxorubicin (hydroxydaunomycin), Oncovin® (vincristine), prednisone
COP	Cytoxan® (cyclophosphamide), Oncovin® (vincristine), prednisone
COX	cyclooxygenase
CR	complete response/ complete remission
CSA	chondrosarcoma
CT	computed tomography
CTCL	cutaneous T cell lymphoma
DFI	disease-free interval
DIC	disseminated intravascular coagulation
DLH	domestic longhaired (cat)
DNA	deoxyribonucleic acid
DSH	domestic shorthaired (cat)
ECG	electrocardiogram/ electrocardiography
EG	eosinophilic granuloma
EMP	extramedullary plasmacytoma
FeLV	feline leukemia virus
FIP	feline infectious peritonitis
FISS	feline injection site sarcoma
FIV	feline immunodeficiency virus
FNA	fine needle aspirate/ aspiration
FPH	feline progressive histiocytosis
FSA	fibrosarcoma
GCMB	granular cell myoblastoma
GGT	gamma-glutamyltransferase
GI	gastrointestinal
GIST	gastrointestinal stromal tumor
Gy	Gray
HA	hyaluronic acid
H & E	hematoxylin and eosin
HO	hypertrophic osteopathy
HPC	hemangiopericytoma
hpf	high power field
HS	histiocytic sarcoma
HSA	hemangiosarcoma
IC	intracavitary
ICC	immunocytochemistry
IHC	immunohistochemistry
IMC	inflammatory mammary carcinoma
IV	intravenous/intravenously
LCH	Langerhans' cell histiocytosis
LGL	large granular lymphoma
L-MTP-PE	liposomal muramyl tripeptide phosphatidylethanolamine
MC	metronomic chemotherapy
MCT	mast cell tumor

MCUP — metastatic cancer of unknown primary
MDB — minimum database
MG — myasthenia gravis
MI — mitotic index
MLO — multilobular osteochondrosarcoma
MM — malignant melanoma
MRI — magnetic resonance imaging
MST — median survival time
MTD — maximum tolerated dose
NSAID — non-steroidal anti-inflammatory drug
OHE — ovariohysterectomy
OMM — oral malignant melanoma
OSA — osteosarcoma
PAHS — periarticular histiocytic sarcoma
PARR — PCR for antigen receptor rearrangements
PCR — polymerase chain reaction
PCV — packed cell volume
PDGFR — platelet-derived growth factor receptor
PEG — percutaneous endoscopically placed gastrostomy
PET — positron emission tomography
PFI — progression-free interval
PFS — progression-free survival
PKD — polycystic kidney disease
PNST — peripheral nerve sheath tumor
PR — partial response/partial remission
PTHrP — parathyroid hormone-related peptide
PU/PD — polyuria/polydipsia
RBC — red blood cell

RT — radiation therapy
RTK — receptor tyrosine kinase
SBC — simple bone cyst
SCC — squamous cell carcinoma
SD — stable disease
SOP — solitary osseous plasmacytoma
SRT — stereotactic radiotherapy
STS — soft tissue sarcoma
SVAP — subcutaneous vascular access port
T3 — thyroxine
T4 — triiodothyronine
TCC — transitional cell carcinoma
TDC — thyroglossal duct cyst
TECA — total ear canal ablation
TECABO — total ear canal ablation and bulla osteotomy
TKI — tyrosine kinase inhibitor
Treg — regulatory T cell
TSH — thyroid stimulating hormone
TVT — transmissible venereal tumor
UA — urinalysis
US — ultrasound
UVB — ultraviolet B (short wave) rays
VD — ventrodorsal
VEGFR — vascular endothelial growth factor receptor
WBC — white blood cell
WHO — World Health Organization

MDB (minimum database)

Dogs: CBC, serum chemistry panel, urinalysis, and thoracic radiographs (3 views)

Cats: CBC, serum chemistry panel, urinalysis, retroviral testing (FeLV, FIV), and thoracic radiographs (3 views)

Broad classification of cases

Note: Some cases appear under more than one category.

Anal/anal gland
56, 98, 121, 133

Cardiovascular
96, 140

Chemotherapy/drugs
12, 57, 58, 158, 161, 162, 170, 187

Dermatologic
11, 26, 41, 53, 71, 74, 91, 92, 93, 99, 105, 137, 147, 160, 181, 185

Endocrine
18, 19, 75, 157, 171, 177

Gastrointestinal
141, 143, 174, 175, 177, 179, 186, 200

Head and neck
46, 115, 116, 126, 132, 157

Hemangiosarcoma
3, 61, 87, 135

Histiocytic diseases
27, 80, 136, 181, 198

Liver/pancreas
9, 35, 54, 70, 94

Lymphoid/hematopoietic
5, 29, 36, 41, 52, 59, 101, 107, 110, 112, 130, 133, 143, 155, 160, 169, 174, 180, 184, 185, 186, 190, 193, 194, 196, 202

Mast cell tumors
11, 17, 62, 77, 120, 123, 147, 188, 199

Melanoma
1, 28, 44, 53, 64, 67, 89, 99, 114, 137, 156, 192

Metastatic disease
45, 63, 87, 102, 117, 146

Miscellaneous
7, 10, 14, 33, 34, 37, 38, 50, 78, 81, 103, 109, 129, 131, 139, 142, 145, 168

Musculoskeletal
13, 16, 21, 24, 25, 39, 43, 45, 60, 72, 73, 90, 113, 124, 126, 132, 138, 150, 163, 183, 192, 201

Nasal/nasal planum
27, 49, 79, 93, 106, 118, 130, 152, 172

Neurologic
30, 90, 149, 173, 182, 190

Ocular/periocular
40, 97, 100, 105, 109, 114, 169

Oral cavity
1, 2, 8, 16, 20, 22, 28, 67, 73, 76, 83, 84, 88, 89, 99, 110, 111, 115, 153, 183, 191

Paraneoplastic syndromes
9, 42, 48, 58, 101, 144, 148, 159, 165, 203

CASE 1 A 12-year-old neutered male Yorkshire Terrier presents because of a recent onset of oral bleeding and a foul odor from the mouth. The patient is otherwise healthy, but has stopped eating and playing with his toys. On physical examination, a large, ulcerated, infected flesh colored mass is present. The peripheral lymph nodes are normal and there are no other significant findings on physical examination. Under anesthesia, the mass is seen to extend from in front of the right canine tooth, crosses the midline past the second incisor tooth on the left, and measures 2.5 × 3 × 2 cm. This radiograph was taken while the patient was under anesthesia (**1**).

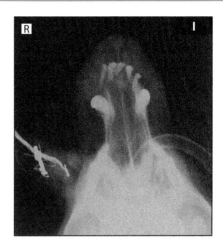

1 What are the radiographic findings?
2 What diagnostic tests should be performed prior to a treatment decision?
3 The biopsy revealed an undifferentiated sarcoma. What further information should be gained from the tissue sample?
4 What further staging tests are recommended in light of the histopathology results?
5 What type of surgery and postoperative therapy are indicated for this patient?

CASE 2 A 9-year-old neutered male Shetland Sheepdog presented after the owner noted a foul odor coming from the mouth and bleeding from the oral cavity (**2a**).

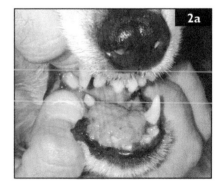

1 What are the primary differential diagnoses for this patient?
2 A biopsy revealed acanthomatous ameloblastoma. What further diagnostic tests should be performed in assessing this patient for treatment?
3 Surgery is the primary recommendation for this patient but the owner is not willing to consider mandibulectomy. What other therapeutic option has the greatest chance for control/cure of disease?

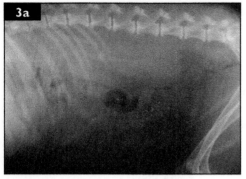

3a

CASE 3 A 12-year-old neutered male Flat Coated Retriever presented for a vague history of intermittent anorexia and weakness in the hind end. Clinical signs were initially thought to be due to arthritis. On physical examination he was noted to have slightly pale mucous membranes and a palpable mid-abdominal mass. Thoracic radiographs were normal. An abdominal radiograph (3a), blood work, and urine specific gravity are shown.

1 Describe the radiograph and blood work. What is the probable anatomic location of the mass and how should this be confirmed?
2 List the differential diagnoses.
3 What further diagnostic tests are indicated to formulate a treatment plan?
4 What is the prognosis for this patient?

Test	Result	Flag	Units	Normal Range
Chemistry Panel				
BUN	48.4	High	mg/dl	9.0–29.0
Creatinine	0.9		mg/dl	0.4–1.4
Phosphorus	4.0		mg/dl	1.9–5.0
Calcium	10.3		mg/dl	9.0–12.2
Corrected Ca	11.2		mg/dl	9.0–12.2
Total Protein	5.7		g/dl	5.5–7.6
Albumin	2.6		g/dl	2.5–4.0
Globulin	2.7		g/dl	2.0–3.6
Alb/Glob Ratio	1.0			
Glucose	109		mg/dl	75–125
Cholesterol	279		mg/dl	120–310
ALT (GPT)	65		U/l	0–120
ALP	112		U/l	0–140
GGT	12		U/l	0–14
Total Bilirubin	0.1		mg/dl	0.0–0.5

Test	Result	Flag	Units	Normal Range
Hematology				
WBC	21.2	High	10³/µl	6.0–17.0
LYM	2.5		10³/µl	1.2–5.0
MONO	2.2	High	10³/µl	0.3–1.5
GRAN	16.5	High	10³/µl	3.5–12.0
LYM%	12.2			
MONO%	10.1			
GRAN%	77.7			
HCT	28.7	Low	%	37.0–55.0
MCV	68.6		fl	60.0–72.0
RDWa	47.7		fl	35.0–53.0
RDW%	15.8		%	11.0–16.0
HGB	10.2	Low	g/dl	12.0–18.0
MCHC	35.6		g/dl	32.0–38.5
MCH	24.4		pg	19.5–25.5
RBC	4.19	Low	10⁶/µl	5.50–8.50
PLT	184	Low	10³/µl	200–500
MPV	8.2		fl	5.5–10.5

Urine specific gravity = 1.025

CASE 4 A 3 cm bleeding and ulcerated mass was noted in the right second mammary gland of a 10-year-old spayed female DLH cat. The mass had been present for up to 2 years, but had recently shown evidence of more rapid growth (**4a**).

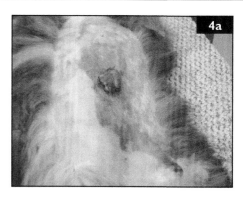

1 What is the likelihood that this mammary mass is malignant?
2 In addition to the MDB, should any further tests be performed?
3 What type of surgery is recommended for this patient?
4 Is postoperative therapy advised?
5 What are the most important prognostic factors for this disease?

CASE 5 A 10-year-old neutered male Standard Poodle developed a mass on the mucocutaneous junction near the lower right canine tooth (**5a, b**). There are also reddened areas along the lips and gum line of the upper jaw and depigmentation/discoloration below the right nostril. He had been sneezing and snorting and an occasional bloody discharge from the nasal cavity was also noted. The physical examination, other than the oral cavity and nasal abnormalities, is normal. A biopsy revealed epitheliotropic lymphoma or "mycosis fungoides". Immunohistochemistry revealed a predominance of CD8+ T cells.

1 What is the natural course of this disease?
2 What additional tests should be performed for staging on this patient?
3 What treatment options are available and what is the prognosis?

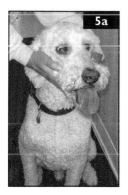
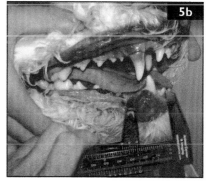

CASE 6 Shown here are lateral (**6a**) and ventrodorsal (**6b**) views of the thorax of a 12-year-old neutered male DSH cat. He was presented for occasional gagging and coughing. The physical examination was normal.

1 What is the abnormality shown in the radiographs?
2 What are the most common differential diagnoses for this patient?
3 How should the diagnosis be confirmed?
4 The ultrasound of the mass (**6c**) and fluid obtained from an FNA (**6d**) are shown. What is the diagnosis?
5 What therapy is indicated?

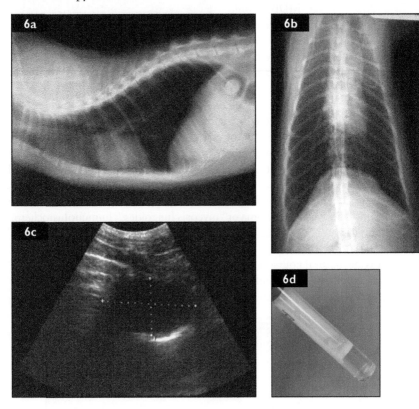

CASE 7 A 5-year-old neutered male DSH cat was presented because of a mass on his back noted within 1 month after vaccination. Approximately 2 months after vaccination, the mass was continuing to grow and the patient had been lethargic and his appetite was decreased. On examination, the patient was febrile (103.5°F; 39.7°C) and had a firm, 3.5 cm subcutaneous mass over the left thoracolumbar area (**7a, b**). The remainder of the physical examination was normal.

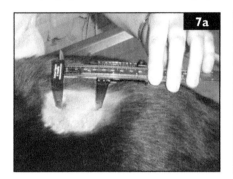
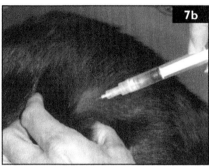

1 What are the major differential diagnoses for this patient?
2 What diagnostic tests can be easily performed to obtain a presumptive diagnosis?
3 What considerations for future vaccination should be made for this patient?

CASE 8 A 9-year-old neutered male German Shepherd Dog mix (34 kg) was noted to have ptyalism. Physical examination revealed this ulcerated and infected caudal mandibular mass (**8**). The mass measured 6 × 4 cm. The left submandibular lymph node was prominent (2 cm).

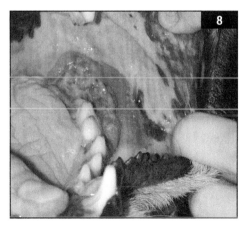

1 What are the differential diagnoses for this patient?
2 What further staging tests should be included in the evaluation of this patient?
3 What treatment options are available for this patient?
4 What is the prognosis for this patient?

CASE 9 A 9-year-old neutered male DSH cat was referred because of a 5-month history of progressing hindlimb muscle wasting, anorexia, weight loss, and intermittent vomiting. Within the past month, alopecia of the whisker pads, lip margins, ventrum, and medial hindlimbs had developed (**9a, b**). The skin appeared erythematous and "glistening" and the hair fell out readily when touched. The feet appeared to be painful owing to changes in the nail beds. The remainder of the physical examination was unremarkable. The patient had not received any medications. The CBC, serum chemistry panel, and urinalysis were within normal limits. Thoracic radiographs were normal. Abdominal ultrasound revealed a 1.5 × 1.2 cm right cranial abdominal mass.

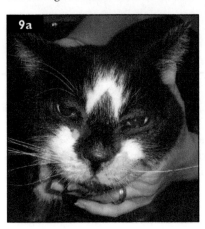
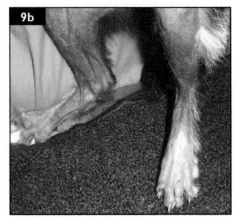

1 Based on the clinical presentation, what are the primary differential diagnoses for the cranial abdominal mass?
2 What is the best way to make a diagnosis and potentially treat this patient?
3 What is the prognosis for this patient?

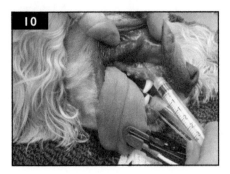

CASE 10

1 What procedure is being performed (**10**)?
2 What are the analgesic benefits?

CASE 11 Cytology from a fine needle aspirate of the hairless cutaneous lesion on the head of this 8-year-old spayed female DSH cat (**11a**) is shown (**11b**). The patient is otherwise healthy with no other lesions noted.

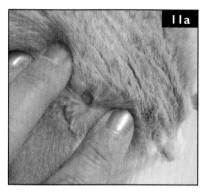
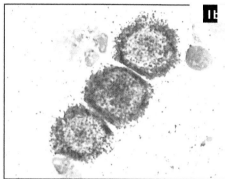

1 What is the cytologic diagnosis?
2 What are the two histologic forms of this disease?
3 How should this patient be managed?
4 What histologic parameter provides the most information regarding the potential for recurrence or metastasis?

CASE 12 The use of lomustine (CCNU) (**12**) for a variety of cancers is becoming increasingly popular. Ease of administration and lower cost of treatment in comparison with most intravenous chemotherapy agents make it a desirable choice for many pet owners.

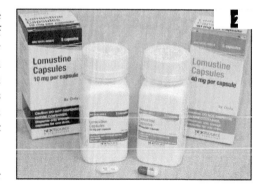

1 What are the indications for using the pictured drug?
2 What is the mechanism of action of CCNU?
3 What are the side effects commonly associated with lomustine and how can they be alleviated?
4 What characteristic does this drug possess that is seen in very few chemotherapeutic agents?

CASE 13 An 11-year-old neutered male Weimaraner presented for an acute onset of non-weightbearing lameness and swelling of the hock (tibiotarsal) joint (**13a, b**). The patient is otherwise clinically normal with no history of penetrating trauma, draining tract wounds, or previous surgery at the site.

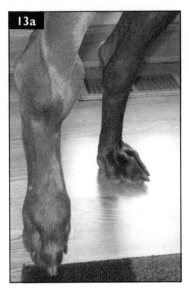
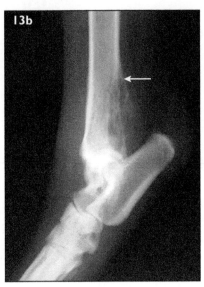

1 Describe the radiographic findings. What specific structure is the arrow pointing to?
2 What are the differential diagnoses?
3 What diagnostic tests are indicated?
4 Describe both definitive and palliative treatment options for this patient.
5 What are negative prognostic indicators for this disease?

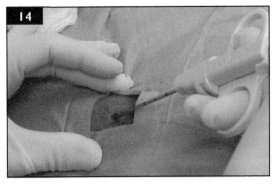

CASE 14

1 What procedure is being shown (**14**)?
2 What are the indications for this procedure?
3 What are the limitations of this procedure?
4 What are the potential complications?

CASE 15 A 3-year-old spayed female chocolate Labrador Retriever was noted to have a small soft mass on the sternum/manubrium area about 6 months prior to presentation. The referring veterinarian clinically diagnosed a lipoma and advised monitoring. The mass continued to grow and a tissue biopsy revealed an undifferentiated sarcoma, with soft tissue osteosarcoma considered likely.

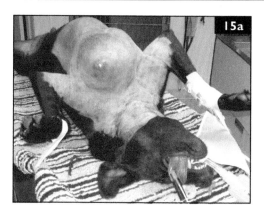

At the time of referral, the mass measured 13 × 14 × 8 cm and was loosely attached to the underlying tissues (**15a**).

1 What immunohistochemical (IHC) stains could help confirm soft tissue osteosarcoma in this patient?
2 In addition to a MDB, what staging tests should be performed?
3 What therapeutic recommendations can be made?
4 What is the probability for metastasis in this patient and what factors are present that indicate a poorer outcome?

CASE 16 An 11-year-old spayed female DSH cat had a 2-month history of sneezing, with a worsening mucopurulent discharge from the right nostril. Symptoms initially resolved with azithromycin but returned 2 months later. On recurrence, the nasal discharge was blood tinged. There was no improvement after a second course of antibiotics. The patient was then referred for a suspected nasal tumor. On physical examination, the right maxilla was slightly swollen and

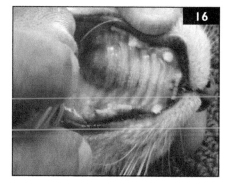

painful to the touch. Ventral deviation of the hard and soft palate was visible on oral examination (**16**). The suspected mass crossed the midline.

1 What is an appropriate diagnostic plan?
2 What therapeutic options can be considered?

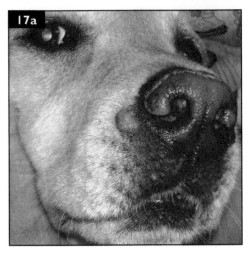

CASE 17 An 8-year-old neutered male Labrador Retriever developed a cutaneous mass on the right muzzle near the nostril (**17a**). It was initially thought to be due to a bug bite and regressed with antihistamine therapy. When growth was again noted, a fine needle aspirate yielded moderately differentiated mast cells. Regional lymph nodes were normal, no other masses were present, and the MDB was normal. Abdominal ultrasound showed no evidence of disease.

1 What therapeutic options offer the best chance of long-term control?
2 How does the location of this tumor impact the prognosis?

CASE 18 Pictured (**18a**) is a CT scan of a 9-year-old spayed female Staffordshire Terrier mix with a suspected thyroid tumor. The owner had noted a small mass approximately 1 year prior to referral that appeared to remain stable until about

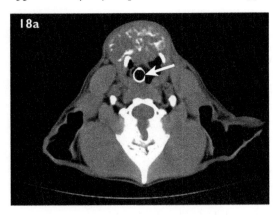

1 month prior to referral. Excessive panting and harsher breathing sounds were noted. On presentation, a firm mass was palpated on the ventral midline of the neck caudal to the larynx. The mass was somewhat moveable but was partially adhered to the underlying structures. An MDB was performed and was normal. A CT scan was advised.

1 Describe the CT findings. What structure is the arrow pointing to?
2 In addition to the MDB, what further staging tests should be performed?
3 What therapies can be considered for this patient?

CASE 19 A 7-year-old neutered male Shih Tzu had a several-month history of bilateral neck masses in the region of the thyroid glands. A fine needle aspirate had been performed and, although very bloody, was suggestive of thyroid carcinoma. On physical examination, the left-sided mass measured 5.5 cm and

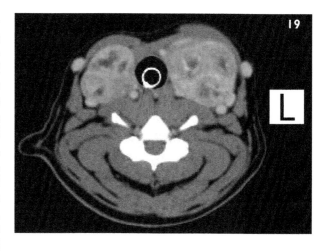

the right 3.8 cm. Both masses were fixed to underlying tissue in the jugular furrow. The patient was otherwise normal. An MDB and thyroid panel (T3, T4, TSH, thyroglobulin autoantibodies) were normal. The CT scan is shown (**19**).

1 Describe the CT scan.
2 What other therapy could be offered for this patient?
3 How common are bilateral thyroid tumors?
4 What is the rate of metastasis seen in bilateral thyroid carcinoma?
5 What potential complications exist for bilateral thyroidectomy?

CASE 20 A 7-year-old neutered male Retriever/Shepherd mix (34 kg) presented because of increasing difficulty eating. The owners noted a large mass on the tongue that seemed to have had an acute onset (**20a**).

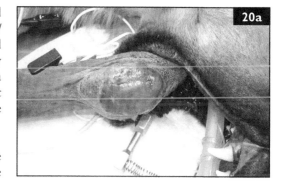

1 Based on the appearance of the mass, what are the differential diagnoses?
2 Is surgery an option?
3 What is the likely outcome for this patient?

11

CASE 21 A 10-year-old neutered male Border Collie mix presented 1 year following a conservative and incomplete surgical excision of a grade I multilobular tumor of bone (formerly known as multilobular osteochondrosarcoma, or MLO). No further treatment was advised at that time. The tumor had regrown to the extent shown in (**21a**). The patient was not able to see, based on the physical obstruction of vision due to the growing tumor. The patient was otherwise healthy and the MDB normal. A CT scan was performed and is shown (**21b**).

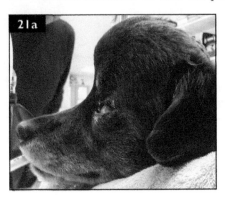

1 Describe the CT scan.
2 What therapeutic options exist for this patient?
3 What are the most important prognostic factors for this type of tumor?

CASE 22 A 9-year-old neutered male Boxer/Shepherd mix developed severe ptyalism and dysphagia. A rapidly growing mass was seen on the ventral aspect of the tongue (**22**). The mass was ulcerated and proliferative, involving the ventral surface of the tongue and the junction of the tongue with the frenulum bilaterally. Full-thickness erosion through the tongue on the left was noted. Submandibular lymph nodes were not palpable and an MDB was unremarkable.

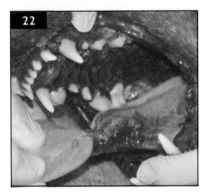

1 What is the most common tumor type observed in the canine tongue?
2 What are the criteria for surgical resection of tongue tumors?
3 Is this patient a candidate for surgery?
4 What is the prognosis for this patient?

CASE 23 A 10-year-old neutered male Shetland Sheepdog mix had a recent onset of hematuria and pollakiuria. He was treated initially for a suspected urinary tract infection. The symptoms resolved, but recurred within 3 weeks of stopping antibiotics. At the time of recurrence of symptoms, the hematuria had worsened. An ultrasound of the bladder was performed (**23**).

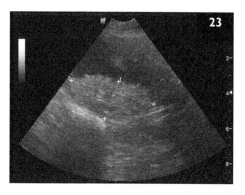

1 Describe the ultrasound findings. What is the likely diagnosis?
2 What staging tests should be performed and how should the diagnosis be confirmed?
3 What procedures should be avoided when attempting to obtain a diagnosis?
4 How should this patient be treated?

CASE 24 A 10-year-old Shepherd mix (37 kg) presented for a painful, swollen third digit on the left front paw. It was initially treated with antibiotics owing to the suspicion of an infection but actually worsened (**24a**). Radiographs were taken, which revealed extreme lysis of P3 and concern for lysis extending into P2 (**24b**).

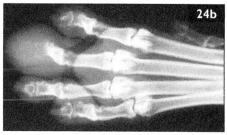

1 What diagnostic and staging tests should be performed on this patient prior to treatment recommendations?
2 What is the most common digital tumor seen in dogs? What are the other differential diagnoses?
3 What therapy is advised and what is the prognosis for this patient?

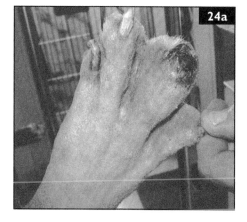

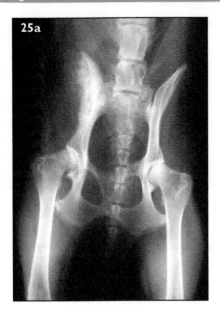

CASE 25 This ventrodorsal radiographic view of the pelvis (**25a**) is from a 10-year-old spayed female mixed breed dog (23 kg), presented for a 1-month history of progressive lameness in the right hindlimb. There was a firm "lump" palpated over the right hip.

1 Describe the radiograph and list the differential diagnoses.
2 What further diagnostic tests should be performed?
3 What therapeutic options are available for this patient and what is the prognosis?

CASE 26 This is the picture of a non-healing surgical wound on a 7-year-old neutered male Coonhound (**26a**). A small (1 cm) mass had been noted on the metatarsal pad approximately 1 year prior to referral. The dog would favor his paw occasionally, but the owner assumed there had been some form of trauma. The mass continued

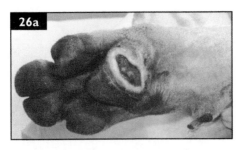

to grow and was approximately 3 cm when the primary care veterinarian attempted an excisional biopsy. Histopathology revealed soft tissue sarcoma, intermediate grade, with all surgical margins showing tumor cells present. The surgical incision dehisced and the patient was referred for further therapy.

1 What further diagnostic tests are necessary in this patient?
2 Assuming localized disease only, what is the best way to control disease or cure this patient?
3 What are the primary concerns with removal of the metatarsal pad in dogs?
4 What non-surgical treatment could be considered?
5 If tumor-free margins are not achieved, what further therapy could be considered?

CASE 27 A 9-year-old spayed female calico cat presented with a 3-month history of crusting and scabbing of the nose (**27**). Pruritus was not observed. The remainder of the physical examination was normal.

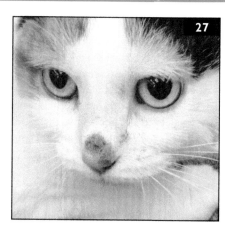

1 What are the differential diagnoses for this lesion?
2 A biopsy was performed and the histopathologic diagnosis was feline progressive histiocytosis (FPH). What is the expected clinical course of this disease?
3 What treatment should be recommended?

CASE 28 An 11-year-old, 22.7 kg mixed breed dog presented for a routine wellness examination. On physical examination, a mass was noted in the hard palate (**28a**, arrows). A fine needle aspirate was performed and the cytology is shown (**28b**). There were no clinical symptoms to report and the patient was thought to be normal. The remainder of the examination was normal.

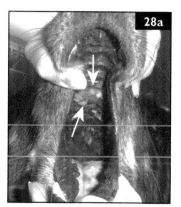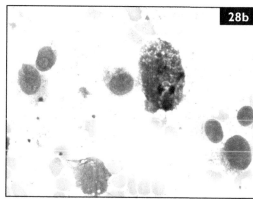

1 Describe the cytology. What is the diagnosis?
2 What further staging tests are important?
3 Describe treatment options.

CASE 29 A 6-year-old spayed female DSH cat was presented for a 1–2-day history of lethargy, weakness, ataxia, and vomiting. She had been urinating outside the litter box and her appetite had been poor. On physical examination, bilateral renomegaly was present. She was also approximately 5% dehydrated. Laboratory abnormalities included BUN >130 mg/dl, creatinine 7.1 mg/dl, phosphorus >16.1 mg/dl, and urine specific gravity 1.016. Thoracic radiographs were within normal limits. An abdominal ultrasound was performed and both kidneys appeared similar (**29a**). There were no other significant findings within the abdomen.

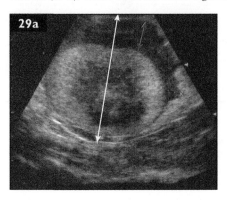
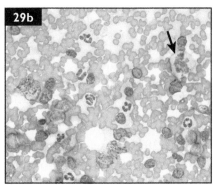

1 Describe the ultrasound findings.
2 An ultrasound-guided FNA of the kidney was performed and cytology is shown (**29b**). What is the clinical diagnosis?
3 Based on the degree of renal failure present, is this patient a reasonable candidate for treatment?
4 What are the possible causes of this patient's ataxia?

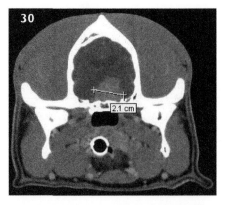

CASE 30 A 5-year-old spayed female Labrador Retriever was referred for oculomotor dysfunction in the right eye. The right eyelid was not closing normally and there was mydriasis in the right eye. A post-contrast CT image is shown (**30**).

1 Describe the lesion seen on CT.
2 What is the cause of the oculomotor dysfunction?
3 What therapy is recommended and what is the prognosis for this patient?

CASE 31 A 16-year-old neutered male DSH cat was presented for an open, ulcerative, infected mass lesion just distal to the right hock (**31**). The MDB was within normal limits and regional lymph nodes were not palpable. On physical examination, the mass extended 360° around the leg. An incisional biopsy

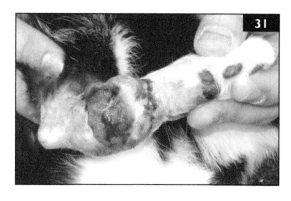

revealed a peripheral nerve sheath tumor of low-grade malignancy. The owner was strongly opposed to amputation of the leg.

1 What therapeutic options should be considered for this patient?
2 What is the long-term prognosis for this patient with treatment?

CASE 32 A 10-year-old spayed female Rottweiler presented for an acute onset of non-weightbearing lameness and pain. Prior to jumping out of a truck, she had been clinically normal.

1 Describe the radiographic findings (**32**).
2 What further diagnostic tests are recommended for this patient?
3 What is the appropriate treatment plan?

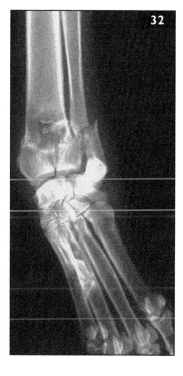

CASE 33 A 10-year-old Golden Retriever undergoing chemotherapy for T cell lymphoma developed proliferative cutaneous lesions near the penis (**33**).

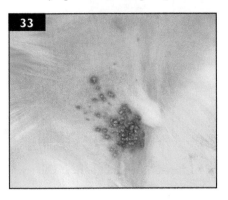

On physical examination, there was no evidence of lymphadenopathy or other abnormalities to suggest the dog was out of remission. He had been on chemotherapy for 1 month (first cycle of induction therapy – week 1: vincristine; week 2: cyclophosphamide; week 3: vincristine; week 4: doxorubicin; with decreasing dosages of oral prednisone) and appeared to go into remission readily. The lesions appeared 7 days post doxorubicin.

1 What diagnostic tests are recommended for this patient?
2 What therapy is indicated?

CASE 34 A 12-year-old spayed female German Shepherd Dog was undergoing a routine yearly examination. The owners reported that she was "slowing down" and that her appetite was slightly decreased. On physical examination, a mid- to cranial abdominal mass was appreciated. Radiographs revealed a mass, which appeared to be associated with the spleen (**34a**).

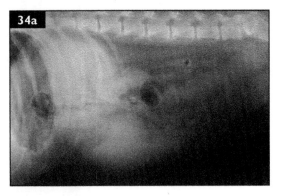

1 What are the differential diagnoses for this patient?
2 Does the patient's breed play a role in determining the most likely diagnosis?
3 What further diagnostic tests should be performed?
4 What is the recommended treatment and the expected prognosis for this patient?

CASE 35 A 13-year-old spayed female mixed breed dog presented for a routine yearly examination. The owner reported that her appetite seemed to be gradually decreasing and a 2 kg weight loss was documented over the past year. Physical examination findings were unremarkable with the exception of a palpable mass in the left cranial quadrant. Blood work was normal with the exception of moderate elevations in ALP and ALT. An abdominal ultrasound revealed a large mass in the left lateral liver lobe (**35a**).

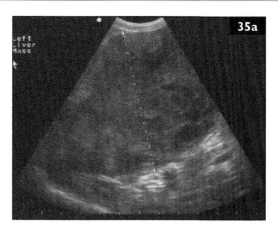

1 What additional diagnostic tests are indicated for this patient?
2 What is the significance of the mass being on the left side?
3 What are the primary rule outs for this mass?
4 Is this patient a poor candidate for surgery because of the large size of the mass?

CASE 36 A 9-year-old neutered male Boxer was noted by the owner to have a rapid onset of submandibular lymphadenopathy. The dog is not showing any other clinical symptoms. On physical examination, his body temperature is normal, heart and lung sounds are normal, but abdominal palpation reveals cranial organomegaly. All of the peripheral lymph nodes are enlarged and measure at least 4 cm (**36**). Blood work was within normal limits.

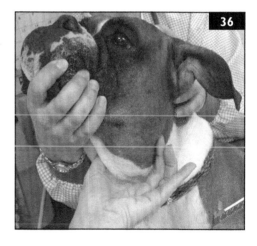

1 What are the likely causes of the lymphadenopathy?
2 What further tests should be performed prior to instituting treatment?
3 What is the likelihood that this patient has T cell lymphoma?

19

CASE 37

1 What device is being placed in this patient (37a–c) and what is it used for?
2 What are the advantages of this device?
3 What are the disadvantages that can be seen?

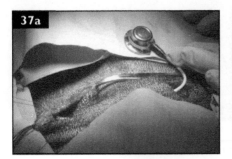

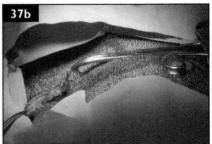

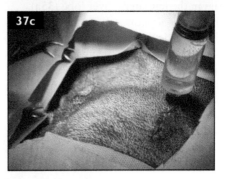

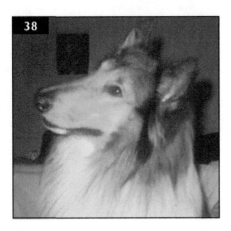

CASE 38

1 What risk factor(s) would exist for increased toxicity to chemotherapy in this patient (38)?
2 What additional tests should be run before planning a chemotherapy protocol?
3 What drugs should be avoided in this patient?

CASE 39 A 9-year-old spayed female Doberman Pinscher developed a forelimb lameness and swelling on the dorsal aspect of the foot (**39a**). She was otherwise healthy with no other significant physical examination findings. An MDB including thoracic radiographs was normal. A biopsy was performed and histopathology confirmed osteosarcoma.

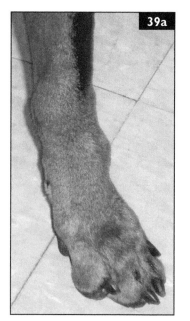
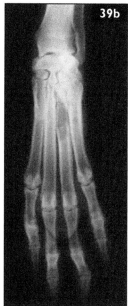
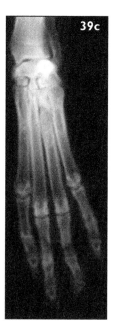

1 Describe the pretreatment (**39b**) and post-treatment (**39c**) radiographs.
2 What curative-intent therapeutic options can be offered to this patient?
3 Describe options for palliative therapy.

CASE 40 A 12-year-old spayed female DSH cat was presented for a routine yearly physical examination. Other than the pictured abnormality (**40**), the physical examination was normal.

1 Describe the abnormality observed.
2 What are the recommendations for this patient?

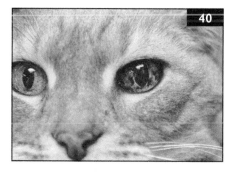

CASE 41 A 9-year-old neutered male Beagle presented with an ulcerated, rapidly growing mass on the ventral aspect of the foot (**41a**). Cytology from a fine needle aspirate of the mass is shown (**41b**).

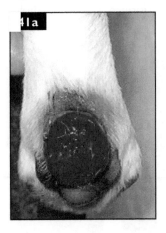
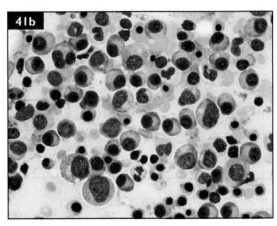

1 Describe the cytologic findings and give a diagnosis.
2 What staging tests should be performed?
3 What are the treatment recommendations for this patient?

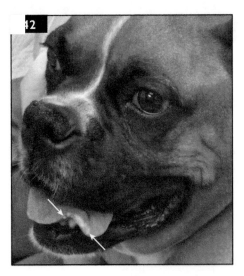

CASE 42 A 6-year-old spayed female Boxer currently undergoing chemotherapy for lymphoma was noted to have tiny white, firm, raised lesions at the lateral tip of the tongue (**42**, arrows) and on the ventral surface of the tongue.

1 Are these lesions consistent with progression of lymphoma?
2 How could these lesions be a result of therapy?
3 What other diagnostic tests should be done on this patient?
4 What is the recommended therapy for these lesions?

CASE 43 A 12-year-old spayed female calico cat had a history of lameness thought to be secondary to a soft tissue injury 1 year prior to presentation. The lameness initially improved with cortisone injections and rest. Three weeks prior to referral, she started limping again. Cortisone and rest did not allow any improvement this time. On physical examination, there was a firm swelling over the mediolateral aspect of the metatarsals (**43a**).

1 Describe the radiographic findings (**43b**).
2 An MDB and a fine needle aspirate of the lesion were performed. The MDB was normal and the cytology slide is shown (**43c**). What is the presumptive diagnosis?
3 What is the recommended treatment and the expected outcome?

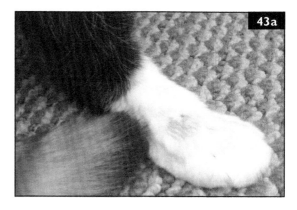

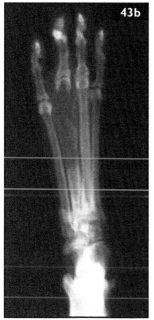

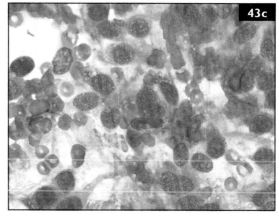

CASE 44 A 13-year-old neutered male Shepherd mix presented after the owner noted a foul odor coming from the mouth and blood in his water bowl after drinking. Physical examination revealed a large, ulcerated infected mass surrounding the

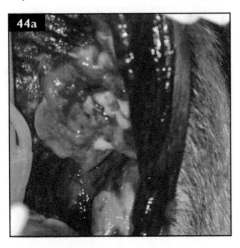

premolars and molars (**44a**). The submandibular lymph node on the ipsilateral side was enlarged.

1 What are the primary differential diagnoses for this mass?
2 The owners only wished to pursue palliative therapy. What would be advised and what diagnostic tests would be necessary prior to instituting palliative therapy?
3 What palliative therapy would most likely have the greatest impact on improving this patient's quality of life?

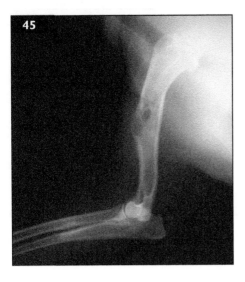

CASE 45

1 Describe the abnormality seen on this radiograph (**45**) of a 12-year-old Labrador Retriever presented for an acute onset of forelimb lameness.
2 What staging tests would be required before further prognostic information can be given?
3 What therapeutic options would be recommended in this case?
4 What tumors are most commonly associated with bone metastasis?

CASE 46 An 11-year-old neutered male Shih Tzu presented with a large mass on the right side of the neck. A biopsy revealed squamous cell carcinoma. CT (**46**) was performed to determine whether surgery was possible and, if not, it was to be used for radiation therapy planning.

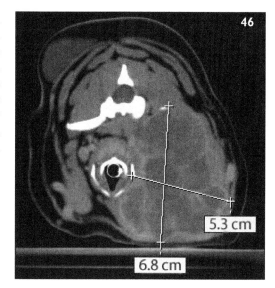

1 Describe the CT findings.
2 Is this a surgical case?
3 What therapy is advised?

CASE 47 A 7-year-old intact female German Shorthaired Pointer presented for an acute onset of lesions in the skin of the caudal abdominal area. She was also reported to be extremely lethargic and anorectic. On physical examination, in addition to the lesions seen in the picture (**47**), multiple subcutaneous masses throughout the mammary chain were noted. The biopsy revealed a grade III mammary

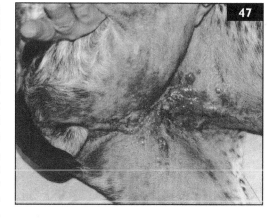

adenocarcinoma with cells suspected to be within the lymphatic vessels. No further treatment was elected at that time.

1 Describe the clinical appearance and likely diagnosis for this patient.
2 What additional diagnostic tests should be performed?
3 Given the clinical appearance of the lesions and histopathology results, what treatment can be considered and what is the prognosis for this patient?

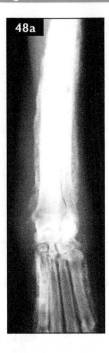

CASE 48

1 Name the disorder noted on the radiograph (48a) of this 10-year-old Golden Retriever that presented for lameness and swelling of the distal limbs (48b).
2 What is the next diagnostic step for this patient?
3 How is this disorder treated?

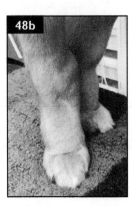

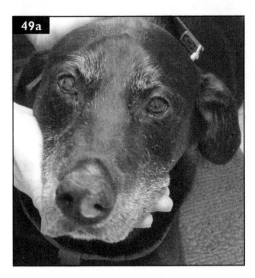

CASE 49 A 14-year-old spayed female black Labrador Retriever presented with a lesion on the nasal planum (49a). On physical examination, the submandibular lymph nodes were not palpable. There were no other significant findings on physical examination.

1 What is the most likely diagnosis, based on the physical examination?
2 What diagnostic tests should be performed?
3 What therapeutic options should be considered?

CASE 50 A 9-year-old spayed female Jack Russell Terrier had a slower than expected recovery from anesthesia following a routine dental prophylaxis. The physical examination was normal except for a grade IV/VI pansystolic murmur heard best on the left side. Radiographs were taken, which revealed a cranial abdominal mass. Abdominal ultrasound confirmed a 6 × 4.5 cm mass of

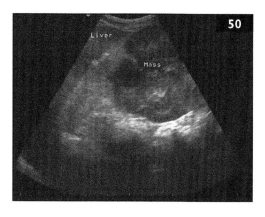

mixed echogenicity that appeared to be associated with the spleen (50). The remainder of the ultrasound was normal.

1 What are the primary differential diagnoses for this mass?
2 What further diagnostic tests should be performed prior to surgical removal of the mass?
3 What prognosis can be given to this pet's owner prior to surgery?

CASE 51 This 8-year-old spayed female Golden Retriever presented with a large recurrent mass of the left tibial tarsal (hock) joint (51). The mass was initially taken out over 2 years prior to this picture. Histopathology at that time revealed hemangiopericytoma (HPC), but there were tumor cells extending to the surgical margins.

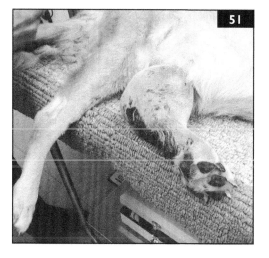

1 Is this patient a good candidate for radiation therapy?
2 What further staging tests are indicated?
3 What treatment is most appropriate for this patient?

CASE 52 This is the lateral radiograph of a 5-year-old neutered male Siamese cat presented for an acute onset of severe dyspnea (**52a**). The cytology obtained from an

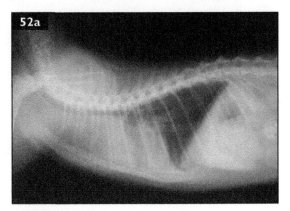

ultrasound-guided aspirate of the mass shown in the radiograph is shown (**52b**).

1 Describe the radiographic and cytologic findings and give the diagnosis.
2 What staging tests and further diagnostic tests should be considered?
3 Is this disease unusual for this age and breed of cat? What is the likely result of retroviral testing in this patient?
4 What treatment is recommended and what are the survival expectations?

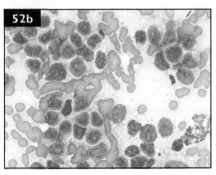

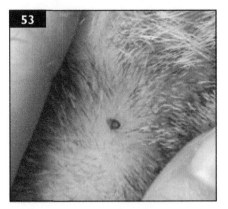

CASE 53 A 12-year-old neutered male DSH cat was presented for evaluation of a small black cutaneous lesion in front of his ear (**53**). The patient was asymptomatic.

1 Based on the clinical appearance, what is the most likely diagnosis?
2 An excisional biopsy was performed, which confirmed a dermal melanoma. What features of the histopathology report are necessary to determine further treatment and outcome for this patient?

CASE 54 A 6 × 4 cm mass was seen in the liver on a monitoring ultrasound 1 year following a lung lobectomy (for primary pulmonary adenocarcinoma). This 10-year-old neutered male DSH cat was asymptomatic, and radiographs of the thorax remained clear. The CBC and serum chemistry panel were unremarkable.

The mass shown (54) was removed; the remainder of the abdomen appeared normal.

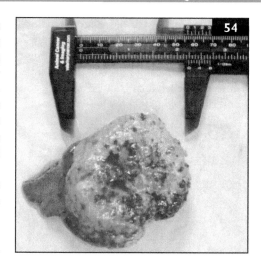

1 Describe the tumor tissue and likely diagnosis.
2 Approximately what percentage of hepatobiliary tumors in cats are benign?
3 What further treatment beyond surgery is recommended?

CASE 55 A 10-year-old neutered male American Bull Terrier presented for a 3-month history of straining to urinate with intermittent frank blood at the end of urination. Antibiotics were initially prescribed but only transient improvement was noted. A rectal examination revealed an enlarged firm prostate. An ultrasound image is shown (55).

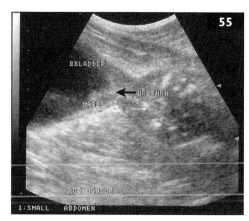

1 Describe the abnormalities on this ultrasound image.
2 Why is prostatic neoplasia the primary differential? This patient was castrated at a young age. How does this affect your diagnostic considerations?
3 How should the diagnosis be confirmed?

CASE 56 A 10-year-old neutered male Miniature Schnauzer mix was noted to be straining to defecate for approximately 2 weeks prior to presentation. There was a small amount of frank blood noted in the stool and on the rectum, but he was otherwise clinically normal. On physical examination, a 3 cm ulcerated mass is noted in the left anal gland (**56a**). A fine needle aspirate of the mass was performed and the cytology is shown (**56b**).

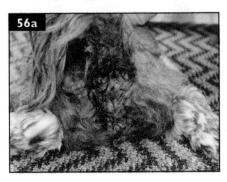
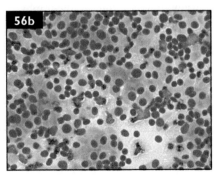

1 Describe the cytology.
2 What are the primary diagnostic considerations?
3 What specific abnormality on a serum chemistry panel has prognostic significance?
4 In addition to the MDB, what further testing should be done to make a definitive diagnosis and stage this patient?

CASE 57 Cyclophosphamide (Cytoxan®) and chlorambucil (Leukeran®) (**57a**) are commonly used in metronomic chemotherapy protocols. Low dose, oral administration of chemotherapeutic agents such as these typically involves sending medications home with pet owners.

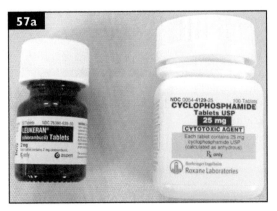

1 What instructions should be provided for owners regarding handling of these medications?
2 Is it safe to cut/split tablets?

CASE 58 An acute onset of polyuria and polydipsia was the only clinical symptom noted in a 12-year-old spayed female Husky. A CBC and serum chemistry panel revealed that all values, including BUN, creatinine, and phosphorus, were within normal limits except for a corrected calcium of 18 mg/dl (reference = 9.0–12.2 mg/dl). A urine specific gravity was 1.027.

1 In considering cancer as an underlying cause for this patient's hypercalcemia, what must a physical examination include?
2 A 1.0 cm mass is detected on digital rectal examination that appears to be within the right anal gland. Cytology from a fine needle aspirate is suggestive of anal sac gland adenocarcinoma (ASGAC). What is the suspected cause of the hypercalcemia?
3 How should this patient be managed?
4 Despite the small size of the primary mass, an ultrasound examination (58) revealed significantly enlarged sublumbar lymph nodes (4.48 × 5.54 cm). How does this affect the treatment approach and the prognosis?
5 What factors are considered negative prognostic indicators?

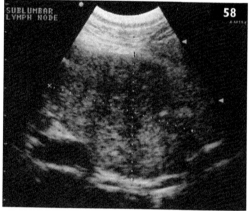

CASE 59 A small gingival mass (59) was an incidental finding on this 9-year-old spayed female Golden Retriever. A conservative excisional biopsy was performed at the time of a routine dental prophy and a plasma cell tumor was diagnosed. There were tumor cells present at the margins of the excisional biopsy.

1 What is the biologic behavior of this tumor in dogs?
2 What further diagnostic tests should be performed?
3 Is any further treatment necessary?

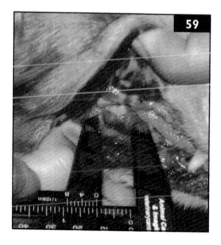

CASE 60 A 5-year-old 14.5 kg spayed female Husky mix was evaluated for a 1-month history of lameness that progressed to a non-weightbearing lameness of the

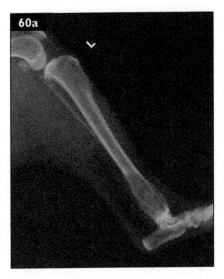

left hindlimb. The pain appeared to have started after she had been playing roughly, leading to the initial concern for trauma. There was minimal soft tissue swelling in the area of the distal tibia. After 2 weeks of non-steroidal anti-inflammatory drug treatment, the lameness was progressive and radiographs were taken (60a).

1 Describe the radiographic lesion.
2 What in this dog's signalment and the radiographic appearance of this lesion would indicate that the lesion is less likely to be osteosarcoma?
3 List the differential diagnoses for this patient and diagnostic recommendations.

CASE 61 A 7-year-old spayed female Norwegian Elkhound presented for evaluation because of a 1-week history of being "less willing to play" and seemingly weak. On physical examination, slightly pale mucous membranes

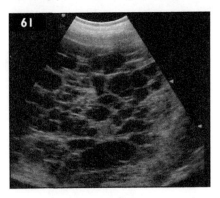

are noted. There is a palpable large mid-abdominal mass. Thoracic radiographs, CBC, and chemistry panel were performed. The only abnormality noted was mild thrombocytopenia (125,000/µl). A large abdominal mass is visualized on ultrasound (61). The mass is cavitary and appears to be effacing the spleen. There is a small amount of peritoneal fluid noted on ultrasound. There is no further disease appreciated on ultrasound.

1 What are the primary differential diagnoses for this mass?
2 What further tests should be performed to complete the preoperative staging?
3 Histopathology revealed hemangiosarcoma (HSA). What treatment should be considered postoperatively and what are the survival expectations?

CASE 62 This is cytology (62) from an ultrasound-guided fine needle aspirate of a diffusely enlarged spleen in a 9-year-old spayed female Boxer presented for recent weight loss and diarrhea. On physical examination, the spleen was palpably enlarged. Blood work and thoracic radiographs were normal. A cutaneous mast cell tumor, low grade, had been completely removed from the lateral thigh over 3 years ago.

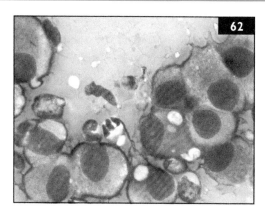

1 What is the cytologic diagnosis?
2 A splenectomy was performed. Histopathology confirmed the diagnosis of poorly differentiated mast cell tumor. What further information can be gained from the tissue sample that will help in making treatment recommendations for this patient?
3 What is the prognosis for this patient?

CASE 63 A 10-year-old spayed female 45 kg mixed breed dog was evaluated for recent weight loss, mild dyspnea, and anorexia. On physical examination, the abdomen was mildly distended and firm. Lung sounds were clear, but there was an abdominal component to the breathing noted. Thoracic radiographs and blood work were normal. On ultrasound, there was moderate

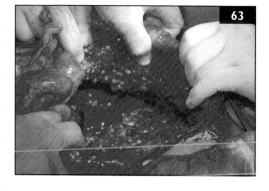

peritoneal effusion and thickened and irregular appearing tissue along all linings. Exploratory surgery was performed and the abdominal cavity is pictured (63).

1 Describe the photograph.
   A fine needle aspirate of several of the masses was suspicious for carcinoma.
2 What is the probable diagnosis?
3 What treatments can be considered and what is the prognosis for this patient with or without treatment?

CASE 64 A 14-year-old spayed female Labrador Retriever had been treated 15 months previously for a stage II oral malignant melanoma (OMM) of the right rostral maxilla (a 2.5 cm mass on the gingiva just behind the right canine tooth) with maxillectomy and the Oncept® melanoma vaccine, but the owners did not choose to continue with the recommended booster vaccinations. The mitotic index of the maxillary tumor was 2 (2 mitotic figures per 10 hpf). She now presented for having difficulty swallowing, but there was no evidence of recurrence of disease noted and thoracic radiographs were normal. On oral examination, a pharyngeal mass was seen, believed to be tonsillar in origin (64).

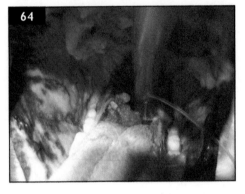

1 What further tests would help in determining a treatment plan?
2 An excisional biopsy revealed an undifferentiated round cell tumor with cells seen at the margins of the surgical sample. What further information from the biopsy can help in determining a more definitive diagnosis and the biologic behavior of this tumor?
3 What treatment options can be considered?

CASE 65 A fine needle aspirate (65) of a mass protruding from the urethral opening was performed on a 10-year-old spayed female West Highland White Terrier that had presented for pollakiuria, stranguria, and hematuria. A firm, distended bladder was palpable. Ultrasound of the abdomen revealed a thickened, irregular urethra and distended bladder, but no obvious evidence of disease within the bladder.

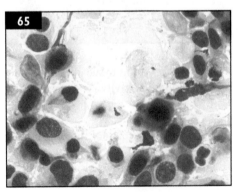

1 Describe the cells seen on cytology.
2 What are the differential diagnoses for this patient?
3 What further diagnostic tests should be performed on this patient?
4 What treatment should be offered?

CASE 66 This is the contrast CT image (**66**) from a 12-year-old neutered male Golden Retriever presented for a recurrent grade II peripheral nerve sheath tumor in the caudal abdominal wall/flank area. The mass had initially been removed with incomplete surgical margins 6 months prior to referral. The mass now measured

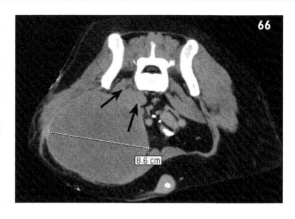

approximately 10 cm on physical examination; it was located in the left flank area but extended onto the caudal abdominal wall and the left hindlimb, causing restriction of movement. Thoracic radiographs and abdominal ultrasound were free of metastatic disease. The tumor was causing restriction of movement and pain for the patient, but he was otherwise healthy. A CT was performed, which revealed a minimally contrast-enhancing mass located in the left caudal abdomen and inguinal area. There are well-defined margins and the mass is within the abdominal wall. The mass is infiltrating into the muscles ventral to the left ilium and sacrum (**66**, arrows). The mass had been removed and histopathology performed 6 months previously.

1 Should this recurrent mass be biopsied?
2 What treatment recommendations can be made for this patient?

CASE 67 A 9-year-old neutered male Labrador Retriever was presented for a mass at the right mucocutaneous junction of the lip (**67a**). There has been an odor noted with occasional bleeding from the mass. The patient was brought in within 1 week of the mass being noted. The mass measured 3 × 1.5 cm, the ipsilateral submandibular lymph node was slightly prominent (<1 cm) and firm, and the remainder of the physical examination was normal.

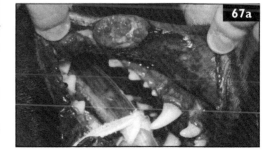

1 What are the differential diagnoses for this lesion?
2 What is the diagnostic approach to this lesion?

35

CASE 68 A 10-year-old spayed female Golden Retriever presented for evaluation of this mass on the left rear tarsal pad (68a). She was noted to be licking at her foot and the mass was first noted at the pictured size. The dog's physical examination was unremarkable with the exception of the mass and a 1 cm left popliteal lymph node. A fine needle aspirate of the mass was performed (68b).

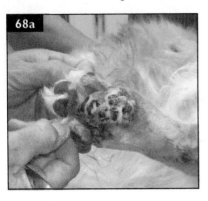

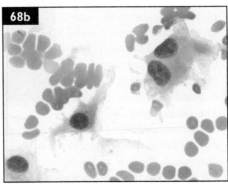

1 What is the clinical diagnosis?
2 What diagnostic tests are indicated?
3 What is the expected biologic behavior of this cancer?
4 Based on the location and size of this mass, complete surgical excision would only be possible with limb amputation. The owners have declined amputation. Describe a treatment plan that does not include amputation.

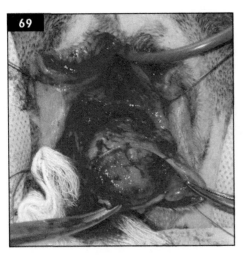

CASE 69 A 6-year-old intact female Boston Terrier presented for straining to urinate and a thick mucoid vaginal discharge. A firm, smooth, round 2 cm mass could be palpated per rectum. On vaginal examination, the mass was noted to be caudal to the urethral papilla. At surgery, the mass appeared discrete and encapsulated (69).

1 List the differential diagnoses for this lesion.
2 What additional therapy is recommended?

CASE 70 A 12-year-old spayed female DSH cat was presented for evaluation of anorexia, weight loss, and lethargy. On physical examination, she was thin but otherwise normal. She was uncomfortable when her abdomen was palpated. An MDB was unremarkable. Abdominal ultrasound revealed an enlarged and irregular pancreas but was otherwise normal. Surgical exploratory was recommended. The entire pancreas was enlarged with firm coalescing nodules throughout (**70a**). An impression smear from a section of the abnormal pancreatic tissue is shown (**70b**).

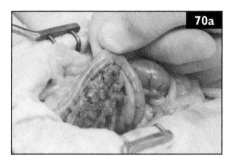
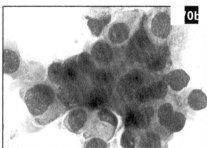

1 Describe the cytology. What is the most common exocrine pancreatic neoplasia in the cat?
2 If cancer is confirmed histologically, what is the likelihood of finding further metastasis in the abdominal cavity?
3 What treatment options are available for this cat?

CASE 71 A raised, cutaneous lesion is found on the dorsum of a cat (**71**). The lesion is firm and does not feel attached to deeper structures. The lesion is pigmented in nature.

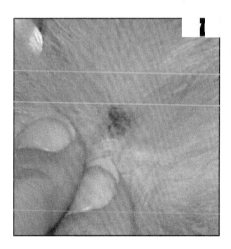

1 What are the most common skin tumors in the cat?
2 Based on its appearance, what is the most likely diagnosis?
3 What diagnostic tests are indicated?
4 What treatment is indicated?

CASE 72 A 12-year-old spayed female Labrador Retriever presented for a 1-month history of an enlarging mass on the left side of the thorax. The patient was otherwise healthy. The only significant biochemical abnormality noted on the MDB was an elevated alkaline phosphatase of 870 U/l (reference, 0–140 U/l). Following the MDB, a biopsy and thoracic CT (**72a**, pre-contrast; **72b**, post-contrast) were performed. A CT-guided aspirate of the mass was performed and the cytology is shown (**72c**).

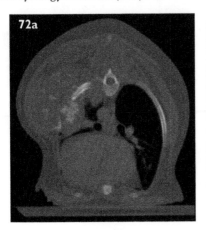

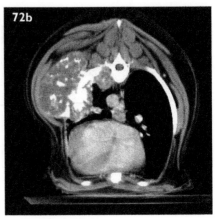

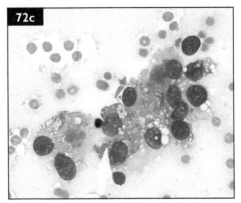

1 Describe the lesion seen on the CT scans.
2 What are the two most common tumors seen arising from the ribs?
3 From the rostral to caudal direction, the mass appeared to be affecting at least three ribs. Is curative intent surgical resection likely in this patient?
4 Histopathology confirmed OSA in this patient. What is the prognosis for this patient? Describe the prognostic significance of the elevated ALP.

CASE 73 The arrows in **73a** point to a firm mass encompassing the left mandible. Within the oral cavity, the mass appeared to cross the midline. The regional lymph nodes were normal and the remainder of the physical examination was normal. Open mouth VD radiographs of the mandible were taken (**73b**).

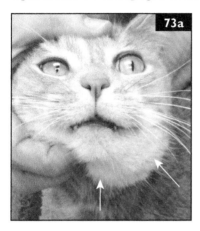

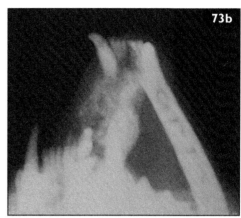

1 What are the two most common tumors seen in the oral cavity of cats?
2 What non-malignant lesions could be present in this cat?
3 Assuming this is a malignant tumor, what diagnostic and therapeutic options are available for this patient?

CASE 74 A 7-year-old neutered male Labrador Retriever is presented for his annual examination. There is a cutaneous wart-like lesion on the top of the patient's head (**74**). The lesion is fluctuant and feels slightly "greasy".

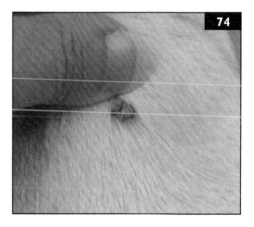

1 What is the clinical diagnosis?
2 What recommendations should be made?

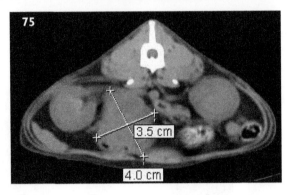

CASE 75 A 16-year-old neutered male DSH cat had a history of poor appetite and weight loss. On abdominal palpation, a cranial abdominal mass was suspected. This patient had a grade III/VI pansystolic heart murmur. The remainder of the physical examination was normal. Serum chemistry panel, CBC, urinalysis, and thoracic radiographs were normal. Electrolyte analysis revealed mildly decreased potassium levels. Echocardiography revealed left ventricular hypertrophy. Blood pressure was 220 mmHg. Ultrasound revealed a cranial abdominal mass near the left kidney. A CT scan was performed (**75**).

1 Describe the CT findings and suggest differential diagnoses.
2 What further diagnostic testing is indicated for this patient?
3 What treatment is recommended?
4 What are survival expectations with treatment?

CASE 76 This 14-year-old neutered male DSH cat had been experiencing ptyalism and dysphagia. There was a foul odor coming from the oral cavity. On

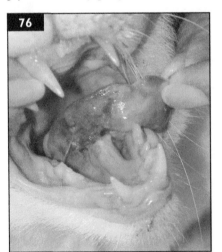

examination, there was a sublingual mass that was friable, proliferative, and ulcerative (**76**). The mass was destroying the tongue tissue and had actually caused a separation of the base of the tongue from the frenulum. A biopsy revealed squamous cell carcinoma (SCC).

1 What is the prognosis and expected metastatic rate of this cancer?
2 Are there any environmental or lifestyle factors that increase the risk of this cancer in cats?
3 What therapies are described for this disease?
4 Develop a palliative therapeutic plan for this cat.

CASE 77 A 10-year-old spayed female Golden Retriever presented for evaluation and possible adjunct therapy for a low-grade mast cell tumor that had been removed from the flank area. The healed surgical incision in the left dorsal flank area measured 3.1 cm (77). An MDB, abdominal ultrasound, and evaluation of the regional lymph nodes revealed no further evidence of mast cell tumor. The mass had initially measured 2 cm in diameter,

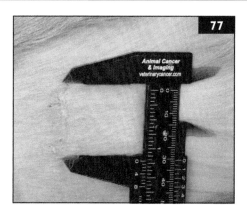

was subcutaneous, and was removed by the referring veterinarian. Histologically, the tumor was considered to be low grade, had 2 mitotic figures per 10 hpf, and the results of the prognostic panel are shown here:

> PCR was **negative** for a *c-KIT* mutation in exon 8.
> PCR was **negative** for a *c-KIT* mutation in exon 11.
> KIT pattern 1, Ki67: 9; AgNORs/cell: 1.5; AgNOR × Ki67: 13.5

1 The mass measured 2 cm. The surgical scar measured 3.1 cm. Is this adequate surgical planning?
2 Interpret the prognostic panel.
3 Does the subcutaneous location of the tumor provide any additional prognostic information?
4 What are the treatment options for this patient?

CASE 78 This is a radiograph taken of a patient undergoing radiation therapy (78a).

1 What type of radiograph is being illustrated?
2 What is the purpose of this radiograph?

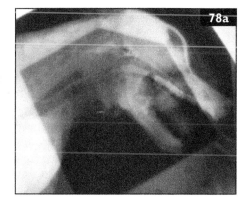

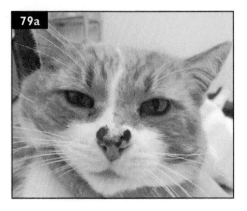

CASE 79 A 12-year-old neutered male domestic medium hair cat presented with ulcerative lesions on the nasal planum (79a). There had been a 1-year history, which initially started with a right-sided dry crust or scab-like lesion with secondary swelling. Over time, it progressed to ulcerative lesions on the entire nose. The MDB and physical examination were normal.

1 What is the most likely diagnosis?
2 What are possible causes or predisposing factors for development of this lesion?
3 What are the most important criteria when considering surgery of the nasal planum?
4 Describe a non-surgical option for the treatment of this patient.

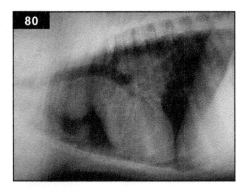

CASE 80 This is the lateral thoracic radiograph (80) from a 10-year-old Golden Retriever that presented for coughing and weight loss. On abdominal palpation, cranial organomegaly was appreciated. The submandibular and prescapular lymph nodes were enlarged. On abdominal ultrasound, two large masses of mixed echogenicity were found in the spleen. Cytology from aspirates of the prescapular lymph node revealed a population of vacuolated round cells. Immunocytochemistry was performed: the cells were CD18+, CD3– and CD79a–. The CBC, chemistry panel, and urinalysis were normal.

1 Describe the thoracic radiograph. Based on the radiograph and physical examination, what is the presumptive diagnosis?
2 What is the interpretation of the ICC and what is the diagnosis?
3 What is the prognosis for this patient?
4 What is the significance of the normal blood work?

CASE 81 A 4-year-old neutered male DSH cat was presented because of the owner's concern about "a change in the appearance of the cat's pupils" (**81**). He was not showing any other clinical symptoms. The pupillary light reflex was normal in the left eye, but minimal on the right. There was some response to light on the medial (nasal) aspect of the right pupil. At times, the owner reports, the eyes will look normal.

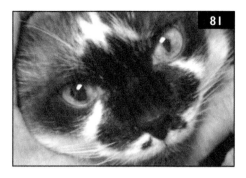

1 Describe the abnormality pictured here.
2 What are the differential diagnoses?
3 What is unique about the feline pupil that allows this abnormality to occur?

CASE 82 A 12-year-old neutered male Shepherd/Dobermann mixed breed dog presented for an acute onset of dyspnea. Mucous membranes were pale pink and the heart rate was increased (160/min). There were no other significant physical examination findings. Radiographs of the thorax revealed significant pleural effusion. Thoracocentesis revealed the pictured fluid (**82a, b**). The fluid was bloody throughout the entire procedure.

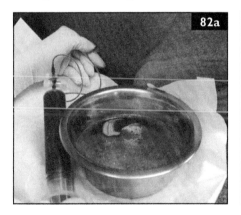
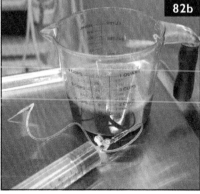

1 What is the significance of the fluid being bloody throughout the thoracocentesis procedure?
2 What diagnostic tests are indicated once the fluid has been removed?
3 List the differential diagnoses for a hemorrhagic pleural effusion.

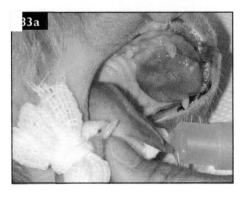

CASE 83 A 12-year-old neutered male DSH cat presented for evaluation of a slowly growing mass on the rostral maxilla/hard palate (**83a**). There had been a several-month history of noting blood in the water bowl and excessive licking at the roof of the mouth prior to the mass being visualized. The mass was very firm and adherent to underlying bone.

1 What are the differential diagnoses for this lesion?
2 What is the likelihood of metastasis?
3 What diagnostic tests should be performed?
4 The tumor extends too far back on the hard palate to be operable. What therapeutic options are available?

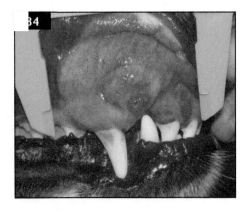

CASE 84 A 5-year-old intact male Golden Retriever was found to have a 1.5 cm mass located above the right upper canine tooth (**84**). An excisional biopsy was performed and histopathology revealed a very low-grade fibrosarcoma, extending to the surgical margins. There were no mitotic figures observed and the pathologist commented that it was difficult to completely rule out a benign fibroma. Based on the relatively benign diagnosis, the owner had been advised that no further treatment would be necessary. Six months later, the patient returned with recurrence of disease that was now closer to 5 cm and wrapped around the bone.

1 What clinical diagnosis does this represent?
2 What was the mistake made in the clinical interpretation of this patient's disease?
3 Based on the current clinical presentation, what further diagnostic evaluation and treatment options are available?
4 What features of this patient's tumor can help predict outcome?

CASE 85 Lateral (**85a**) and VD (**85b**) thoracic radiographs were taken of a 10-year-old spayed female DLH cat that presented for a 2-week history of coughing/gagging. An ultrasound-guided fine needle aspirate was also performed (**85c**).

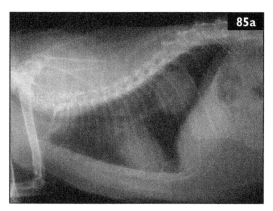

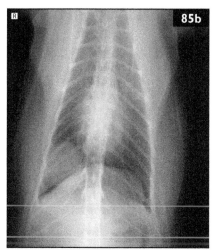

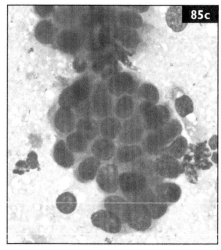

1 Describe the radiographs and list the differential diagnoses.
2 Describe the cytology.
3 What additional diagnostic tests should be performed?
4 What treatment is indicated and what are the most important prognostic indicators for this patient?

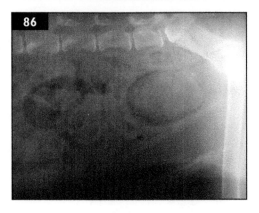

CASE 86 This is a lateral abdominal radiograph (**86**) from a 5-year-old neutered male German Shepherd Dog mix that was referred for a suspected bladder tumor. This dog had initially presented for an acute onset of hematuria. The patient had been missing for several days. When he returned he was lethargic and appeared painful in the abdomen. When he strained to urinate, the urine was blood-tinged with several small blood clots noted. The primary care veterinarian took this radiograph and submitted a free-catch urine sample for a bladder tumor antigen (BTA) test. The results were positive.

1 Describe the radiograph.
2 Explain the interpretation of the BTA test in this patient.
3 What are the differential diagnoses for this patient?

CASE 87 This is a lateral thoracic radiograph (**87**) of a 12-year-old spayed female German Shepherd Dog that presented for a 2-month history of weight loss and a 2-week history of lethargy and coughing. On physical examination, the patient was thin and there was a slight abdominal component to the breathing. The body temperature was normal as were peripheral lymph nodes

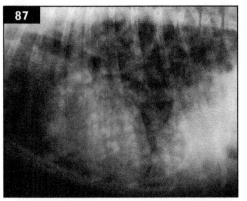

and abdominal palpation. Blood work (CBC and chemistry panel) was within normal limits.

1 Describe the radiograph and give the differential diagnoses.
2 In addition to the MDB, an abdominal ultrasound was performed and was normal. What further testing is indicated in order to differentiate between malignancy and a non-neoplastic cause?

CASE 88 A 10-year-old neutered male German Shepherd Dog was presented for an acute onset of severe dyspnea and wheezing. The only abnormality noted prior to the onset of dyspnea was several days of difficulty swallowing. A lesion was seen on oral examination (**88**).

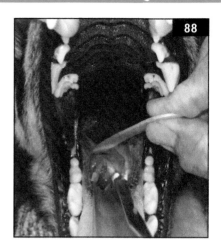

1 Describe the lesion.
2 List the differential diagnoses.
3 Surgical debulking was performed because of the severe clinical symptoms. A biopsy revealed squamous cell carcinoma. What is the recommended treatment?
4 What is the prognosis for this patient?

CASE 89 This is the cytology (**89a**) from a fine needle aspirate of the darkly pigmented mass noted in the rostral mandible between the canine teeth of a 10-year-old spayed female Golden Retriever (**89b**). The mass was an incidental finding on routine examination; it measured 1 × 1 cm and had a broad-based attachment to the lower jaw.

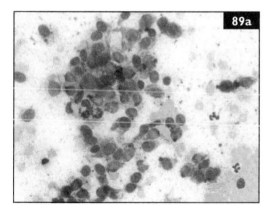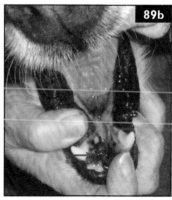

1 What is the diagnosis?
2 What further tests need to be performed before treatment can be recommended?
3 What treatment has the greatest chance for long-term survival?
4 What is the prognosis for this patient?

CASE 90 This is the CT image (90a) from a 14-year-old neutered male Rottweiler presented for an acute onset of lethargy and apparent back pain.

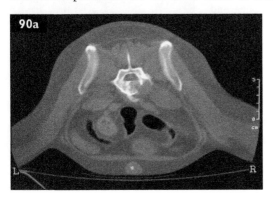

Other than pain being easily elicited when the lumbar spine area was palpated, the physical examination was normal. Thoracic radiographs and blood work were normal. Radiographs of the abdomen were taken and a suspicious area of lysis was noted on the ventral lumbar spine at L6. A CT scan was performed.

1 Describe the CT image and list the differential diagnoses.
2 What is the most common primary vertebral body tumor diagnosed in the dog?
3 What further testing is indicated?
4 What treatments are indicated? Given the patient's age, the owners did not wish to pursue surgery. What palliative options could be considered for this patient?

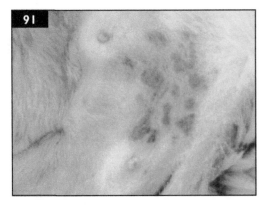

CASE 91 A 14-year-old spayed female DSH cat presented for an acute onset of erythema and edema in the caudal abdominal area. She was constantly licking at the area. She appeared very painful. On physical examination, she was febrile (103.8°F; 39.9°C). There were multiple ulcerated areas on her abdomen (91). On careful palpation of the mammary tissue, a large (3 × 3 cm) firm subcutaneous mass was palpated in association with one of her caudal mammary glands. The skin felt warm to the touch and there was moderate edema in her hindlimbs.

1 What is the diagnostic plan?
2 What does the clinical presentation suggest?
3 What is this patient's prognosis and how should treatment be approached?

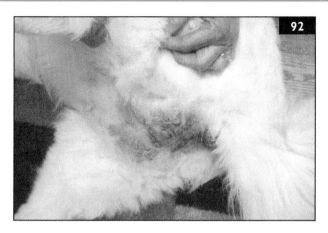

CASE 92 A 10-year-old spayed female American Eskimo was evaluated because of irritation and crusting in the perineal region (92). She was treated conservatively for several weeks for a suspected moist dermatitis. She was healthy otherwise and, other than an elevated WBC of 22,000/µl, the MDB was normal.

1 Describe the lesions pictured.
2 Biopsies were taken in different areas of the perineum and all areas confirmed basal cell carcinoma (BCC). What treatment should be considered?

CASE 93 A 13-year-old neutered male DSH cat was evaluated for erythema and alopecia on the dorsum of the nose (93a). Alopecia had been noted over the past 2 years, but the area was becoming more reddened and "irritated". There were no clinical symptoms or other abnormal physical examination findings. A skin biopsy was performed, which revealed actinic keratitis (actinic carcinoma in situ).

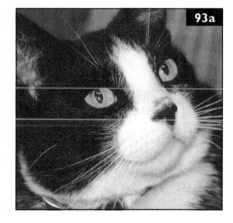

1 What is the probable cause of this lesion?
2 What is the natural progression of disease?
3 How should this patient be managed?
4 If the lesion progresses to SCC, what treatment is advised?

CASE 94 This 13-year-old cat (94a) presented for a 2 kg weight loss over approximately 1 year. There had been a 1-month history of poor appetite and occasional gagging thought to be due to hairballs. A CBC was normal and a serum chemistry panel revealed a BUN of 75 mg/dl, creatinine of 4.0 mg/dl, and mild elevations in ALT, ALP, and gamma-glutamyltransferase (GGT). Ultrasound of the abdomen was performed and an image of the liver is shown (94b).

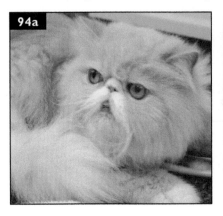
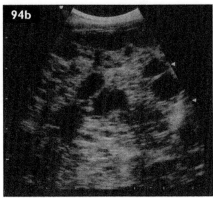

1 What is the primary differential diagnosis for the findings on liver ultrasound?
2 What is a possible cause of the azotemia and how should this be evaluated?
3 What treatment should be considered?

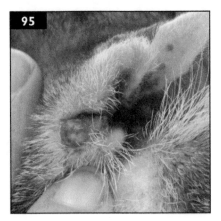

CASE 95 A 12-year-old neutered male DSH cat is evaluated for shaking his head, scratching at his right ear, with blood occasionally noted after scratching (95). He had been non-responsive to topical and systemic antibiotics.

1 Describe the lesions noted in the ear.
2 What are the primary differential diagnoses for this cat's lesions?
3 In addition to the MDB, what testing should be done to determine the course of treatment?
4 If these lesions are malignant, what treatment is recommended and what is this cat's prognosis?

CASE 96 A 10-year-old spayed female mixed breed dog presented for a recent onset of lethargy and one episode of collapse. She was also noted to be somewhat weak in the hindlimbs. On physical examination, her heart sounds were muffled and the heart rate was 160/min. There were no other abnormalities noted.

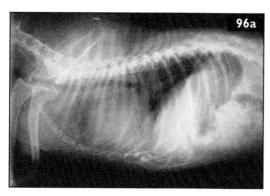

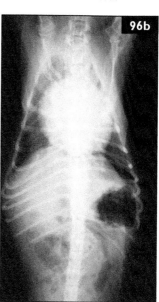

1 Describe the radiographs (96a, b) and give a clinical diagnosis.
2 What are the most common causes for the radiographic findings?
3 What further diagnostic tests are indicated?
4 What is the likelihood of making a diagnosis based on the tests performed (listed in 3). What further non-invasive tests could be performed to help make a diagnosis?
5 What therapy is advised?

CASE 97 A 12-year-old spayed female Cocker Spaniel is noted to have an acute onset of significant swelling in the left third eyelid (nictitans). There is also a mucoid discharge from the eye (97).

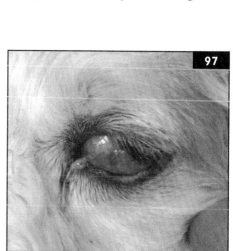

1 What does this picture suggest?
2 What is the recommended work-up for this patient?
3 What are the differential diagnoses for this patient?
4 What therapy is indicated?

51

CASE 98 The red arrow in **98** points to the rectal opening of a 9-year-old neutered male Golden Retriever mix. The black arrows outline a 6 × 4 cm

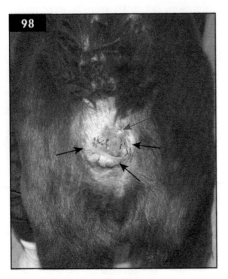

anal gland mass. An incisional biopsy was performed and revealed anal sac gland adenocarcinoma (ASGAC). An MDB was normal.

1 What staging tests are indicated for this patient?
2 Surgical removal was accomplished to relieve obstructive symptoms; however, as expected given the large size of the tumor, margins showed tumor cells still present. What adjunctive therapy should be considered postoperatively and what is this patient's prognosis?
3 What side effect can be expected with postoperative therapy?

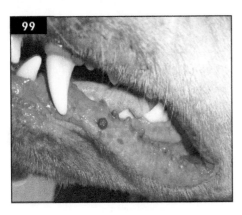

CASE 99 A 0.5 cm pigmented, pedunculated mass was noted on the lip near the mucocutaneous junction in a 7-year-old neutered male Labrador Retriever (**99**). The patient is clinically normal. An excisional biopsy was performed which revealed melanoma, low grade, with 1–2 mitotic figures per 10 hpf. The margins of the surgical specimen were free of tumor cells, and were at least 5 mm wide.

1 What staging tests should be performed?
2 What further treatment is indicated?
3 How does the location of this lesion affect its biologic behavior?

CASE 100 A 12-year-old neutered male Beagle mix was presented for acute onset of pain on opening his mouth and an elevated third eyelid (**100a**). An ocular examination was normal except that the eye did not retropulse normally into the socket. There was no response to a 2-week course of broad-spectrum antibiotics.

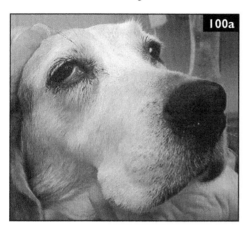
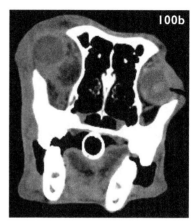

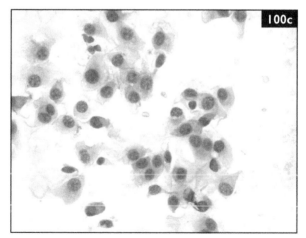

1 What are the differential diagnoses for this patient?
2 What further diagnostics should be performed?
3 A CT image (**100b**) and cytology from a fine needle aspirate (**100c**) obtained at the time of the CT scan are shown. What is the diagnosis?
4 Describe treatment options for this patient.

CASE 101 A 7-year-old spayed female mixed breed dog presents for an acute onset of facial swelling (**101a**). The only abnormality noted by the owner prior to the facial swelling was a 2-week history of PU/PD. On physical examination, generalized lymphadenopathy and cranial organomegaly are noted. An abdominal ultrasound (**101b**), fine needle aspirate of an enlarged lymph node (**101c**), blood work, and urinalysis are ordered.

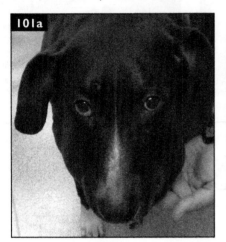

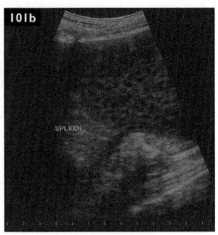

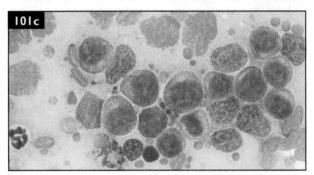

Test	Result	Flag	Units	Normal Range
WBC	45.1	High	10³/µl	6.0–17.0
LYM	3.1		10³/µl	0.9–5.0
MONO	2.5	High	10³/µl	0.3–1.5
GRAN	39.5	High	10³/µl	3.5–12.0
LYM%	6.9			
MONO%	5.4			

Continued

Test	Result	Flag	Units	Normal Range
GRAN%	87.7			
HCT	40.9		%	37.0–55.0
MCV	67.3		fl	60.0–72.0
RDWa	51.8		fl	35.0–53.0
RDW%	18.5	High	%	12.0–17.5
HGB	14.0		g/dl	12.0–18.0
MCHC	34.3		g/dl	32.0–38.5
MCH	23.1		pg	19.5–25.5
RBC	6.08		$10^6/\mu l$	5.50–8.50
PLT	367		$10^3/\mu l$	200–500
MPV	8.1		fl	5.5–10.5
pH	7.346			7.330–7.450
Na	148.3		mmol/l	139.0–151.0
K	4.01		mmol/l	3.80–5.30
Cl	105.6		mmol/l	102.0–120.0
Ca^{2+} ionized	2.381	High	mmol/l	1.120–1.420
BUN	47.1	High	mg/dl	9.0–29.0
Creatinine	0.8		mg/dl	0.4–1.4
Phosphorus	4.8		mg/dl	1.9–5.0
Calcium	>15.3	High	mg/dl	9.0–12.2
Corrected Ca	Unable to measure		mg/dl	9.0–12.2
Total Protein	7.0		g/dl	5.5–7.6
Albumin	4.3	High	g/dl	2.5–4.0
Globulin	2.7		g/dl	2.0–3.6
Alb/Glob Ratio	1.6			
Glucose	158	High	mg/dl	75–125
Cholesterol	231		mg/dl	120–310
ALT (GPT)	110		U/l	0–120
ALP	127		U/l	0–140
GGT	10		U/l	0–14
Total Bilirubin	0.1		mg/dl	0.0–0.5

Urine specific gravity = 1.048, urinalysis normal.

1 What is the clinical syndrome shown in the picture of this patient?
2 Describe the ultrasound and cytology findings.
3 What significant abnormality is noted in the blood work and how does this impact the patient's treatment and prognosis? What further testing is indicated before treatment is initiated?
4 How should this patient be managed?

CASE 102 This is the CT scan (**102**) from a 10-year-old neutered male Labrador Retriever that was previously diagnosed with osteosarcoma in the right proximal

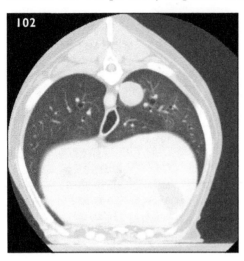

tibia. He underwent amputation and carboplatin chemotherapy. Exactly 1 year following amputation, radiographs were taken for monitoring purposes, which revealed a solitary lesion in the dorsal lung field on the left lateral view.

1 What further diagnostic tests are indicated?
2 Are there any surgical options available for this patient?
3 What is the prognosis for this patient if this is metastatic disease?

CASE 103 A 10-year-old spayed female Doberman Pinscher mix was presented for a yearly geriatric examination. She was clinically normal. As part of this very thorough veterinarian's geriatric examination, thoracic radiographs and abdominal

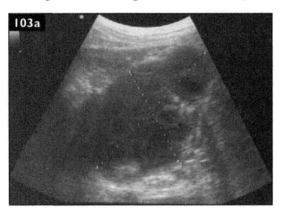

ultrasound were performed (**103a**). There was a mass imaged that measured 6.5 × 10.2 cm and appeared to be between the liver and the stomach shadow, but it was difficult to determine which structure it was attached to. An ultrasound-guided fine needle aspirate was performed and yielded only peripheral blood and scattered macrophages. An MDB was normal.

1 What recommendations should be made to this pet's owner?
2 Based on the dog's age and the appearance of this mass on ultrasound, cancer was suspected. What are other considerations?

CASE 104 This is the CT scan (**104**) of a 7-year-old neutered male Bernese Mountain Dog that was presented for a large mass in the inguinal region. The mass was extending onto the prepuce. On palpation, the mass appeared to be firm and fixed to underlying tissues. An MDB was normal. Cytology was poorly cellular with several mesenchymal cells noted. An incisional biopsy confirmed a soft tissue sarcoma, grade I.

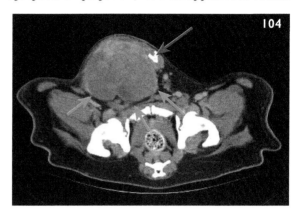

1 The blue arrows outline the mass. What does the red arrow point to?
2 What treatment is recommended?
3 What is the prognosis for this patient?

CASE 105 A 12-year-old spayed female DSH cat presented for a several-year history of periocular scabs. More recently, there was evidence of ulceration of the lower eyelid (**105a**). An impression smear of a biopsy taken from the lower eyelid is shown (**105b**). There are also pinpoint scabby areas over the dorsum of the nose.

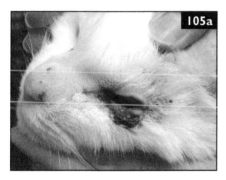 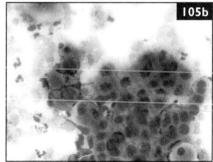

1 Describe the cytology and give a presumptive diagnosis.
2 What is the recommended staging for this patient and the likelihood of metastasis?
3 What therapeutic options are available?

CASE 106 These are images from the CT scan (**106a,** scout film; **106b,** corresponding slice in a "bone window"; **106c,** same slice in a "head and neck window") from a 10-year-old neutered male Bearded Collie that presented for a several-week history of unilateral right-sided nasal bleeding. He was otherwise normal.

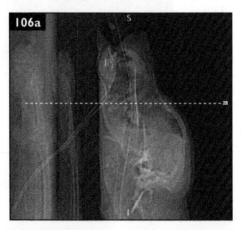

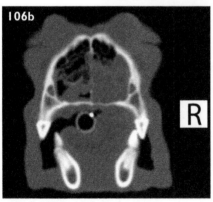

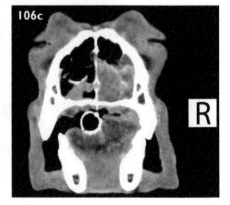

1 Describe the CT findings.
2 What clinical signs are most commonly associated with nasal neoplasia?
3 How should this patient be evaluated prior to biopsy?
4 What procedures can be used for biopsy?
5 What is the recommended treatment for this patient and the expected prognosis?

CASE 107 A 5-year-old spayed female DSH cat is evaluated for lameness of the left hindlimb and a firm swelling in the tarsus. The cat was initially treated symptomatically with antibiotics with no improvement. Subsequently the limb became diffusely swollen and firm (107a) and the popliteal and inguinal lymph nodes (107b) were also enlarged. The remainder of the examination is normal. An MDB is performed and blood work, urinalysis, thoracic radiographs, and FeLV/FIV status are all normal. A fine needle aspirate of the inguinal lymph node is performed. Radiographs of the tibiotarsal joint showed no obvious bony changes. Cytology from an aspirate of the enlarged inguinal lymph node is shown (107c).

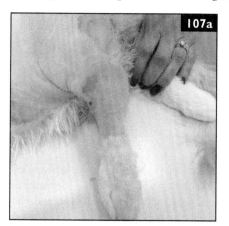
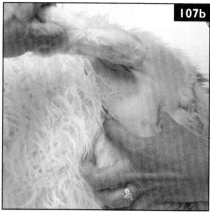
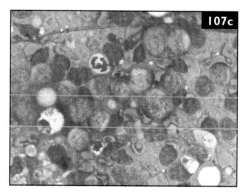

1 Describe the cytologic findings.
2 Based on the presumptive diagnosis, what further diagnostics are indicated?
3 What treatment is advised?

CASE 108 A 7-year-old intact male Boxer is evaluated for an asymptomatic, visible enlargement of the left scrotum (108). A testicular mass is palpable.

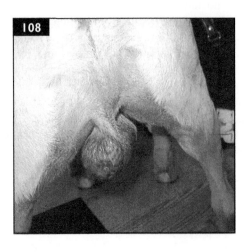

1 List the differential diagnoses for this clinical presentation.
2 Which of the common testicular tumors in dogs produce estrogen and what are the clinical manifestations of excess estrogen production?
3 Based on the photograph alone, is this mass more likely to be malignant or benign?
4 What diagnostic tests are indicated for this patient and why?
5 What are the treatment options?

CASE 109 A 12-year-old neutered male Great Dane mix had a slowly growing mass over the left eye (109a). It was first noted almost 1 year ago and had been aspirated several times yielding only fat. The mass was firm and appeared fixed to underlying tissues on palpation. It was causing a physical obstruction to vision and the patient could barely open the eye because of the mass. An MDB including thoracic radiographs was within normal limits.

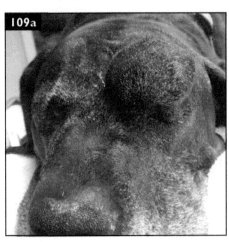

1 Should an incisional biopsy or an excisional biopsy be performed and why?
2 How should this patient be further assessed?
3 A new FNA was performed and again yielded fat, but scattered mesenchymal cells were also noted. What are the differential diagnoses?
4 How can this dog be treated?

CASE 110 An 8-year-old neutered male mixed breed dog (30 kg) was noted to have a focal swelling in the lower jaw. He would yelp in pain when playing with toys and was not taking treats as he normally would. On physical examination, there is a firm mass arising from the mid-mandible whose surface was smooth (**110**). The

mass measured 4 × 2.5 × 2.5 cm. The regional lymph nodes were not palpable, and the remainder of the physical examination was normal.

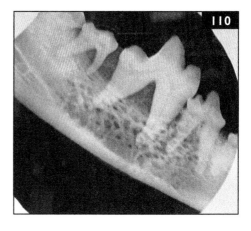

1 Describe the radiographic changes.
2 A fine needle aspirate of the mass was taken. It yielded large pleomorphic round cells with occasional plasmacytoid differentiation. Based on the radiographic appearance and cytology, what further diagnostic tests are indicated before a treatment decision is made?
3 The owner has declined mandibulectomy as a treatment option. What other therapy can be offered?

CASE 111 A 7-year-old neutered male German Shepherd mix was evaluated for swelling in the left maxillary area. Other than the maxillary swelling and

a depigmented and ulcerated area surrounding the caudal molars (**111**), the physical examination was normal.

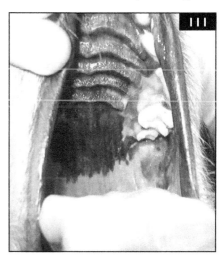

1 What diagnostic tests should be performed?
2 List the most common tumors of the oral cavity in the dog.
3 Based on the photograph, what parameters are visible that indicate that surgery is a consideration?
4 This dog was diagnosed with an intermediate-grade fibrosarcoma. What treatment is indicated and what is the likelihood that this cancer will spread?

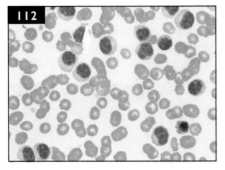

CASE 112 This is the CBC and peripheral blood smear (**112**) from a 10-year-old neutered male Golden Retriever, taken at the time of a routine wellness examination. There were no reported clinical symptoms.

1 What is the presumptive diagnosis?
2 What staging tests are indicated?
3 How is the definitive diagnosis made?
4 Describe treatment options and prognosis for this patient.

Test	Result	Flag	Units	Normal Range
Hematology (HemaTrue)				
WBC	51.9	High	10³/µl	6.0–17.0
LYM	24.4	High	10³/µl	0.9–5.0
MONO	9.7	High	10³/µl	0.3–1.5
GRAN	17.8	High	10³/µl	3.5–12.0
LYM%	46.9			
MONO%	18.7			
GRAN%	34.4			
HCT	37.4		%	37.0–55.0
MCV	65.1		fl	60.0–72.0
RDWa	47.4		fl	35.0–53.0
RDW%	17.7	High	%	12.0–17.5
HGB	13.0		g/dl	12.0–18.0
MCHC	35.0		g/dl	32.0–38.5
MCH	22.7		pg	19.5–25.5
RBC	5.74		10⁶/µl	5.50–8.50
PLT	50	Low	10³/µl	200–500
MPV	7.4		fl	5.5–10.5

Test	Result	Flag	Units	Normal Range
Chemistry (DRI-CHEM)				
BUN	18.8		mg/dl	9.0–29.0
Creatinine	0.8		mg/dl	0.4–1.4
Phosphorus	3.7		mg/dl	1.9–5.0
Calcium	10.0		mg/dl	9.0–12.2
Corrected Ca	10.2		mg/dl	9.0–12.2
Total Protein	7.0		g/dl	5.5–7.6
Albumin	3.3		g/dl	2.5–4.0
Globulin	3.6		g/dl	2.0–3.6
Alb/Glob Ratio	0.9			
Glucose	112		mg/dl	75–125
Cholesterol	142		mg/dl	120–310
ALT (GPT)	84		U/l	0–120
ALP	60		U/l	0–140
GGT	13		U/l	0–14
Total Bilirubin	0.1		mg/dl	0.0–0.5

CASE 113 The 10-year-old neutered male Weimaraner pictured here (**113a**) had limb radiographs taken (**113b**) for his 6-month recheck examination following treatment for cancer.

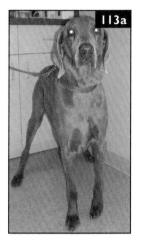 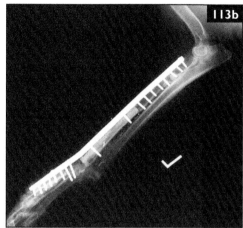

1 Describe the radiograph shown and the procedure that was performed.
2 What was the probable diagnosis?
3 When is this procedure indicated?
4 How does the prognosis for this patient differ from that of patients undergoing amputation?

CASE 114 This is the left eye of a 13-year-old spayed female chocolate Labrador Retriever mix (**114**). She had a history of cataracts and vision was already poor, but seemed worse in the left eye.

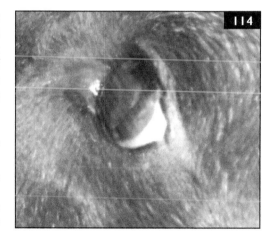

1 Describe the abnormality within the eye.
2 What recommendations can be made to the pet owner?
3 What criteria are used to determine malignant behavior?

CASE 115 A 12-year-old neutered male large mixed breed dog presented because of the development of a large, firm mass below the right ear (**115a**, arrows). The owner reported that the mass seemed to develop quickly over a 2-week period, but was preceded by noticeable halitosis.

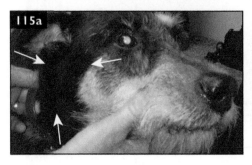
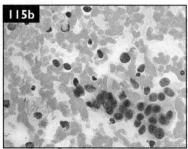

1 What are the differential diagnoses for this patient?
2 Cytology from a fine needle aspirate revealed the cells pictured (**115b**); what is your presumptive diagnosis?
3 What further diagnostics are indicated?
4 What treatment is recommended?
5 What is this patient's prognosis?

CASE 116 An 8-year-old spayed female Giant Schnauzer presented for evaluation of a visible mass in the left ear canal (**116**, arrow). The mass was obliterating the ear canal and growing onto the pinna. The patient had been treated for chronic ear infections in the ear for at least 8 months prior to the mass being visualized. The remainder of the physical examination, including the submandibular lymph nodes and the right ear, was normal.

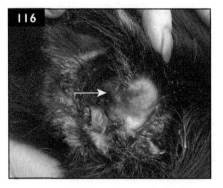

1 What are the differential diagnoses for this lesion?
2 In addition to the MDB, what diagnostic tests should precede treatment?
3 What is the prognosis for this patient and how does the type of surgery performed affect the prognosis?
4 In addition to the presence of lymph node or lung metastasis, what are the negative prognostic indicators for this type of tumor?

CASE 117 A 10-year old neutered male Labrador Retriever presented for a 3-month history of diminishing appetite and a 3 kg weight loss. On physical examination, the only abnormal finding was that the dog was thin. An MDB was performed and the lateral thoracic radiograph is shown (**117**).

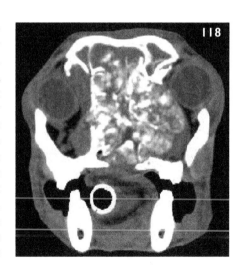

1 Describe the radiograph.
2 What are the differential diagnoses?
3 What diagnostic tests should be performed?
4 What is meant by "metastatic cancer of unknown primary" and how should it be treated?

CASE 118 This is the CT scan (**118**) of a 6-year-old neutered male Border Collie mix that was presented for a 2–3-month history of nasal discharge, which was initially mucoid but progressed to epistaxis. The owner had also noted swelling between the eyes. On physical examination, the right submandibular lymph node was approximately 3 cm and firm. There was a firm swelling over the right maxilla and rostral frontal bones. On intraoral examination there was a mass visible near the midline in the caudal hard palate. The right eye was slightly exophthalmic.

1 Prior to the CT scan, what diagnostic tests should be performed?
2 Describe the CT scan.
3 What is the clinical stage of disease?
4 A biopsy confirmed an undifferentiated carcinoma and cytology of the submandibular lymph node confirmed metastatic carcinoma. What are the negative prognostic indicators in this case?

CASE 119 A 9-year-old intact female Golden Retriever is presented for evaluation due to a recent history of stranguria and constant licking at the vaginal area. On careful examination of the perineal area, a thickened area is palpated (**119**, blue arrows) and a smooth, firm area visualized below the vaginal opening (**119**, white arrow).

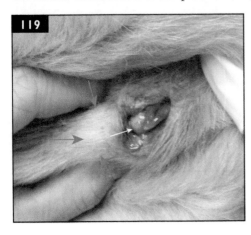

1 How should this patient be evaluated?
2 What information from the signalment helps in making a presumptive diagnosis?
3 What further diagnostic tests are indicated?
4 What is the recommended treatment and the prognosis for this patient?

CASE 120 A 9-year-old neutered male mixed breed dog was evaluated 6 months after an inguinal tumor had been removed. The histologic diagnosis was a "grade II" mast cell tumor removed with narrow margins (approaching 1 mm in some sections). No further treatment or diagnostics were pursued at that time. Now there is a visible thickening of the previous incision line with associated erythema (**120**). There is a second mass palpable deep to the visible mass that measures approximately 1.5 × 1.5 cm.

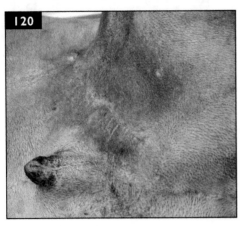

1 What could have been done differently at the time of the first surgery?
2 What diagnostic tests are indicated in this patient?
3 What is a potential tumor-related cause of the erythema noted?
4 Describe treatment options for this patient.

CASE 121 A 10-year-old intact male Old English Sheepdog had a 6-month history of a slowly growing mass on the anus (**121a**). At presentation, the mass measured 3 × 3 × 2 cm; it appeared circumscribed and did not appear to be firmly attached to underlying tissues. There had been no significant clinical signs until recently, when a small amount of frank blood was noted periodically on defecation. Cytology from an FNA is shown (**121b**, low power 100×; **121c**, high power 500×).

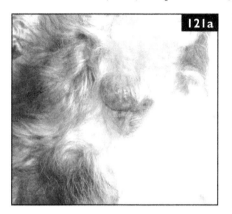
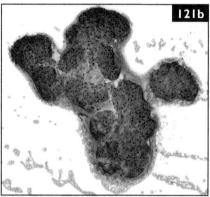
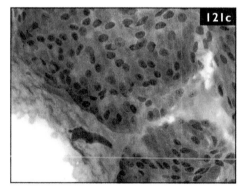

1 What is the presumptive clinical diagnosis?
2 Describe the cytologic appearance.
3 If this dog had been neutered, how would that change the presumptive clinical diagnosis?
4 What are the treatment recommendations and expected outcome?

CASE 122 A 10-year-old neutered male Golden Retriever presented 6 days after initiating chemotherapy for stage IVa lymphoma, B cell, high grade. On the first day of chemotherapy, he received vincristine and started oral prednisone as per the University of Wisconsin Madison Canine Lymphoma protocol. He had early infiltration of the lymphoma into the spleen noted on ultrasound. His blood work was normal. His lymph node measurements at the time of diagnosis were as follows:

Node	Left (cm)	Right (cm)
Submandibular	5	4
Prescapular	4	3.5
Axillary	1.5	1.5
Inguinal	2	3
Popliteal	2.5	3

Six days later, he started to feel lethargic and was warm to the touch. The left submandibular lymph node appeared larger to the owner and there was concern about lack of response to chemotherapy. On presentation, he was quiet, but responsive. His temperature was 104.5°F (40.3°C). The lymph node measurements were as follows:

Node	Left (cm)	Right (cm)
Submandibular	7	<1
Prescapular	Not palpable	<1
Axillary	Not palpable	Not palpable
Inguinal	Not palpable	Not palpable
Popliteal	1	1

1 Because the left submandibular lymph node is larger, is it safe to assume that the clinical symptoms 6 days after initiating chemotherapy are due to progressive lymphoma?

2 Should this patient be treated with chemotherapy today, given the concern about progressive disease?

3 A CBC was performed and yielded the following results:

What is the clinical assessment and what further diagnostics are indicated?

Test	Result	Flag	Units	Normal range
WBC	32.1	High	10³/µl	6.0–17.0
LYM	2.2		10³/µl	0.9–5.0
MONO	1.7		10³/µl	0.3–1.5
GRAN	28.2	High	10³/µl	3.5–12.0
LYM%	6.9			
MONO%	5.4			
GRAN%	87.7			
HCT	38.2		%	37.0–55.0
PLT	225		10³/µl	200–500
MPV	8.1		fl	5.5–10.5

CASE 123 A 2-year-old neutered male Shar Pei developed what was initially thought to be an acute swelling from a bug bite. Initially he was treated with diphenhydramine and prednisone and the swelling resolved. Approximately 1 week after stopping these medications, the swelling started again and reached the pictured severity within 2 weeks (**123**). Fine needle aspirates revealed sheets of mast cells.

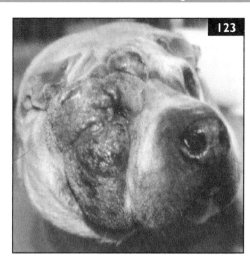

1 What diagnostic tests should be performed?
2 What is known about mast cell tumors in the Shar Pei breed?
3 What treatment recommendations can be made?

CASE 124 A 10-year-old spayed female Labrador Retriever was noted to have a "swollen" caudal left thigh. The swelling was diffuse and firm but did not appear to be causing any clinical signs. On physical examination, there were no abnormalities other than the swelling noted. Multiple fine needle aspirates revealed only blood and fat. On ultrasound, normal muscle with excessive fat was seen. A radiograph of the limb showed no obvious bony changes.

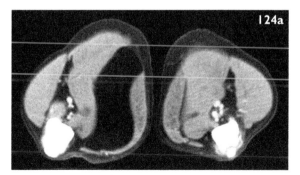

1 Based on the evaluation thus far, what are the differential diagnoses?
2 A post-contrast CT scan of the hindlimbs is shown (**124a**). Describe the scan.
3 What treatments are advised and why?

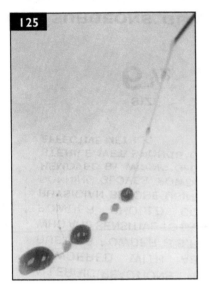

CASE 125 An 8-year-old spayed female chocolate Labrador Retriever was noted to be losing weight with apparent abdominal distension. An MDB was within normal limits. An abdominal ultrasound was performed and a mass found in the spleen. An ultrasound-guided aspirate of the splenic mass was performed (**125**).

1 Describe the character of the material obtained from FNA of the splenic mass. On cytology, malignant spindle cells with a proteinaceous background were observed. What is the likely diagnosis?
2 What treatment is indicated?
3 What feature of the histopathology will help determine this patient's prognosis?

CASE 126 This is the CT scan of a 12-year-old 25 kg neutered male mixed breed dog presented for evaluation of pain on opening his mouth (**126**). No obvious

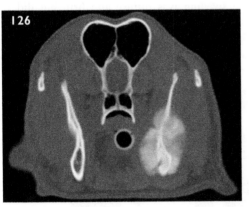

masses were palpated, but there was the impression that the right jaw felt slightly larger than the left. An MDB including thoracic radiographs was normal. Because the physical examination findings were not clear, a CT scan was recommended. He was otherwise healthy.

1 Describe the CT scan.
2 What are the differential diagnoses for this lesion?
3 A biopsy was performed, which confirmed multilobular tumor of bone. What important information from the histopathology is necessary in order to predict outcome? With complete surgical removal, what are the expectations for this patient?

CASE 127 A 9-year-old neutered male Labrador Retriever presented with a 6-week history of progressively worsening lameness of the left forelimb. Knuckling at the carpus was seen. On physical examination, muscle atrophy of the left shoulder area was noted and thickening deep in the left axillary region was suspected. There was significant pain on palpation. The remainder of the physical examination was normal. Radiographs failed to reveal a cause of the lameness. A CT scan was performed and the post-contrast image is shown (**127a**).

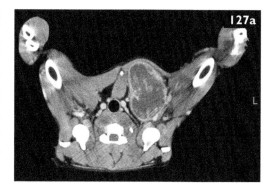

1 Describe the CT findings and possible diagnosis.
2 What diagnostic tests should be performed?
3 What type of surgery would be recommended?

CASE 128 A 12-year-old neutered male Labrador Retriever presented with a firm mass palpated in the region of the caudal mandible on the right. The mass was first noted when the patient appeared to be having difficulty eating. There were no further abnormalities noted on physical examination.

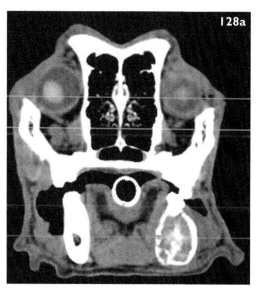

1 What diagnostic tests are necessary to determine whether further treatment is indicated?
2 What is evident on the CT scan (**128a**)?
3 What treatment is advised?
4 With clean surgical excision, what are survival expectations?
5 What are favorable prognostic indicators for oral cavity osteosarcoma in dogs?

CASE 129 A 14-year-old neutered male DSH cat initially presented for a 6-month history of an intermittent gagging cough and progressive dyspnea. On physical examination, a mass was noted cranial to the thoracic inlet. It was fluctuant in nature. When it was aspirated, a blood tinged fluid was removed, and as a result, the mass went down considerably in size and clinical symptoms improved. When the mass started to grow again, the patient started regurgitating food approximately once per day. Thoracic radiographs were taken and the pulmonary parenchyma appeared normal. Blood work was normal with the exception of a slightly elevated WBC. A CT scan was performed and is shown (**129a**, pre-contrast; **129b**, post-contrast). A fine needle aspirate with ultrasound guidance and cytology revealed a fluid of low cellularity, with RBCs, macrophages, rare squamous epithelial cells, and a proteinaceous background.

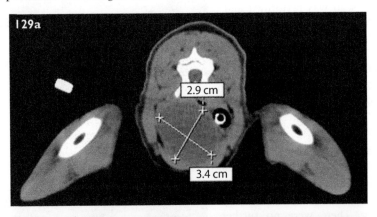

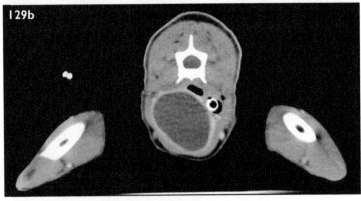

1 What are the differential diagnoses for this patient?
2 What is the cause and the biologic behavior of this lesion?

CASE 130 A 14-year-old neutered male DSH cat was evaluated for a 1-month history of sneezing and nasal discharge. The discharge was first noted coming from the right nostril and was serosanguineous in nature. After several weeks, it was also noted to be coming from the left side. As the sneezing episodes became more frequent and severe, the discharge was becoming increasingly bloody. Following a normal MDB, a CT scan was performed (**130a**). A swab of the right nasal cavity was performed and the cytology is shown (**130b**).

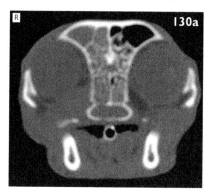 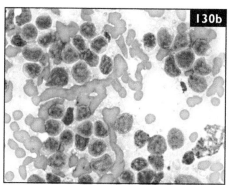

1 Describe the CT and cytology findings.
2 What is the diagnosis?
3 Is a tissue biopsy necessary?
4 What treatment should be recommended and what are the survival expectations with treatment?
5 What are the most important prognostic factors for cats with nasal lymphoma?

CASE 131 A 10-year-old neutered male Golden Retriever was prescribed postoperative radiation therapy for an incompletely excised soft tissue sarcoma of the lateral caudal forelimb. This is the appearance of the radiation site after 13 of the 18 prescribed fractions of radiation therapy (**131a**).

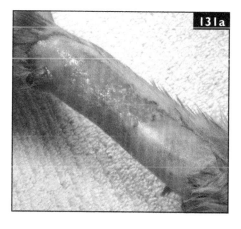

1 What is being illustrated in this photograph?
2 How should this patient be medically managed?

CASE 132 This is the post-contrast CT scan at the level of the caudal maxilla/orbit (**132a**) of a 9-year-old neutered male white Boxer that presented for a firm swelling

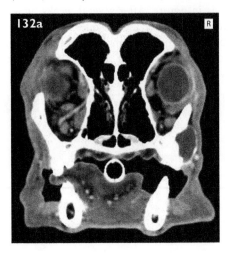

in the right maxilla. Examination of the oral cavity under anesthesia was normal.

1 Describe the CT findings.
2 A fine needle aspirate was performed and a proteinaceous fluid with evidence of mild hemorrhage was identified. In addition, there were occasional macrophages, neutrophils, and lymphocytes present. What is the clinical diagnosis?
3 What treatment is advised?

CASE 133 A 6-year-old neutered male Weimaraner presented for a 1-month history of straining to defecate. Two weeks prior to presentation, a mass was noted protruding from the rectum (**133a**). There were no other clinical symptoms. A fine needle aspirate of the mass was performed, which yielded the cytology shown (**133b**).

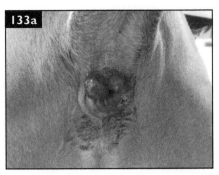
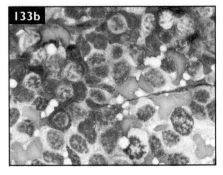

1 What is the clinical diagnosis?
2 What further staging tests should be performed?
3 Assuming regional disease without evidence of distant disease, what is the prognosis for this patient?

CASE 134 A 7-year-old neutered male German Shorthaired Pointer was found to have a palpable caudal abdominal mass on routine yearly physical examination. There were no symptoms observed. An abdominal ultrasound was performed and the only abnormality noted was within the bladder (**134a**, arrow = apex of bladder). The MDB was normal but there were increased red and white blood cells on a urinalysis from a free-catch sample.

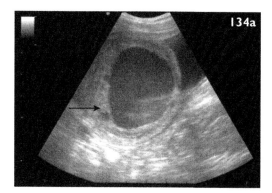

1 Describe the ultrasonogram.
2 What further tests would be indicated?
3 Is this patient a surgical candidate?
4 Does the gross appearance of the tumor give any indication about diagnosis?

CASE 135 A 12-year-old neutered male Italian Greyhound had what initially appeared to the owner to be a bruise under the left forearm. It was thought to be due to trauma when playing with another dog at home. Within 2 weeks, the bruised area had significantly widened and a mass developed. At presentation, the mass measured 10 × 6 × 4 cm (**135**). An MDB was normal. Fine needle aspirates were performed and consisted primarily of peripheral blood with an occasional mesenchymal cell present. An incisional biopsy revealed subcutaneous hemangiosarcoma.

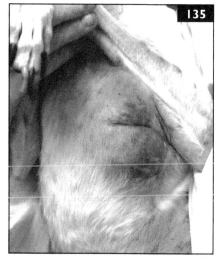

1 How does the biologic behavior for this lesion differ from hemangiosarcoma that occurs internally?
2 This lesion is too large and broad based to achieve a complete surgical excision. What therapy should be considered?
3 What factors are believed to be negative prognostic indicators for subcutaneous HSA?

CASE 136 These are the abdominal ultrasound images (**136a**, the splenic mass measured 7.0 × 4.8 cm; **136b**, the left medial iliac lymph node measured 2.0 × 2.0 cm) for an 8-year-old neutered male Golden Retriever that was evaluated for lethargy (reluctance to go for walks) and poor appetite. On physical examination, a firm mass could be palpated in the cranial ventral abdomen. There were no other significant findings. Blood work revealed a hematocrit of 30.7% (reference, 38.3–56.5%) and reticulocyte count of 91 × 10^3/µl (normal 10–110 × 10^3/µl). All other values, including platelets, were normal. Thoracic radiographs were normal.

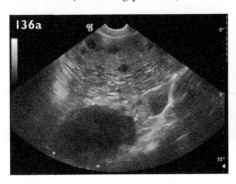
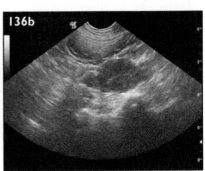

1 Describe the ultrasound.
2 An ultrasound-guided FNA of the spleen was performed and revealed a population of atypical histiocytic cells. What is a presumptive diagnosis?
3 How should the diagnosis be confirmed?
4 How should this patient be treated?

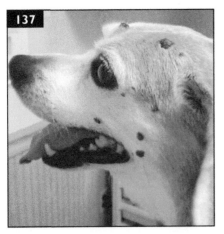

CASE 137 A 9-year-old spayed female Beagle presented for evaluation of multiple cutaneous pigmented lesions, all arising in areas of haired skin (**137**). They had remained unchanged for over a year. The patient was otherwise healthy with no significant abnormalities on physical examination. The lesions appeared to be limited to the head. A biopsy of two of the lesions revealed melanocytomas with a mitotic index of <1.

1 What is the prognosis for this patient?
2 What treatment options are available?

CASE 138 An 8-year-old neutered male DSH cat presented for a 2–3-week history of inappetence, weight loss, and a swollen toe. On physical examination he was febrile (103.5°F; 39.7°C) and had a swollen distal second digit of the right forefoot (**138a**). Infection was suspected. After a 10-day course of antibiotics, the toe improved slightly, but the mass was still present. A radiograph of the foot showed osteolysis of P3. A fine needle aspirate of the swollen toe is shown (**138b**).

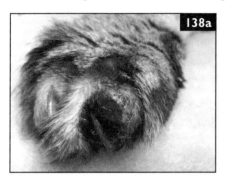

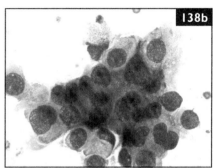

1 What is the cytologic diagnosis?
2 What diagnostic tests are indicated next?
3 What is the likely explanation for the clinical findings?
4 What is the prognosis for this patient?

CASE 139 This is a picture of a surgical specimen (**139a,** courtesy of Dr. Matti Kiupel, MSU DCPAH). An incompletely excised soft tissue sarcoma was re-excised in order to obtain clean margins.

1 What is being illustrated in this picture?
2 If this were a canine soft tissue sarcoma, what width of microscopic margins is required to be confident that a clean surgical margin has been achieved?

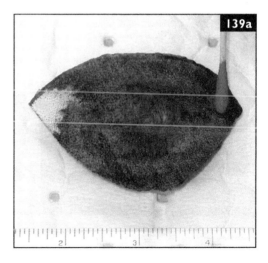

CASE 140 A 9-year-old spayed female Labrador Retriever was presented for a gagging cough that was progressing, but had been noted up to a year earlier. There

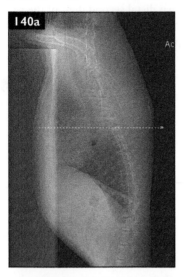

had also been a change in the sound of her bark. The symptoms had initially been attributed to laryngeal paralysis. Radiographs were performed and a mass was displacing the trachea dorsally and causing widening of the cranial mediastinum. The pulmonary parenchyma and vasculature appeared normal. The cardiac silhouette was also normal. The MDB and abdominal ultrasound were normal. An echocardiogram confirmed an 8 × 9 cm homogeneous, encapsulated mass, which was associated with the ascending aorta. Cardiac function was normal. The following images are from a CT scan. In the survey CT image of the thorax (**140a**) the dotted line corresponds to the CT images shown. Figure **140b** shows the "thorax" window. Figure **140c** is at same level as in **140b** in a "lung window".

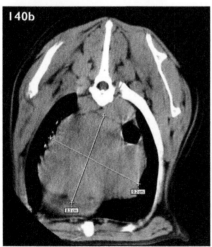

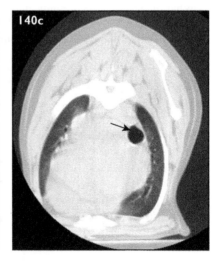

1 What is the anatomic location and character of the mass? What is the arrow pointing to in **140c**?
2 List the differential diagnoses for this mass. What tumor is most likely and why?
3 What further diagnostic tests should be performed?
4 What treatment should be considered for this patient?

CASE 141 A 13-year-old neutered male Siamese cat presented for a 4-month history of anorexia, vomiting, and weight loss. On physical examination, there was a palpable mid-abdominal mass. He was approximately 5% dehydrated. There were no other abnormalities. Ultrasound revealed a 4 cm mass associated with the small intestine. There were five enlarged mesenteric lymph nodes ranging in size from 0.6 × 0.4 cm to 1.5 × 1.0 cm. Thoracic radiographs revealed an enlarged sternal lymph node. CBC and chemistry panel were normal and FeLV and FIV were negative.

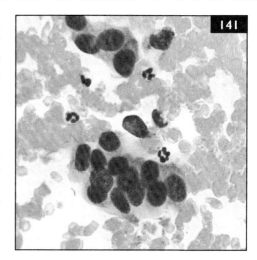

1 An ultrasound-guided FNA of the intestinal mass was performed and the cytology is shown (**141**). What is the cytologic diagnosis?
2 How does the presence of the enlarged lymph nodes affect survival expectations?
3 This patient was taken to surgery for resection and anastomosis of the primary tumor and removal of the lymph nodes. What significant prognostic factors can be obtained from the histopathology results?
4 What is the significance of this patient's breed?

CASE 142 Thoracic radiographs were taken (**142**) of a 10-year-old spayed female DLH cat as part of a yearly geriatric wellness exam. The patient's physical examination is normal. A CBC, chemistry panel, and urinalysis were normal.

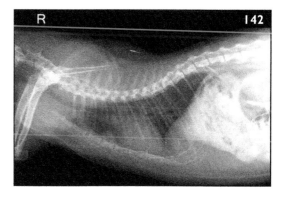

1 Describe the radiograph.
2 Could this be considered a variation of normal?
3 What structures do the sternal nodes receive drainage from?
4 What further diagnostics are indicated?

CASE 143 An 8-year-old spayed female Chihuahua mix presented for anorexia of 3 weeks' duration. Her weight was 4.5 kg on presentation, which represented a 1 kg weight loss since her last examination 6 months prior. On physical examination, she was thin and had several palpable masses within the abdomen. The remainder of the examination was normal. Blood work and urinalysis were normal. A thoracic radiograph and images from an abdominal ultrasound are shown (143a–c).

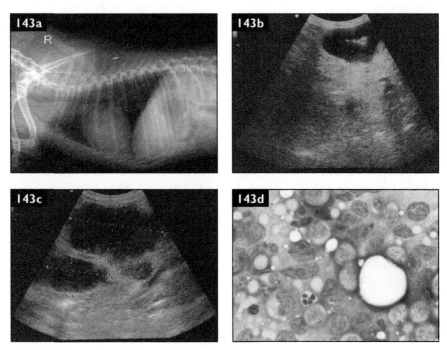

1 What abnormalities are noted on the thoracic radiograph?
2 Figure **143b** shows a cross section of the small intestine and **143c** is an image of the mid-abdomen. Describe these ultrasound images.
3 Figure **143d** shows the cytology obtained from an ultrasound-guided aspirate of the mesenteric lymph nodes. What is the diagnosis?
4 What further tests are indicated?
5 What is the treatment and prognosis for this patient?

CASE 144 These are the lateral (**144a**) and VD (**144b**) radiographs at initial presentation of a 12-year-old neutered male German Shepherd mix that presented for a 2-week history of coughing. The owner noted that the dog was losing weight, and records documented that he had lost 5 kg in the previous 4 months. He also appeared to be weaker in the hindlimbs. In addition to the cough, there had been several episodes of vomiting a clear fluid. On physical examination he was thin. Increased respiratory sounds were noted on expiration.

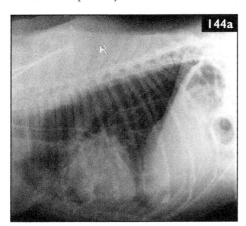
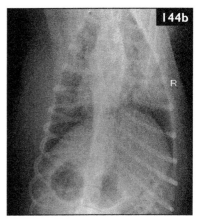
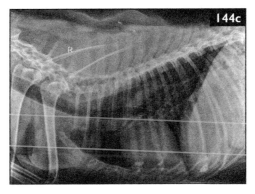

1 What is the radiographic diagnosis?
2 Another radiograph (**144c**) was taken following a 2-week course of antibiotics. What is the revised radiographic diagnosis?
3 What are the differential diagnoses?
4 How is the megaesophagus related to the anterior mediastinal mass?
5 What further diagnostic tests should be performed?
6 What are the potential treatment options?

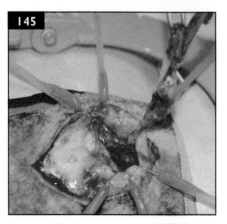

CASE 145 A 4-year-old spayed female DSH cat presented for a subcutaneous lump on the midline over the caudal lumbar spine. The mass was fixed to underlying tissue. An MDB was normal. Fine needle aspirates of the mass yielded sebaceous material and were considered non-diagnostic. An excisional biopsy was performed (**145**). At the time of surgery, the mass was found to be attached to a stalk, which appeared to be extending to the depth of the spinal column.

1 What does this mass likely represent?
2 What are the possible complications that can occur if the external portion of the mass were to rupture?

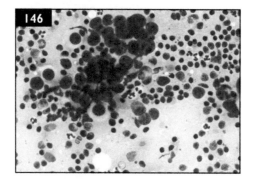

CASE 146 This is the cytology (**146**, 500× oil immersion) from an FNA taken from the submandibular lymph node of an 11-year-old neutered male Spaniel mix that had been losing weight for several weeks. The owner reported that the dog sounded congested at home and had experienced several episodes of gagging. The submandibular lymph nodes were bilaterally enlarged (1.5 cm) and firm. There were no other abnormalities found on examination. Thoracic and abdominal radiographs were normal. Blood work was unremarkable.

1 What does the cytology reveal?
2 What is the probable cause of the lymphadenopathy and what should be done to evaluate this patient further?

CASE 147 Figure (**147a**) is a photograph of a 6-year-old neutered male DSH cat that developed two subcutaneous masses on the left forelimb. Two weeks after the initial masses were noted, the disease had progressed and at least eight new masses were noted on the opposite forelimb and neck (**147b**). A fine needle aspirate was performed on one of the masses, which confirmed mast cell tumor.

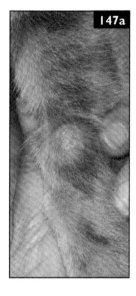 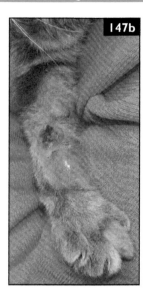

1 What further staging tests should be performed?
2 What is the prognostic value of histopathology?
3 Do cats possess mutations in *c-KIT* as seen in dogs? Is evaluation of cytoplasmic KIT labeling beneficial in cats?
4 What are negative prognostic indicators for mast cell tumors in cats?
5 What treatment should be considered for this patient?

CASE 148 A 12-year-old spayed female DSH cat presented when it was noted that the right third eyelid was prolapsed. Her appetite had been decreased for several days. On physical examination, the right pupil was miotic, the third eyelid was prolapsed, and the eye was enophthalmic (**148**). There were no other physical abnormalities.

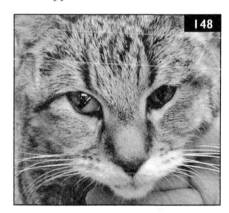

1 What does this picture demonstrate?
2 What are the differential diagnoses for this abnormality?
3 What diagnostic tests are indicated?

CASE 149 An apparently healthy 7-year-old neutered male Golden Retriever collapsed while playing with the other dogs in the household and it was assumed

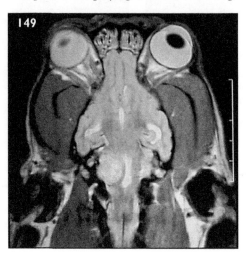

he had been playing too roughly and had been knocked over by another dog. Later in the same week, he was walking across the kitchen floor, appeared ataxic, and collapsed again. He remained conscious (no evidence of seizure-like activity) but it took several minutes for him to stand up. On physical examination, the heart and lungs were normal. There was a slight decrease in conscious proprioception in the hindlimbs. An MDB revealed no clinical abnormalities. An abdominal ultrasound was normal.

1 What are the possible causes for collapse?
2 How should this patient's work-up proceed?
3 Based on the T1-weighted post-contrast MRI findings (**149**, courtesy of Dr. Michael Wolf, Diplomate ACVIM [Neurology]), what treatments can be considered?
4 What is the prognosis for this patient?

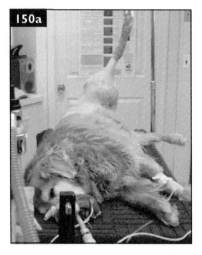

CASE 150 A large mass was noted in the left rear thigh of a 10-year-old spayed female Golden Retriever (**150a**). It had been growing slowly for over a year, but only recently started to cause the dog discomfort and lameness. Multiple fine needle aspirates in different regions of the mass yielded only fat. Radiographs of the limb showed fat density throughout the thigh.

1 What is the probable diagnosis?
2 What further work-up is indicated?
3 What is the best treatment for this patient?

CASE 151 Shown are CT scans (thorax window, post-contrast [**151a**] and lung window, at caudal aspect of the mass, post-contrast [**151b**]) from a 13-year-old spayed female Shih Tzu that was evaluated for an intermittent gagging cough. She was otherwise normal clinically. Thoracic radiographs showed an anterior thoracic mass. An MDB was otherwise normal. An abdominal ultrasound was also performed and was unremarkable. Cytology from a CT-guided FNA of the mass is shown (**151c**).

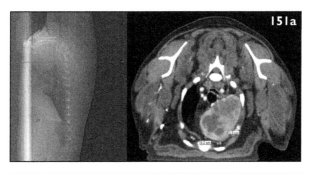

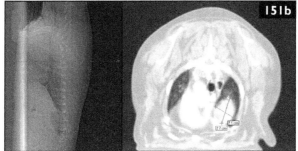

1 Describe the CT images.
2 What is the cytologic diagnosis?
3 What are the differential diagnoses for this patient's mass?
4 This patient was taken to surgery and a right cranial lung lobe mass was found to be infiltrating into the mediastinum. The tumor was removed and the histologic diagnosis was well-differentiated

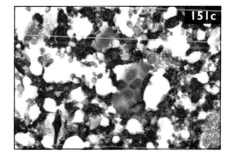

papillary carcinoma with clean margins. What are the negative prognostic indicators for dogs with primary lung tumors?

CASE 152 A 15-year-old neutered male DSH cat presented for evaluation of a right-sided nasal discharge, sneezing, and apparent pain on the right side of the face. On physical examination, there was a low-grade heart murmur. There was a serosanguineous discharge noted from the right nostril with thickening over the right frontal sinus. The right eye was not able to be retropulsed. There was no evidence of lymphadenopathy. The remainder of the physical examination was normal. The MDB was also normal. Shown is a non-contrast CT scan from the largest part of the mass (**152a**) and cytology from a CT-guided fine needle aspirate (**152b**).

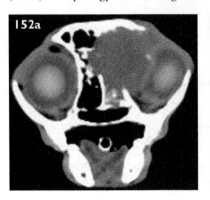
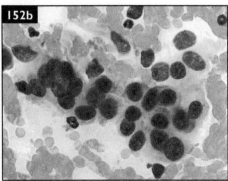

1 Describe the CT scan and list the differential diagnoses for this lesion.
2 What is the cytologic diagnosis?
3 What further diagnostic tests should be performed?
4 What treatment options can be offered?

CASE 153 A 2.5-year-old neutered male Long Haired Dachshund is pictured (**153**). A tongue mass was noted incidentally by the owner when the dog was panting. A biopsy

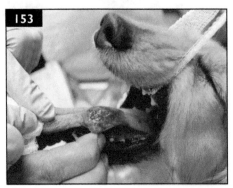

was performed and histologically the mass was an undifferentiated round cell tumor. Immunohistochemistry was performed: CD79a, CD3, and CD18 were negative; CD45 was positive.

1 What is the interpretation of the IHC results?
2 The tumor goes to the midline. Is surgery an option?
3 What further diagnostics should be performed?

CASE 154 A clinically normal 8-year-old neutered male DSH cat was found to have a palpably enlarged left kidney on routine yearly examination (**154**).

1 What are the differential diagnoses for this patient?
2 What diagnostic tests should be done?

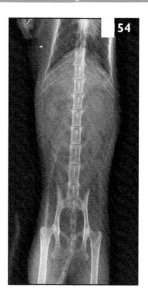

CASE 155 A 10-year-old neutered male Golden Retriever is presented for generalized lymphadenopathy. When node enlargement was first noted 1 week prior, the patient was asymptomatic. Over the last week, the nodes were increasing in size rapidly and now he was vomiting, dehydrated, very lethargic, and had pale mucous membranes. Thoracic radiographs showed sternal and hilar lymphadenopathy, and abdominal ultrasound revealed an enlarged

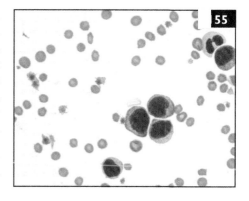

mottled spleen and mesenteric and sublumbar lymphadenopathy. Cytology of the lymph node was consistent with lymphoma. The peripheral blood smear is shown (**155**).

1 What stage of disease is represented in this patient?
2 What further diagnostics should be recommended?
3 What factors in this patient's case are associated with a poorer prognosis?

CASE 156 This is the Canine Transdermal Device used to administer the Oncept®
canine melanoma vaccine (**156a, b**).

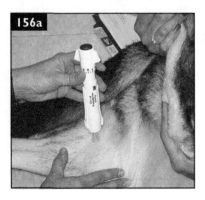

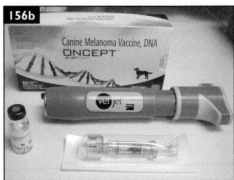

1 What is the purpose of using a transdermal device to deliver this vaccine?
2 What are the major side effects noted when using this type of device?

CASE 157 A 10-year-old spayed female mixed breed dog was having difficulty
swallowing. A large, firmly fixed midline mass was palpated in the neck. The lateral
neck radiograph (**157a**) and cytology from an FNA of the mass (**157b**) are shown.
The cytology was very bloody, but clumps of the cells pictured here were seen at
the feathered edge of the slide.

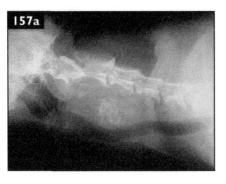

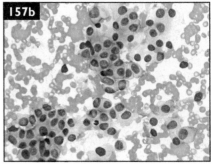

1 What is the most likely diagnosis?
2 In addition to the MDB, what diagnostic tests are advised?
3 What dictates the treatment decision?
4 What treatment options can be considered?

CASE 158 In **158a**, doxorubicin (Adriamycin®) is being drawn up for use in a dog with hemangiosarcoma. A Class II chemotherapy vertical laminar flow hood is being used, but additional precaution is being taken.

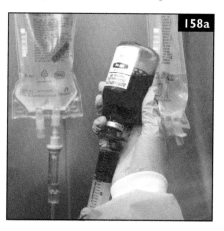

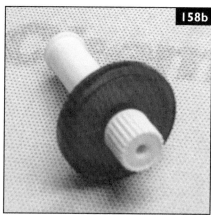

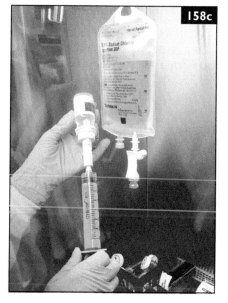

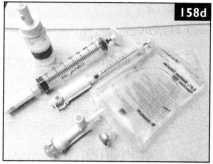

1 What is the name of the object shown in **158a** and **158b**?
2 What major contamination risk is this object attempting to overcome?
3 What are the devices shown in **158c** and **158d** and what are their advantages?

CASE 159 An 8-year-old neutered male Shih Tzu was evaluted for polyuria/polydipsea of approximately 2–3 months' duration. Most recently, he had started to lose weight and had a poor appetite. The physical examination was normal. The MDB was normal except for an ionized calcium of 2.2 mmol/l. Abdominal ultrasound was unremarkable. Parathyroid hormone, ionized calcium, and PTH-related peptide (PTHrP) were evaluated:

Procedure	Results	Reference range	Units
Parathyroid hormone	3.90	0.50–5.80	pmol/l
Ionized calcium	2.20 H	1.25–1.45	mmol/l
Parathyroid hormone-related peptide	0.0	0.0–1.0	pmol/l

1 What are the causes of hypercalcemia in dogs?
2 What is the interpretation of these results?
3 What further diagnostic tests should be performed?
4 How should this dog be treated?
5 What are the complications of treatment?

CASE 160 A 6-year-old spayed female American Bulldog was evaluated for a 6-month history of cutaneous lesions initially believed to be due to bacterial dermatitis. She was pruritic, but this appeared to be well controlled with diphenhydramine. The skin lesions were generalized, but worse in the caudal abdominal and inguinal area. The lesions varied in appearance and included focal areas of depigmentation and scaling, plaque-like lesions with erosions and crusting (160). There was also diffuse erythema noted. The remainder of the physical examination was unremarkable. Lymphadenopathy was not present. A skin biopsy was performed and confirmed epitheliotropic lymphoma (cutaneous T cell lymphoma [CTCL] or mycosis fungoides). Immunohistochemistry confirmed CD8+ T cells.

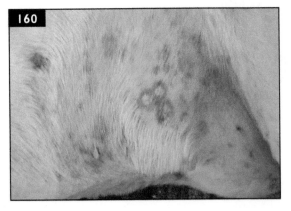

1 What further diagnostic tests should be considered prior to treatment?
2 What treatment and supportive care should be recommended?
3 What is the prognosis for this patient?

CASE 161 Many pet owners have received chemotherapy themselves or have watched friends and relatives undergo cancer treatment and have great concern over the potential for side effects. Hair loss is one of those side effects that raises significant concerns among pet owners. Figure **161a** shows a Giant Schnauzer mix undergoing chemotherapy; **161b** shows loss of feathering in a Golden Retriever receiving doxorubicin chemotherapy.

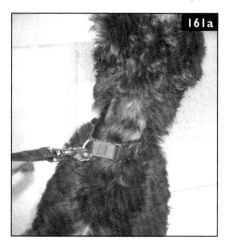
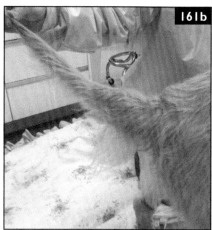

1 Name the breeds of dog that are more susceptible to chemotherapy-related hair loss.
2 What hair loss patterns are seen in cats undergoing chemotherapy?
3 What chemotherapy agents are more likely to cause hair loss?

CASE 162 Adriamycin® (doxorubicin HCl) is a commonly used chemotherapeutic agent in human and veterinary medicine. It is pictured (**162**) with a chemotherapy dispensing pin.

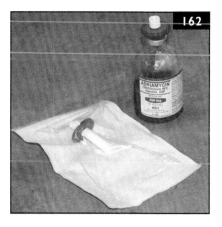

1 What are the primary side effects of doxorubicin seen in dogs?
2 How do the side effects of doxorubicin seen in cats differ from those in dogs?

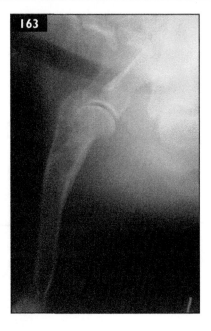

CASE 163 A 9-year-old spayed female mixed breed dog weighing 10 kg presented for an acute onset of left forelimb lameness. A firm, painful swelling was noted at the level of the proximal humerus. A radiograph of the limb was taken (**163**). Thoracic radiographs, CBC, chemistry panel, and urinalysis were normal.

1 Describe the radiograph and give the differential diagnoses.
2 What further diagnostic tests are indicated?
3 A biopsy revealed osteosarcoma, low grade. What treatment recommendations should be made?
4 How is the prognosis for this patient different from that of the majority of dogs diagnosed with osteosarcoma?

CASE 164 A 32 kg Golden Retriever mix was presented following an excisional biopsy of a tumor on the lateral aspect of the elbow (**164**). The diagnosis was a grade II soft tissue sarcoma with tumor cells extending to the lateral and deep margins. The owners did not wish to pursue either more surgery or postoperative radiation therapy. The following chemotherapy protocol was prescribed:

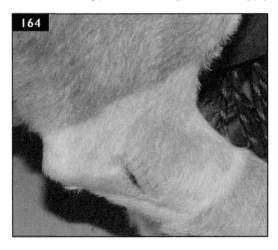

- Cyclophosphamide 15 mg once daily
- Piroxicam 10 mg once daily.

1 Describe the type of chemotherapy protocol that this represents.
2 In what cancers in dogs and cats has this type of chemotherapeutic regimen been evaluated?

CASE 165 A 9-year-old spayed female Pit Bull mix presented for a 2-week history of rapid weight loss (5.5 kg) in the face of a good appetite. On physical examination, in addition to the profound weight loss and muscle wasting, peripheral lymph nodes were enlarged (**165**, arrow points to left prescapular lymph node). Further diagnostic tests including an MDB, abdominal ultrasound, and cytology of multiple lymph nodes yielded a presumptive diagnosis of lymphoma.

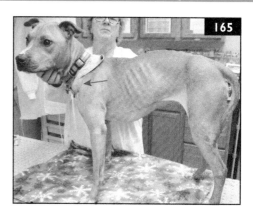

1 The history and clinical appearance of this patient are suggestive of what paraneoplastic syndrome?
2 How common is this syndrome in pets with cancer?
3 How does the presence of this syndrome affect this patient's prognosis?
4 What is sarcopenia?

CASE 166 A 12-year-old intact female Shih Tzu was evaluated for constipation, stranguria, vaginal discharge, and abdominal distension. A large caudal abdominal mass was palpated, but the remainder of the examination was unremarkable. The MDB including thoracic radiographs was normal. Abdominal ultrasound revealed a large homogeneous mass that measured 10.9 × 6.9 × 11.8 cm. The mass appeared to be displacing

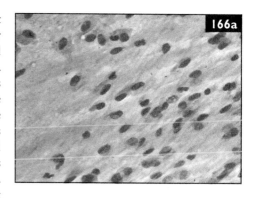

the bladder and colon laterally and other organs cranially. An ultrasound-guided FNA of the mass was performed and the cytology is shown (**166a**).

1 Describe the cytology and give a preliminary diagnosis.
2 What are the differential diagnoses?
3 What further tests are indicated in order to determine the best treatment plan?
4 What is the best course of treatment?

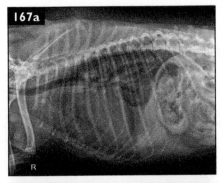

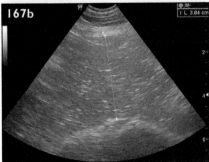

CASE 167 This (**167a**) is a radiograph taken of a 9-year-old spayed female Border Collie that presented for a recent onset of a non-productive cough that was noted at least 4–5 times daily. There had been a history of up to 2 years of an occasional cough that was thought to be due to allergies. The patient was otherwise healthy, had a good appetite, and was showing no other clinical symptoms. Other than muffled heart sounds, the physical examination was normal. The MDB was normal. An ultrasound of the heart and surrounding structures was performed. Cardiac function was normal and an ultrasound of tissue near the heart is shown (**167b**).

1 Describe the radiograph and ultrasound.
2 What further diagnostics are indicated for this patient?
3 What treatment is advised?
4 What is the patient's prognosis?

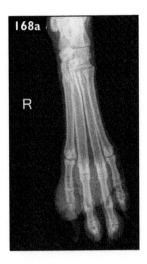

CASE 168 This is the radiograph of the right rear foot of a 9-year-old neutered male Rottweiler that presented for lameness and a painful swollen second digit (**168a**). The right popliteal lymph node was firm and measured 2 cm; the left popliteal node was normal. An MDB including thoracic radiographs was normal.

1 What are the radiographic findings?
2 What are the differential diagnoses for this patient?
3 What additional tests should be performed?
4 What is the treatment and prognosis for this patient?

CASE 169 A 10-year-old Giant Schnauzer mix presented for a 3-day history of hyphema (hemorrhage into the anterior chamber). The hyphema was bilateral, but more obvious in the left eye (**169a**). There was no history of trauma. The remainder of the physical examination was unremarkable except for a palpable (1.0 cm) left submandibular lymph node. Thoracic radiographs were normal. The spleen was moderately enlarged and mottled in appearance. A CBC and chemistry panel were normal with the exception of increased globulins (10 mg/dl). A fine needle aspirate of the submandibular node was performed and the cytology is shown (**169b**).

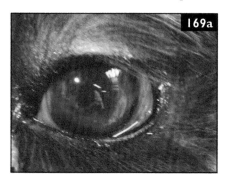
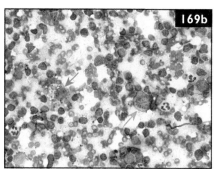

1 Describe the cytology.
2 What further diagnostic tests should be performed?
3 What are the differential diagnoses for hyphema and hyperglobulinema?
4 What is a possible mechanism of the hyphema?

CASE 170 A 12-year-old spayed female Rottweiler and a 12-year-old neutered male DSH cat were both diagnosed with osteosarcoma of the proximal humerus. Both patients had normal MDBs with no evidence of metastasis. Both patients had forelimb amputations. Cis-platin is one of the drugs used for the treatment of osteosarcoma (**170**).

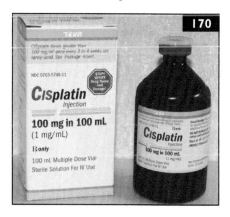

1 Describe how the treatment plans would differ between these two patients.
2 What are the primary toxicities associated with cis-platin use in dogs and in cats?
3 What is the administration protocol for cis-platin?

CASE 171 A 12-year-old neutered male Yorkshire Terrier collapsed while going for a walk. There had been no prior clinical symptoms noted. The dog's owner thought it was due to hot weather and, because the dog got up within a minute,

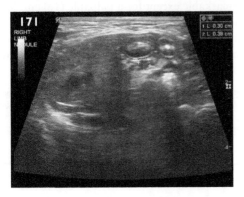

was not initially concerned. One week later, he collapsed again, but this time had a seizure. On physical examination, other than lenticular sclerosis in both eyes (OU), he appeared healthy. There were no cardiac murmurs or arrhythmias noted. Mucous membranes were pink and moist, and capillary refill time was <1 second. However, during the examination the dog was excited, became ataxic, and collapsed.

1 What are the differential diagnoses for this patient?
2 In addition to the MDB, an abdominal ultrasound was performed. The ultrasound image of the region of the pancreas is shown (**171**). A 0.30 × 0.38 cm hypoechoic nodule is seen within the right limb of the pancreas. What further diagnostic tests are indicated?
3 The blood glucose at the time of collapse was 40 mg/dl. What further tests should be performed based on this finding?
4 How is the diagnosis of insulinoma made?
5 List the prognostic indicators for insulinoma in the dog.

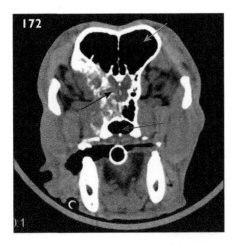

CASE 172 This is a CT scan (**172**) of the head at the caudal aspect of the nasal cavity of a 12-year-old spayed female Golden Retriever that presented for inappetence and right-sided epistaxis.

1 What structure is the blue arrow pointing to?
2 What structure is the black arrow pointing to?
3 What is the red arrow pointing to?
4 Describe the CT scan. What is the significance of the changes seen at the tip of the black arrow?

CASE 173 A 4-year-old spayed female black Labrador Retriever presented for suspected back pain. She had not been as active as normal over the previous several weeks and had stopped jumping up on furniture. A shortened stride and narrow hindlimb gait were noted. She was also experiencing muscle tremors in the shoulder area. On physical examination, she was bright, alert, and responsive. She had decreased hindlimb and tail tone. Mild lumbosacral pain was appreciated with deep palpation of the lumbosacral region of the spine. The neurologic examination revealed normal postural reactions, decreased flexion of both hocks, pseudo-hyperreflexia of both patellas. An L4–S2 myelopathy was suspected. An MDB and abdominal ultrasound were within normal limits (**173a**, T2-weighted image; **173b**, T1-weighted image). An MRI of the spine was performed (**173c**) and, at the same time, cerebrospinal fluid (CSF) was obtained. (Images courtesy Dr. Michael Wolf DACVIM [Neurology]).

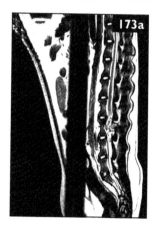

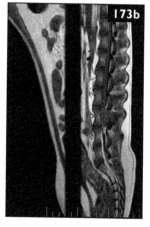

Cytology of the cisternal CSF

Color: colorless

Clarity: slightly cloudy

WBC (CSF): 0

RBC (CSF): 1 (high)

Protein: 35 mg/dl (normal for cisternal, ≤30 mg/dl)

Description: The cytospin preparations lacked overt nucleated cellularity with occasional anucleate keratinocytes, erythrocytes, and glove powder crystals present.

---

1 Describe the lesion seen on MRI.
2 What are the differential diagnoses for this lesion?
3 How should a definitive diagnosis be obtained?
4 What treatment options should be considered and what is this patient's prognosis?

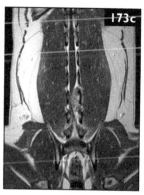

CASE 174 A 9-year-old neutered male DSH cat was evaluated for vomiting, lethargy, and weight loss. On physical examination, there was a firm palpable mid-abdominal mass approximately 5 cm in diameter. Mucous membranes were pale and slightly tacky. FeLV and FIV were negative. On ultrasound, a 5 × 4 cm mass was seen associated with the small intestine. Several mesenteric lymph nodes were noted, measuring 2 cm or less. The echogenicity of the liver and spleen was mottled, suggestive of infiltrative disease. Shown is the cytology from an ultrasound-guided aspirate of the intestinal mass (**174**).

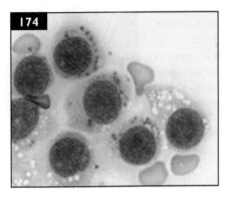

1 What is the cytologic diagnosis?
2 What further diagnostic tests are indicated to make a definitive diagnosis and stage the patient?
3 What is the prognosis for this patient?

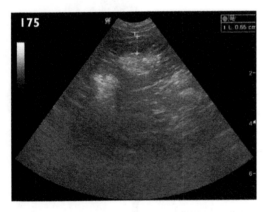

CASE 175 A 12-year-old neutered male Chow Chow was presented for anorexia, weight loss, and intermittent dark, tarry stools. Other than melena noted on rectal examination, the physical examination was normal. The hematocrit was 28%. The mild anemia appeared regenerative on evaluation of the blood smear. The remainder of the CBC and the serum chemistry panel were normal. Thoracic radiographs were normal. An ultrasound image of the stomach is shown (**175**). Approximately 75% of the stomach wall appeared to be abnormal.

1 What is seen on the ultrasound image?
2 What are the primary differential diagnoses?
3 How should a definitive diagnosis be obtained?
4 What is the prognosis for this patient?

CASE 176 A 10-year-old neutered male DSH cat presented for dyspnea with an abdominal component to breathing. He had lost almost 1 kg since last being weighed almost 1 year previously. He was also reported to be lethargic and several episodes of regurgitation had been noted. An MDB was performed. Other than a significant lymphocytosis of 8,000/µl, the results of the MDB were normal. FeLV/FIV status was negative. VD and lateral thoracic radiographs (**176a, b**) and an ultrasound image at the level of the heart (**176c**) are shown. An ultrasound-guided FNA was performed and revealed a mixed population of cells consisting mostly of small lymphocytes, with occasional epithelial cells and mast cells noted.

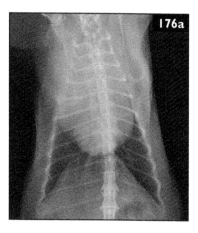

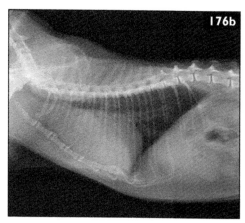

1 Describe the radiographs and ultrasound.
2 List the differential diagnoses for a mass in this location.
3 What diagnosis is most likely based on the testing performed thus far?
4 What further diagnostic tests can provide a definitive diagnosis and establish extent of disease?
5 What are the treatment options for this patient?
6 List the positive and negative prognostic indicators for this disease.
7 What paraneoplastic syndromes can be seen in cats with this diagnosis?

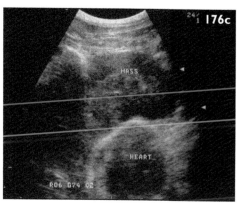

CASE 177 A 7-year-old neutered male 26 kg mixed breed dog was evaluated after several months of symptomatic therapy for chronic vomiting with occasional frank blood. There was also intermittent diarrhea with melena. He had lost approximately 3 kg since symptoms started and was becoming increasingly more lethargic. He initially improved with metoclopramide, famotidine, and a bland diet, but symptoms returned.

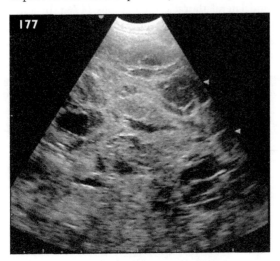

On physical examination, he was noted to have an elevated heart rate (160/min), elevated temperature (103.7°F; 39.8°C), and appeared to be painful on palpation of the cranial abdomen. Thoracic and abdominal radiographs were unremarkable. An abdominal ultrasound was performed and a diffusely thickened gastric wall and prominent rugal folds were noted. Several mesenteric lymph nodes were noted to be enlarged (ranging from 1 cm to 2 cm in diameter). There were multiple hypoechoic lesions in the liver ranging in size from 0.5 cm to 2 cm (**177**) The hematocrit was 24%, WBC 32,000/µl, and platelets 230,000/µl. The serum chemistry panel is shown. Endoscopy was performed and revealed several gastric ulcers.

Test	Result	Flag	Units	Normal Range
Chemistry (DRI-CHEM)				
BUN	52.0	High	mg/dl	9.0–29.0
Creatinine	1.0		mg/dl	0.4–1.4
Phosphorus	3.3		mg/dl	1.9–5.0
Calcium	9.8		mg/dl	9.0–12.2
Corrected Ca	9.9		mg/dl	9.0–12.2
Total Protein	5.0	Low	g/dl	5.5–7.6
Albumin	2.1	Low	g/dl	2.5–4.0
Globulin	2.9		g/dl	2.0–3.6
Alb/Glob Ratio	0.72			
Glucose	111		mg/dl	75–125
Cholesterol	305		mg/dl	120–310
ALT (GPT)	140	High	U/l	0–120
ALP	180	High	U/l	0–140
GGT	16	High	U/l	0–14
Total Bilirubin	0.3		mg/dl	0.0–0.5

1 What further diagnostic tests are indicated?
2 There is evidence of metastatic disease on ultrasound. Would surgery be indicated?
3 What is Zollinger–Ellison syndrome and how should it be medically managed?
4 What is the prognosis for this patient?

CASE 178 A 16-year-old spayed female DLH cat had a 2-year history of mild azotemia. Three weeks prior to presentation, there was concern that she was hiding a lot. There were no other clinical symptoms. Thoracic and abdominal radiographs were normal. On ultrasound, a lesion was noted on the right kidney. Blood work, an ultrasound image of the right kidney (**178a**), and cytology of an ultrasound-guided FNA (**178b**) are shown.

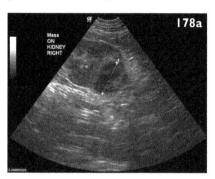
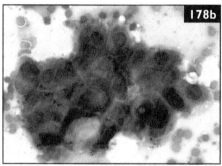

Test	Result	Flag	Units	Normal Range
Hematology (HemaTrue)				
WBC	9.6		10³/µl	5.5-19.5
LYM	0.9	Low	10³/µl	1.8-7.0
MONO	0.4		10³/µl	0.2-1.0
GRAN	8.3		10³/µl	2.8-13.0
LYM%	10.1			
MONO%	3.7			
GRAN%	86.2			
HCT	32.0		%	25.0-45.0
MCV	44.1		fl	39.0-50.0
RDWa	32.1		fl	20.0-35.0
RDW%	19.5	High	%	13.5-18.0
HGB	12.2		g/dl	8.0-15.0
MCHC	38.2		g/dl	31.0-38.5
MCH	16.9		pg	12.5-17.5
RBC	7.25		10⁶/µl	5.00-11.00
PLT	333		10³/µl	200-500
MPV	9.4		fl	8.0-12.0

Test	Result	Flag	Units	Normal Range
Chemistry (DRI-CHEM)				
BUN	39.4	High	mg/dl	15.0-32.0
Creatinine	2.5	High	mg/dl	0.8-1.8
Phosphorus	3.8		mg/dl	2.6-6.0
Calcium	10.0	High	mg/dl	8.8-11.9
Total Protein	7.4		g/dl	6.0-8.0
Albumin	3.4		g/dl	2.3-3.5
Globulin	4.0		g/dl	2.8-4.8
Alb/Glob Ratio	0.9			
Glucose	147	High	mg/dl	70-130
Cholesterol	223	High	mg/dl	70-200
ALT (GPT)	35		U/l	0-85
ALP	42		U/l	0-90
GGT	<10		U/l	0-10
Total Bilirubin	<0.1		mg/dl	0.0-0.5

1 Describe the ultrasound and cytology findings. What is the presumptive diagnosis?
2 What is the treatment of choice for primary renal tumors?
3 What is recommended for this patient?

CASE 179 A 12-year-old neutered male Beagle/German Shepherd mix was presented for an acute onset of bleeding from the rectum. His appetite had been decreased for a few weeks but this was initially attributed to the recent addition of another pet to the household. The physical examination was normal with the exception of frank blood dripping from the rectum (**179a**). On rectal examination, the anal sacs were normal. Immediately after the rectal examination, a large amount of partially clotted blood was eliminated (**179b**).

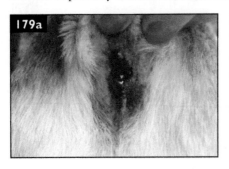 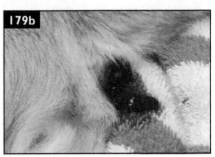

1 What are the differential diagnoses for hematochezia in this patient?
2 What is the likely cause for the blood being eliminated immediately after the rectal examination?
3 What diagnostic tests should be pursued next?
4 What are the most common malignancies found in the rectum?
5 A rectal pull-through surgery was advised for this patient. What complications can be associated with this type of surgery?

CASE 180 A 10-year-old neutered male DSH cat presented for lethargy and poor appetite. The physical examination was normal. An MDB was normal with the exception of the CBC. The hematocrit was 73%, the hemoglobin 23.1 g/dl (reference, 8.0–15.0), and RBC count 16.46 × 10^6/μl (reference, 5.00–11.00). The patient's serum protein was normal.

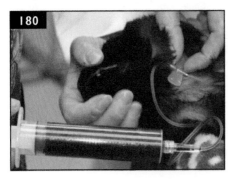

1 What procedure is being illustrated here (**180**)?
2 What are the differential diagnoses for this patient?
3 What further diagnostic tests are indicated?
4 How should this patient be managed?

CASE 181 This is the ventral abdomen of a 3-year-old spayed female Golden Retriever that presented for evaluation of a suspected zoonotic dermatitis (181). She had returned from vacation in an area with a significant tick population and was noted to have small, flat black spots on the skin that were suspected to be secondary to tick bites. She was treated with Frontline® (fipronil), but the lesions progressed from small flat lesions to raised growths, with some open and oozing. In addition to the multiple skin lesions noted, moderate peripheral lymphadenopathy (nodes ranged from 1 to 3 cm) was noted. Skin biopsies showed nodules that appeared like non-regressing histiocytomas. Immunohistochemical staining revealed the following: CD3–; E-cadherin+.

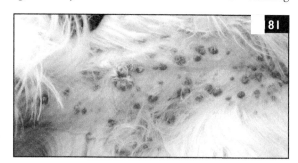

1 What is the diagnosis?
2 What further diagnostics should be performed?
3 What is the cause of this disease?
4 How should this patient be managed?

CASE 182 Shown are a plain radiograph (182a) and a post-contrast CT scan (182b) from a 10-year-old neutered male Golden Retriever that presented for an acute onset of a firm lump over the left zygomatic arch. The lump felt bony, with temporal and masseter muscle atrophy noted. The blink reflexes were normal bilaterally. The physical examination was otherwise normal.

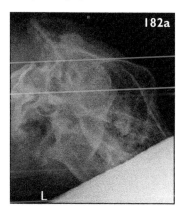

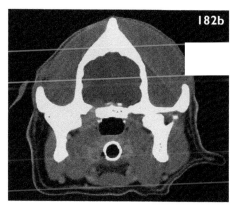

1 Describe the radiograph and CT scan.
2 What are the differential diagnoses for this lesion?

103

CASE 183 A 16-year-old neutered male Poodle presented for evaluation of a firm swelling of the left maxilla (**183a, b**). The patient had recently undergone a dental prophy and tooth extraction for what was believed to be a tooth root abscess. There was no improvement after the extractions and 2 weeks of antibiotics, and the swelling worsened. Given the patient's age, the owner did not wish to pursue definitive treatment such as curative intent radiation, surgery, or chemotherapy, but wanted to pursue an appropriate palliative approach.

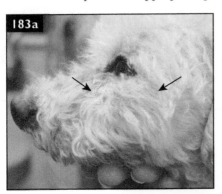
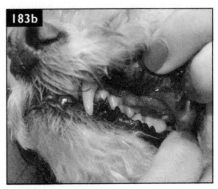

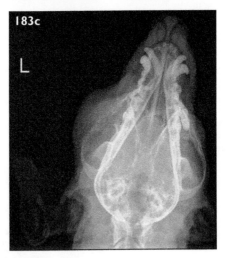

1 Describe the radiograph (**183c**).
2 What are the differential diagnoses for this lesion?
3 What palliative options could be recommended?

CASE 184 This is routine blood work performed as part of a yearly examination for a 10-year-old neutered male Labradoodle. He was experiencing no clinical symptoms except a slight increase in the amount of water he was drinking. This was attributed by the owner to recent hot weather. He was bright, alert, active, and had not lost any weight. There is an elevated globulin level, which was determined to be a monoclonal gammopathy through serum electrophoresis.

Test	Result	Flag	Units	Normal Range
Hematology (HemaTrue)				
WBC	5.3	Low	10³/µl	6.0–17.0
LYM	1.5		10³/µl	0.9–5.0
MONO	0.5		10³/µl	0.3–1.5
GRAN	3.3	Low	10³/µl	3.5–12.0
LYM%	28.1			
MONO%	9.8			
GRAN%	62.1			
HCT	29.7	Low	%	37.0–55.0
MCV	58.0	Low	fl	60.0–72.0
RDWa	46.3		fl	35.0–53.0
RDW%	20.5	High	%	12.0–17.5
HGB	11.5	Low	g/dl	12.0–18.0
MCHC	38.7	High	g/dl	32.0–38.5
MCH	22.4		pg	19.5–25.5
RBC	5.12	Low	10⁶/µl	5.50–8.50
PLT	123	Low	10³/µl	200–500
MPV	7.4		fl	5.5–10.5

Test	Result	Flag	Units	Normal Range
Chemistry (DRI-CHEM)				
BUN	27.7		mg/dl	9.0–29.0
Creatinine	1.3		mg/dl	0.4–1.4
Phosphorus	4.4		mg/dl	1.9–5.0
Calcium	>15.3	High	mg/dl	9.0–12.2
Corrected Ca	****		mg/dl	9.0–12.2
Total Protein	>11.0	High	g/dl	5.5–7.6
Albumin	3.6		g/dl	2.5–4.0
Globulin	****		g/dl	2.0–3.6
Alb/Glob Ratio	****			
Glucose	122		mg/dl	75–125
Cholesterol	201		mg/dl	120–310
ALT (GPT)	176	High	U/l	0–120
ALP	34		U/l	0–140
GGT	10		U/l	0–14
Total Bilirubin	<0.1		mg/dl	0.0–0.5

VitalPathClient:				
pO₂	32.7	Low	mmHg	80.0–100.0
sO₂(c)	65.6		%	
pCO⁻	34.1	Low	mmHg	35.0–45.0
CHCO⁺	22.7		mmol/l	
pH	7.441			7.330–7.450
BEecf	–1.4		mmol/l	
BE	–0.7		mmol/l	
Na	154.7	High	mmol/l	139.0–151.0
K	4.23		mmol/l	3.80–5.30
Cl	113.0		mmol/l	102.0–120.0
AG	23.3		mmol/l	
Ca²⁺	1.52	High	mmol/l	1.25–1.43

1 What are the differential diagnoses for a monoclonal gammopathy?
2 What further diagnostic tests should be performed?
3 What criteria need to be met to make a diagnosis of multiple myeloma?
4 What treatment and prognosis can be provided for this pet?
5 What are the negative prognostic indicators?

CASE 185 This is the VD thoracic radiograph (**185a**) and photograph (**185b**) of a 9-year-old neutered male Beagle mix that presented for an acute onset of multiple generalized subcutaneous lesions (initially thought to be due to an allergic reaction) and a gagging cough. On physical examination, he was bright and alert and appeared to be feeling normal. There were more than a hundred 0.5–1 cm subcutaneous raised lesions, a grade IV/VI pansystolic heart murmur, and generalized lymphadenopathy. Cytology from an FNA of one of the subcutaneous masses is shown (**185c**). A CBC revealed a mild anemia (PCV 29%) and thrombocytopenia (58,000/µl), confirmed on a blood smear. Serum chemistry values, including calcium, were within normal limits.

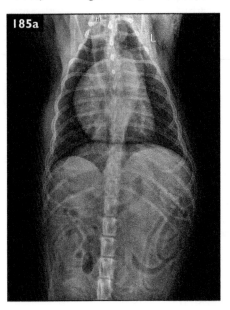

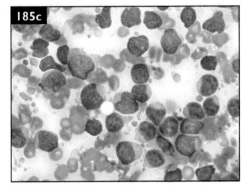

1 What is the diagnosis?
2 Describe the radiograph. What is the probable cause of the cough?
3 What further diagnostics should be performed?
4 What is the stage of disease and how does it affect the prognosis?
5 Describe a treatment plan for this patient taking into consideration the blood work.

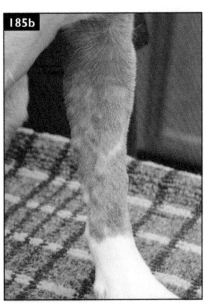

CASE 186 This is the ultrasound image of the stomach wall (**186**) of a 9-year-old neutered male DSH cat presented for inappetence, vomiting, and fever (103.5°F, 39.7°C). The remainder of the ultrasound was normal with the exception of a single 0.9 × 1.0 cm regional lymph node. A fine needle aspirate of the stomach wall was performed with ultrasound guidance and

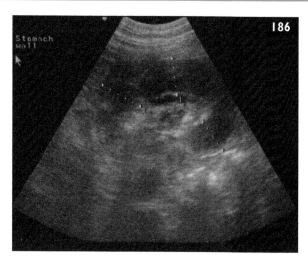

revealed a monomorphic population of medium to large lymphocytes. Thoracic radiographs were normal and blood work unremarkable.

1 Based on the ultrasound appearance and cytology description, what is the diagnosis and stage of disease?
2 What is the most common type of lymphoma diagnosed in the stomach of cats?
3 What are the best indicators of prognosis for this form of lymphoma?

CASE 187 Palladia® (toceranib phosphate) is a tyrosine kinase inhibitor recently approved for use in dogs (**187**).

1 What is the mechanism of action of this drug?
2 What are the indications for using Palladia®?
3 While this drug is not considered to be a chemotherapeutic agent, significant toxicities can be associated with its use. Describe the potential side effects and the management of these side effects.
4 What safety precautions do pet owners need to be aware of when giving their pets Palladia®?

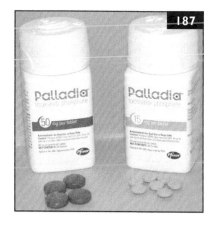

CASE 188 A 12-year-old spayed female Pug presented for evaluation of a 6.5 × 5 × 2 cm cutaneous mass on the left lateral neck (**188a**). The mass was reported to have been first noted as a small (2 cm) lesion over 4 years prior, but diagnosis and treatment were not pursued at that time. A fine needle aspirate was performed and the cytology is shown (**188b**). The patient was otherwise clinically normal.

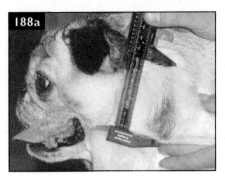 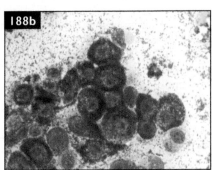

1 What is the diagnosis?
2 What factors seen in these photographs help predict the biologic behavior of this tumor?
3 What further diagnostic tests should be performed in order to develop a treatment plan?

CASE 189 A 12-year-old neutered male DSH cat presented for evaluation of a recently noted mass over the right thigh and flank area (**189**). The mass measured 6 cm in length and was firmly attached to the underlying tissues. A portion of the mass was involving the tissues of the abdominal wall and extended distally to the stifle joint. A fine needle aspirate was performed and results revealed a soft tissue sarcoma. The physical examination was otherwise normal.

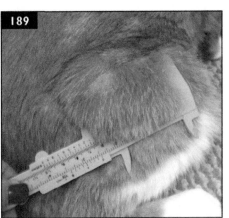

1 What further information should be obtained from the clinical history?
2 What diagnostic tests are indicated?
3 What treatment options should be offered?

CASE 190 A 6-year-old spayed female Golden Retriever presented for a several-day history of lethargy, inappetence, and drooping of the left lip (190a). There was no sensory response on the left lip, the left blink and menace response were absent, and there was crusting of the nasal opening on the left consistent with facial nerve paralysis. The submandibular lymph nodes were prominent (1.5 cm bilaterally). There were no other abnormalities noted. Thoracic and abdominal radiographs were normal. A CBC and blood smear (190b) are shown. A serum chemistry panel was within normal limits.

Test	Result	Flag	Units	Normal Range
Hematology (HemaTrue)				
WBC	47.4	High	$10^3/\mu l$	6.0–17.0
LYM	27.8	High	$10^3/\mu l$	0.9–5.0
MONO	7.9	High	$10^3/\mu l$	0.3–1.5
GRAN	11.7	High	$10^3/\mu l$	3.5–12.0
LYM%	37.6			
MONO%	16.6			
GRAN%	45.8			
HCT	36.2	Low	%	37.0–55.0
MCV	66.3		fl	60.0–72.0
RDWa	50.0		fl	35.0–53.0
RDW%	17.3%			12.0–17.5
HGB	14.2		g/dl	12.0–18.0
MCHC	39.3	High	g/dl	32.0–38.5
MCH	26.1	High	pg	19.5–25.5
RBC	5.46	Low	$10^6/\mu l$	5.50–8.50
PLT	184	Low	$10^3/\mu l$	200–500
MPV	8.3		fl	5.5–10.5

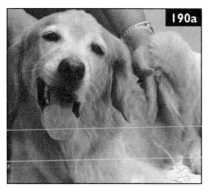

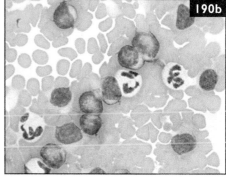

1 What is the presumptive diagnosis?
2 What further diagnostics are needed to confirm the diagnosis?
3 What are the possible reasons for the facial nerve paralysis?
4 How should this patient be treated?

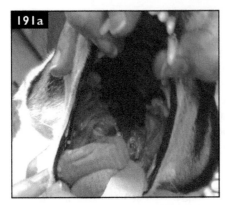

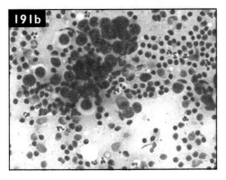

CASE 191 This is the oral cavity of a 10-year-old neutered male mixed breed dog that started losing weight in the face of a good appetite (191a). He sounded congested and would occasionally act as though he were gagging. The submandibular lymph nodes were bilaterally enlarged and measured approximately 2 cm each. The remainder of the physical examination was normal. An MDB was performed and was normal. Shown here is the cytology from a fine needle aspirate of a submandibular lymph node (191b).

1 What abnormality is noted in the oral cavity?
2 Describe the cytology of the submandibular node.
3 What is the most likely diagnosis?
4 What treatment options can be offered?
5 What is the prognosis for this patient?

CASE 192 A 10-year-old neutered male Golden Retriever was noted to have a 1.5 cm interdigital mass on the right forefoot (192). The mass was surgically removed and reported to be a malignant melanoma with clean but narrow (<2 mm) surgical margins. The mitotic index was 7 and malignant cells were considered to be of intermediate malignancy. The right prescapular lymph node was palpable and measured 2 cm. A fine needle aspirate was performed and cytology was consistent with a reactive node.

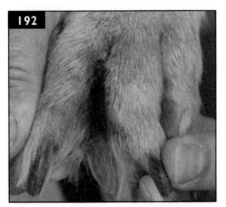

1 What further diagnostic/staging tests are indicated and why?
2 Describe a treatment plan for this patient.
3 What is this patient's prognosis?

CASE 193 A 9-year-old neutered male Bengal cat was evaluated for anorexia and weight loss of approximately 3 months' duration. Other than significant splenomegaly, the remainder of the physical examination was normal. On abdominal ultrasound, the spleen was enlarged, diffusely hypoechoic, and mottled. The laboratory work performed is shown (**193**).

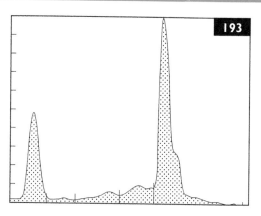

1 What is the interpretation of the protein electrophoresis?
2 What are the differential diagnoses for this patient?
3 What further tests should be done to help make a definitive diagnosis?
4 What treatment is indicated?

Protein electrophoresis, serum		
Total protein	11.5 (High)	6.6–7.8 g/dl
Albumin	2.85	2.1–3.3 g/dl
Globulin	8.65 (High)	2.6–5.1 g/dl
Alpha 1	0.20	0.2–1.1 g/dl
Alpha 2	0.67	0.4–0.9 g/dl
Beta 1	1.11 (High)	0.3–0.9 g/dl
Gamma 1	6.66 (High)	0.3–2.5 g/dl

CASE 194 A 14-year-old spayed female black Labrador Retriever mix was previously diagnosed with stage IVa multicentric lymphoma. She underwent chemotherapy with the University of Wisconsin-Madison Canine Lymphoma protocol. After completion of the protocol, she remained in clinical remission for 11 months at which time a mid-abdominal mass was palpated. Staging (MDB, thoracic radiographs, abdominal ultrasound) was performed. A large splenic mass identified on ultrasound is shown (**194**). An ultrasound-guided FNA confirmed lymphoma relapse. She had no clinical symptoms.

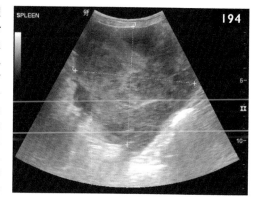

1 Is this patient a good candidate for further chemotherapy?
2 What chemotherapy recommendations should be made?

CASE 195 Shown are ultrasound images (**195a**, left kidney; **195b**, bladder) from a 10-year-old neutered male Beagle mix that presented because of hematuria and pollakiuria. The cytology (**195c**) obtained from a traumatic catheterization of the bladder is also shown.

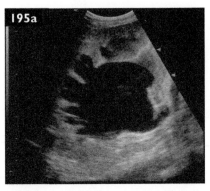

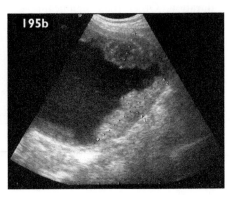

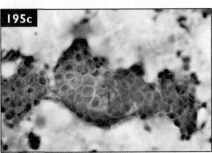

1 What is the presumptive diagnosis?
2 What other staging/diagnostic tests are important in the assessment of this patient?
3 What measures can be taken to help prevent further damage to the kidney?

CASE 196 A 10-year-old neutered male Boxer was presented owing to a sudden onset of increased thirst. The physical examination was normal. A CBC showed a mild anemia (29% hematocrit, hemoglobin 10 g/dl), increased WBC (148,370/µl), neutrophils (6,200/µl), lymphocytes (133,340/µl), and platelets (76,000/µl). The chemistry panel, including calcium, was normal. Thoracic radiographs were normal. On abdominal ultrasound the spleen was moderately enlarged, but no obvious masses or infiltrative disease could be appreciated. Flow cytometry revealed a CD21 lymphocytosis, but the size of the lymphocytes was "borderline" between small and large. There were no CD34+ cells noted.

1 What is the diagnosis for this patient?
2 What is the significance of the size of the lymphocytes?
3 What does the lack of CD34+ cells mean?
4 What treatment should be offered?

CASE 197 A 10-year-old neutered male Labrador Retriever presents with a 2-week history of lethargy and an acute onset (over the previous 2 days) of dyspnea. The patient is healthy otherwise and the physical examination is unremarkable. There is no significant history such as trauma or previous surgeries. An MDB is performed and the thoracic radiograph is shown (**197a**). Thoracocentesis yielded the fluid shown here (**197b**). An abdominal ultrasound was also unremarkable.

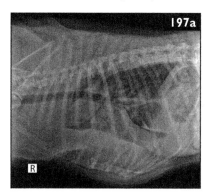
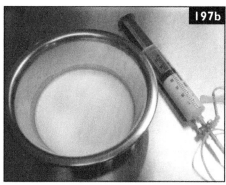

Cytology of Fluid*

Pre-Centrifugation Color: White
Pre-Centrifugation Character: Cloudy
Post-Centrifugation Color: White
Post-Centrifugation Character: Cloudy
Specific Gravity: Unable to read due to fluid character
Total Protein: Unable to read due to fluid character
Nucleated Cells 2290/µl
PCV <2%

Clinical Chemistry

Cholesterol fluid: 100 mg/dl (serum cholesterol: 300 mg/dl)
Triglyceride fluid: 1803 mg/dl (serum triglyceride: 145 mg/dl)

Microscopic Description

Submitted direct smears, as well as direct smears and concentrated preparations from submitted pleural fluid were examined. Submitted direct smears consisted of moderate to large amounts of thick proteinaceous material and cells were not spread well enough for detailed evaluation. Direct smears made from submitted fluid consisted of moderate amounts of thick proteinaceous material in which low numbers of cells were distributed. Concentrated preparations were highly cellular and besides a scant amount of blood consisted of large numbers of small lymphocytes with low numbers of plasma cells, moderate numbers of macrophages and mesothelial cells, moderate numbers of neutrophils, low numbers of mast cells, and a rare eosinophil. Moderate numbers of macrophages contained low numbers of discrete, clear cytoplasmic vacuoles, and few contained large numbers of small, clear cytoplasmic vacuoles. No organisms or atypical cell populations were seen.

* Analysis done at Michigan State University, Clinical Pathology Department.

1 Describe the thoracic radiograph and fluid obtained on thoracocentesis.
2 Based on the appearance of the fluid, what are the primary considerations? The analysis of the fluid is shown. What is your diagnosis?
3 What are the next diagnostic steps following the fluid analysis?

CASE 198 Shown are VD (198a) and lateral (198b) thoracic radiographs of a 7-year-old neutered male Miniature Schnauzer presented for an acute onset of lethargy, vomiting, and apparent discomfort in the abdomen or hips when being picked up. Following identification of the thoracic mass on radiographs, the patient was referred for a CT scan to determine whether the thoracic mass was surgical. The CBC, serum chemistry panel, and urinalysis were normal. A primary lung tumor was suspected.

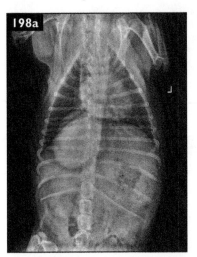

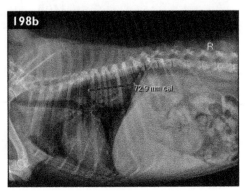

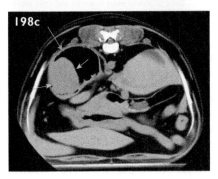

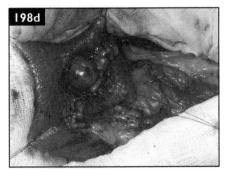

1 What additional tests should be performed prior to a CT scan?
2 A CT image at the level of the stomach is shown (198c, orange arrow indicates stomach wall, green arrows point to mass). In addition to the solitary thoracic mass, a mass in the gastric wall was confirmed. FNA of the lung mass was attempted but was non-diagnostic. What should be done to obtain a definitive diagnosis?

3 The symptoms attributable to the gastric mass predominated; therefore an exploratory laparotomy was performed in order to remove the gastric mass. There was a well-circumscribed mass in the gastric wall (**198d**). Histopathology revealed an undifferentiated round cell tumor. CD3 and CD79a were negative and CD18 was positive. What is the diagnosis?

4 What is the suggested course of treatment and the prognosis for this patient?

CASE 199 A 10-year-old neutered male Jack Russell Terrier had been initially presented 6 months previously for a locally aggressive mast cell tumor over the left elbow. A biopsy revealed a grade III (Patnaik)/high grade (Kiupel) MCT. The regional lymph node was normal. The tumor was negative for both *c-KIT* mutations (exons 8 and 11) and was KIT pattern 2. Given the high grade and locally aggressive nature of the tumor, amputation was elected. Chemotherapy (vinblastine, CCNU, and prednisone) was used postoperatively. At the time of the fourth cycle of vinblastine and CCNU, the patient was reported to have had a poor appetite for approximately 1 week. The CBC and chemistry panel were normal. There was no evidence of local recurrence of disease and the remainder of the physical examination was normal. An ultrasound image of the spleen (**199a**) and cytology from a fine needle aspirate of the spleen (**199b**) are shown. The spleen was only minimally enlarged.

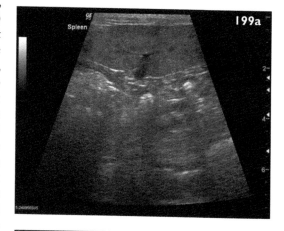

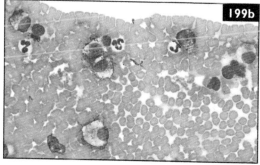

1 What is the diagnosis?
2 What further diagnostic tests are indicated?
3 What treatment should be considered for this patient?

CASE 200 This is the abdominal radiograph (200a) of a 9-year-old neutered male Soft Coated Wheaten Terrier that presented for a 1-month history of tenesmus, weight loss, and intermittent melena. On physical examination, a mid-abdominal mass, approximately 5 cm, was palpable. An MDB was performed. Thoracic radiographs were normal. Blood work and an abdominal ultrasound image (200b, arrow points to duodenum) are shown.

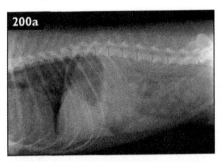

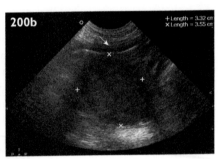

Test	Result	Flag	Units	Normal Range
Hematology (HemaTrue)				
WBC	4.8	Low	10³/µl	6.0–17.0
LYM	2.6		10³/µl	1.2–5.0
MONO	0.4		10³/µl	0.3–1.5
GRAN	1.8	Low	10³/µl	3.5–12.0
LYM%	53.6			
MONO%	7.6			
GRAN%	38.8			
HCT	33.4	Low	%	37.0–55.0
MCV	65.2		fl	60.0–72.0
RDWa	54.9	High	fl	35.0–53.0
RDW%	20.8	High	%	11.0–16.0
HGB	11.6	Low	g/dl	12.0–18.0
MCHC	34.7		g/dl	32.0–38.5
MCH	22.6		pg	19.5–25.5
RBC	5.12	Low	10⁶/µl	5.50–8.50
PLT	66	Low	10³/µl	200–500
MPV	8.3		fl	5.5–1

Test	Result	Flag	Units	Normal Range
Chemistry (DRI-CHEM)				
BUN	20.1		mg/dl	9.0–29.0
Creatinine	1.0		mg/dl	0.4–1.4
Phosphorus	3.3		mg/dl	1.9–5.0
Calcium	9.8		mg/dl	9.0–12.2
Corrected Ca	9.9		mg/dl	9.0–12.2
Total Protein	6.3		g/dl	5.5–7.6
Albumin	3.4		g/dl	2.5–4.0
Globulin	2.9		g/dl	2.0–3.6
Alb/Glob Ratio	1.2			
Glucose	111		mg/dl	75–125
Cholesterol	305		mg/dl	120–310
ALT (GPT)	33		U/l	0–120
ALP	72		U/l	0–140
GGT	16	High	U/l	0–14
Total Bilirubin	0.3		mg/dl	0.0–0.5

1 Describe the findings on abdominal radiographs, blood work, and ultrasound.
2 What further tests should be performed?
3 A surgical exploratory was performed. A lobulated, firm mass was found associated with the anti-mesenteric border of the proximal duodenum opposite

the pancreatic duct. The mass was well encapsulated. A marginal resection was performed owing to the proximity of the mass to the pancreatic duct. Histopathology was consistent with a soft tissue spindle cell sarcoma. There was a normal thin rim of connective tissue microscopically, but clean margins could not be confirmed. What are the diagnostic considerations?

4 How would results of immunohistochemistry be helpful in this patient?

5 What is the prognosis for this patient?

CASE 201 An 8-year-old spayed female Rottweiler presented for lameness of the left forelimb that was believed to be a result of playing roughly with another dog. Rest and a non-steroidal anti-inflammatory medication were prescribed. The lameness improved for several weeks, but then started to worsen. A firm swelling was noted once the lameness returned (**201a**). On physical examination, there was no evidence of lymphadenopathy or other abnormalities. A radiograph of the elbow (**201b**) and cytology from a fine needle aspirate of the swelling around the joint (**201c**) are shown.

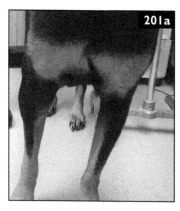

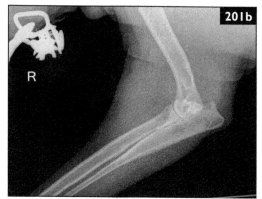

1 Interpret the radiograph and cytology.

2 What are the differential diagnoses for this patient?

3 What further diagnostics should be performed?

4 What is this patient's prognosis?

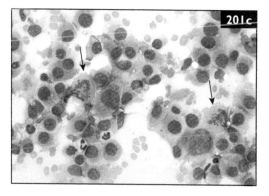

CASE 202 A 16-year-old neutered male DSH cat presented for evaluation of a suspected renal mass. He had an acute onset of facial twitching, ataxia, and stumbling. On physical examination, the kidneys were palpably enlarged and painful. There was hypersensitivity on the left side of the face and loss of conscious proprioception in the left hindlimb. An MDB was performed. The thoracic radiographs were normal and the FeLV and FIV status negative. The ultrasound, blood work, and urine specific gravity are shown. The ultrasound image of the left kidney is shown (**202a**). The right kidney appeared similar.

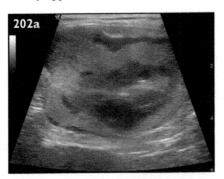

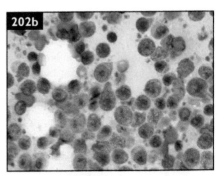

Test	Result	Flag	Units	Normal Range
Hematology (HemaTrue)				
WBC	26.2	High	10³/μl	5.5–19.5
LYM	1.6	Low	10³/μl	1.8–7.0
MONO	1.6	High	10³/μl	0.2–1.0
GRAN	23.0	High	10³/μl	2.8–13.0
LYM%	6.2			
MONO%	6.0			
GRAN%	87.8			
HCT	40.2		%	25.0–45.0
MCV	50.9	High	fl	39.0–50.0
RDWa	39.0	High	fl	20.0–35.0
RDW%	19.3	High	%	13.5–18.0
HGB	15.0		g/dl	8.0–15.0
MCHC	37.4		g/dl	31.0–38.5
MCH	19.0	High	pg	12.5–17.5
RBC	7.89		10⁶/μl	5.00–11.00
PLT	252		10³/μl	200–500
MPV	8.6		fl	8.0–12.0

Test	Result	Flag	Units	Normal Range
Chemistry (DRI-CHEM)				
BUN	36.1	High	mg/dl	15.0–32.0
Creatinine	2.1	High	mg/dl	0.8–1.8
Phosphorus	5.4		mg/dl	2.6–6.0
Calcium	11.4		mg/dl	8.8–11.5
Total Protein	7.3		g/dl	6.0–8.0
Albumin	3.3		g/dl	2.3–3.5
Globulin	4.0		g/dl	2.8–4.8
Glucose	85		mg/dl	70–130
Cholesterol	93		mg/dl	70–200
ALT (GPT)	30		U/l	

Urine specific gravity was 1.045 with no abnormalities noted.

1 Describe the ultrasound findings.
2 Based on the ultrasound alone, what are the differential diagnoses for this patient?
3 Cytology obtained from an FNA of this renal mass is shown (202b). What is your diagnosis?
4 What impact does the azotemia have on predicting outcome for this patient?
5 How do the neurologic symptoms relate to this cancer?
6 How has this disease changed over time?
7 What is this patient's prognosis?

CASE 203 A 12-year-old neutered male Rottweiler was presented for evaluation of exercise intolerance. The owner described the episodes as progressive, profound weakness following spurts of normal activity. At the time of physical examination, he would walk normally for several minutes then, with no obvious respiratory difficulty, would collapse (203). Other than collapsing, there were no abnormal physical examination findings. A CBC, chemistry panel, and urinalysis were normal. Thoracic radiographs revealed a cranial mediastinal mass. Abdominal ultrasound and echocardiogram were normal.

1 What is the association between the clinical symptoms and the mediastinal mass?
2 What further diagnostic tests should be performed?
3 What preoperative management should be instituted?

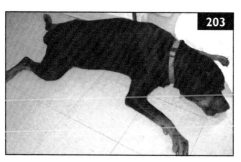

CASE 1

1 What are the radiographic findings? There is a soft tissue density on the right maxilla, with lysis of the maxilla. The right third incisor is separated from the maxilla and the remaining incisors on the right also appear to be loosening.

2 What diagnostic tests should be performed prior to a treatment decision? An MDB to rule out metastasis, careful evaluation of local lymph nodes, and tissue biopsy. Lymph node evaluation should not be limited to physical examination for size or fine needle aspiration and cytology alone. In one report, 40% of dogs with normal-sized lymph nodes had microscopic evidence of metastatic disease, therefore excisional biopsy is recommended for histologic evaluation.

3 The biopsy revealed an undifferentiated sarcoma. What further information should be gained from the tissue sample? Since amelanotic melanoma is a consideration for this patient, immunohistochemistry (IHC) to include Melan-A and S-100 should be performed. In this patient, both were positive, indicating melanoma.

4 What further staging tests are recommended in light of the histopathology results? Abdominal ultrasound should be included in the staging of this patient because of the aggressive metastatic nature of oral malignant melanoma. CT scanning should also be considered to determine the extent of localized disease for surgical or radiation planning.

5 What type of surgery and postoperative therapy are indicated for this patient? The tumor crosses the midline on oral examination. A rostral maxillectomy would be required to achieve local control, but good cosmetic and functional results would be difficult to obtain because the surgical margin would have to be caudal to the canine teeth. Radiation therapy can be considered for patients with tumors that are inoperable, those that undergo surgery but the margins are not microscopically tumor-free, or for patients whose owners elect not to pursue definitive surgery. A variety of hypofractionated radiation protocols have been described. Radiation dosages of 6–9 Gy fractions given once weekly for six treatments, for a total dosage of 24–36 Gy, have been reported to result in 53–69% complete response rates and 25–30% partial response rates. Distant metastasis is the primary cause of death in these patients. Melanoma has typically been a chemotherapy-resistant tumor (carboplatin: 28% response rate in dogs with non-resectable malignant melanoma in one study), therefore recent efforts to control metastatic disease have centered on immunotherapy. A newly developed xenogeneic human DNA tyrosinase vaccine appears to be safe and is recommended by the manufacturer in locoregionally controlled (i.e. following surgery or radiation therapy) stage II and III canine oral melanoma. In one report of 58 dogs with stage II or III oral malignant melanoma (MM) undergoing surgery and vaccination, the results supported the safety and efficacy of the vaccine as adjunctive treatment. Another study of 30 dogs with similarly staged MM failed to support the efficacy of the vaccine.

Answers

References

Boston SE, Xiaomin L, Culp WTN *et al.* (2014) Efficacy of systemic adjuvant therapies administered to dogs after excision of oral malignant melanomas: 151 cases (2001–2012). *J Am Vet Med Assoc* 245:401–407.

Grosenbaugh DA, Leard AT, Bergman PJ (2011) Safety and efficacy of a xenogeneic DNA vaccine encoding for human tyrosinase as adjunctive treatment for oral malignant melanoma in dogs following surgical excision of the primary tumor. *Am J Vet Res* 72:1631–1638.

Koenig A, Wojcieszyn J, Weeks BR *et al.* (2001) Expression of S100a, vimentin, NSE, and melan A/MART-1 in seven canine melanoma cell lines and twenty-nine retrospective cases of canine melanoma. *Vet Pathol* 38(4):427–435.

Liptak JM, Withrow SJ (2013) Cancer of the gastrointestinal tract. Oral tumors. In: Withrow SJ, Vail DM, Page RL, editors, *Small Animal Clinical Oncology*, 5th edition. St. Louis, Elsevier Saunders, pp. 381–399.

Murphy S, Hayes AM, Blackwood L *et al.* (2005) Oral malignant melanoma – the effect of coarse fractionation radiotherapy alone or with adjuvant carboplatin therapy. *Vet Comp Oncol* 3:222–229.

Ottnod JM, Smedley RC, Walshaw R *et al.* (2013) A retrospective analysis of the efficacy of Oncept vaccine for the adjunct treatment of canine oral malignant melanoma. *Vet Comp Oncol* 11(3):219–229.

Rassnick KM, Ruslander DM, Cotter SM *et al.* (2001) Use of carboplatin for treatment of dogs with malignant melanoma: 27 cases (1989–2000). *J Am Vet Med Assoc* 218: 1444–1448.

Williams LE, Packer RA (2003) Association between lymph node size and metastasis in dogs with oral malignant melanoma: 100 cases (1987–2001). *J Am Vet Med Assoc* 222: 1234–1236.

CASE 2

1 What are the primary differential diagnoses for this patient? Squamous cell carcinoma, malignant melanoma, fibrosarcoma, odontogenic tumor (acanthomatous ameloblastoma, fibromatous epulis, ossifying epulis) are the primary differential diagnoses.

2 A biopsy revealed acanthomatous ameloblastoma. What further diagnostic tests should be performed in assessing this patient for treatment? Acanthomatous ameloblastoma is a locally invasive benign tumor arising from the tooth root. It has a tendency to destroy bone aggressively at the localized site, but does not metastasize to distant sites. Plain radiography can be used to determine extent of bony involvement, although care must be taken in using radiography alone to plan surgical resection as it may underestimate disease present. Greater than 50% of the cortical bone needs to be destroyed before becoming radiographically evident. CT scanning appears to be a better tool to evaluate extent of disease. A CT scan becomes even more important when tumors occur in the maxilla, because of underlying structures such as the nasal cavity and orbit. Wide surgical excision is potentially curative, but involves removing underlying bone. Marginal surgical resection results in high local recurrence rates. Rostral mandibulectomy would have the greatest chance for a cure, but based on the extent of disease in this patient, removal of up to 50% of the lower jaw would be necessary – the owner declined this option.

3 Surgery is the primary recommendation for this patient but the owner is not willing to consider mandibulectomy. What other therapeutic option has the greatest chance for control/cure of disease? Radiation therapy (RT) has the greatest chance for long-term control/cure of this tumor type for patients not undergoing surgery. Eighty-five percent of patients treated with RT are tumor-free at 1 year post-RT and 80% are tumor-free at 3 years. Malignant transformation in the irradiated field has been reported in 5–18% of dogs, occurring years after treatment. Orthovoltage radiation had the highest risk and megavoltage radiation the lowest. Although this risk is low, it needs to be taken into consideration for younger patients. Intralesional chemotherapy (bleomycin) has been described as having efficacy. This patient had an excellent response to RT but a second malignant tumor developed more than 3 years post-RT at the radiation site. While mandibulectomy would have again been an option, the owner chose to repeat a full course of RT.

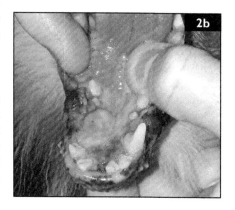

Follow up/discussion

This is the 2-week post-RT appearance of this patient's tumor (**2b**). Post radiation therapy, the tumor is almost gone. The tissue visualized here remained stable. It was biopsied and confirmed scar tissue with no evidence of malignant cells.

References

Bostock DE, White RA (1987) Classification and behavior after surgery of canine epulides. *J Comp Pathol* **97**:197–206.

Kelly JM, Belding BA, Schaefer AK (2010) Acanthomatous ameloblastoma in dogs treated with intralesional bleomycin. *Vet Comp Oncol* **8**:81–86.

Mayer MN, Anthony JM (2007) Radiation therapy for oral tumors: canine acanthomatous ameloblastoma. *Can Vet J* **48**:99–101.

Théon AP, Rodriguez C, Griffey S *et al.* (1984) Analysis of prognostic factors and patterns of failure in dogs with periodontal tumors treated with megavoltage irradiation. *J Am Vet Med Assoc* **184**:826–829.

White RAS, Gorman NT (1989) Wide local excision of acanthomatous epulides in the dog. *Vet Surg* **1**:12–14.

CASE 3

1 Describe the radiographs and blood work. What is the probable anatomic location of the mass and how should this be confirmed? The arrows (**3b**) point

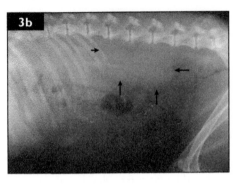

to a large mass located ventral to the lumbar spine causing ventral deviation of the colon, raising suspicion for a retroperitoneal mass. The surgical clips present were from surgery earlier in life to remove an intestinal foreign body. There is an elevated WBC and mild anemia and thrombocytopenia. The BUN is elevated in the face of a normal creatinine. This raises concern for possible gastrointestinal bleeding, early renal insufficiency, or dehydration. An ultrasound was performed. The mass had multiple cavitary areas with anechoic fluid and appeared to lie within the retroperitoneal space.

2 List the differential diagnoses. Hemangiosarcoma (most likely in this case, based on ultrasound appearance and blood work), osteosarcoma, leiomyosarcoma, peripheral nerve sheath tumors, hemangiopericytoma, and other soft tissue sarcomas have been reported to arise in the retroperitoneal space. Retroperitoneal abscesses can also occur but the ultrasound appearance is not consistent with an abscess and the patient is not febrile.

3 What further diagnostic tests are indicated to formulate a treatment plan? Complete staging for this patient should include thoracic radiographs, an echocardiogram (to rule out atrial masses and/or pericardial effusion that could be suggestive of an atrial or heart base mass), coagulation profile, and a CT scan for surgical planning. A reticulocyte count and evaluation of the blood smear are indicated to determine the nature of the anemia (i.e. regenerative vs. non-regenerative). Surgery or CT, or ultrasound-guided aspirate or biopsy, is necessary to obtain a definitive diagnosis. This patient was diagnosed through surgery to have hemangiosarcoma.

4 What is the prognosis for this patient? Retroperitoneal hemangiosarcoma carries a very poor prognosis. In one study that evaluated all types of retroperitoneal tumors, surgical excision and chemotherapy were used and median survival times were 37.5 days. One patient that had a grade II leiomyosarcoma was still alive at >400 days. In another study, three patients with retroperitoneal hemangiosarcoma were treated with palliative dosages of RT and had more favorable outcomes. All three patients had both RT and chemotherapy. One patient that survived 258 days did not have surgery, one patient that survived 408 days did not have surgery, and the one patient that did have surgery survived 500 days. The two that did not undergo surgery had measurable reduction in tumor size.

References
Hillers KR, Lana SE, Fuller CR *et al.* (2007) Effects of palliative radiation therapy on nonsplenic hemangiosarcoma in dogs. *J Am Anim Hosp Assoc* **43**:187–192.
Liptak JM, Dernell WS, Ehrhart EJ *et al.* (2004) Retroperitoneal sarcomas in dogs: 14 cases (1992–2002). *J Am Vet Med Assoc* **224**:1471–1477.

CASE 4
1 What is the likelihood that this mammary mass is malignant? In cats, 85–95% of mammary gland masses are malignant. They are usually very aggressive and have a high metastatic rate. The majority of tumors are carcinomas (approximately 86%) and less than 1% are sarcomas (the remainder are other rare tumor types or benign). Of the carcinoma group, approximately 90% are adenocarcinoma and 10% carcinoma.

2 In addition to the MDB, should any further tests be performed? Thoracic radiographs as part of the MDB are extremely important because of the high metastatic rate. An abdominal ultrasound is also recommended owing to the potential for spread to intra-abdominal lymph nodes or the liver.

3 What type of surgery is recommended for this patient? Unilateral radical mastectomy (**4b–4d**) has been associated with a significantly increased survival time when compared with more conservative surgeries (i.e. lumpectomy) in cats. There is no lymphatic connection between the left and right mammary chains, so bilateral radical mastectomy is usually only indicated if there is disease present in both chains. However, recent studies indicate that there may be a survival advantage to bilateral radical mastectomy. In 37 cats treated with surgery and

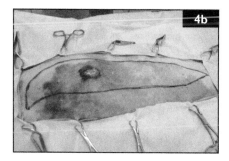
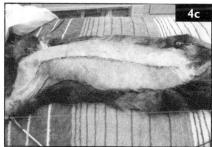

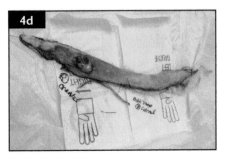

doxorubicin chemotherapy, extent of surgery was prognostic. Patients undergoing bilateral radical mastectomy and doxorubicin chemotherapy had median survival times of 917 days, those that had unilateral radical mastectomies had MSTs of 348 days, and cats having regional mastectomies had MSTs of 428 days. This finding was interesting because earlier studies had demonstrated that the type of surgery had no effect on survival time but did impact disease-free interval. It is often difficult to perform a bilateral radical mastectomy in one surgical procedure, especially in cats with less loose skin to work with. Surgery can be performed in two procedures, called a "bilateral staged radical mastectomy". Following a rest of several weeks after the first surgery, the second side is then done.

4 Is postoperative therapy advised? Given the aggressive nature of mammary cancer in cats, chemotherapy is generally recommended. However, there appears to be no consensus on the value of chemotherapy postoperatively. Doxorubicin based protocols are most commonly used. With postoperative doxorubicin, MSTs were reported to be approximately 448 days in one study. WHO Stage III patients had MSTs of 4–6 months with surgery alone, whereas cats similarly staged that underwent surgery and doxorubicin chemotherapy were reported to have an MST of 416 days. Other studies have shown no benefit to adjuvant doxorubicin based protocols. Aggressive feline mammary tumors have higher expression of COX-2, making the use of COX-2 inhibitors attractive. However, one recent study reported no advantage to the use of meloxicam in addition to surgery and doxorubicin chemotherapy, but further studies are warranted.

5 What are the most important prognostic factors for this disease? The following factors have been associated with a poor prognosis in cats with mammary gland tumors:

- Tumor size (>3 cm).
- Higher stage (presence of lymph node or distant metastasis).
- Higher histologic grade tumors (poorly differentiated; high mitotic, AgNOR, or Ki67 indices; vascular or lymphatic invasion).
- Conservative surgery (regional vs. unilateral or bilateral radical mastectomy).

WHO Clinical Staging System for Feline Mammary Tumors

T: Primary		
T_1: <2 cm maximum diameter		
T_2: 2–3 cm maximum diameter		
T_3: >3 cm maximum diameter		
N: Regional lymph nodes		
N_0: No histologic evidence of metastasis		
N_1: Histologic evidence of metastasis		
M: Distant metastasis		
M_0: No evidence of distant metastasis		
M_1: Evidence of distant metastasis		
Stage grouping		
Stage I	T_1	N_0	M_0
Stage II	T_2	N_0	M_0
Stage III	T_3	N_0 or N_1	M_0
Stage IV	Any T	Any N	M_1

Source: MacEwen EG, Withrow SJ (2001) Tumors of the mammary gland. In: Withrow SJ, MacEwen EG, editors, *Small Animal Clinical Oncology*, 3rd edition. New York, WB Saunders, pp. 467–473.

References
McNeill CJ, Sorenmo KU, Shofer FS *et al.* (2009) Evaluation of adjuvant doxorubicin-based chemotherapy for the treatment of feline mammary carcinoma. *J Vet Intern Med* 23:123–129.
Morris J (2013) Mammary tumours in the cat. *J Fel Med Surg* 15:391–400.
Novosad CA, Bergman PJ, O'Brien MG *et al.* (2006) Retrospective evaluation of adjunctive doxorubicin for the treatment of feline mammary gland adenocarcinoma: 67 cases. *J Am Anim Hosp Assoc* 42:110–120.
Seixas F, Palmeira C, Pires MA *et al.* (2011) Grade is an independent prognostic factor for feline mammary carcinomas: a clinicopathological and survival analysis. *Vet J* 187:65–71.
Viste JR, Myers SL, Singh B *et al.* (2002) Feline mammary adenocarcinoma: tumor size as a prognostic indicator. *Can Vet J* 43:33–37.

CASE 5

1 What is the natural course of this disease? Epitheliotropic lymphoma, also known as mycosis fungoides, most commonly presents as a multicentric disease and is better termed cutaneous T cell lymphoma (CTCL). Rarely, dogs can present with disease limited to the oral cavity, but oral cavity disease is often a component of more generalized disease. In early phases of this disease, there is a mild lymphocytic infiltrate into the epidermis and follicular epithelium, which can resemble any non-specific allergic reaction or mild dermatitis. Subtle erythema, scaling, and mild alopecia can be seen. Pruritus is often present, so early stages are commonly misdiagnosed. These early stages can last extended periods of time (in people they will last decades). As the disease progresses, more typical intraepidermal microabscesses (Pautrier's micropustules) begin to form. As the disease worsens, the intraepidermal masses become ulcerated, crusted, and alopecic. All phases of the disease can occur as solitary or multifocal lesions. The tumor development can be slow and often disease has been present for several years prior to an actual diagnosis.

2 What additional tests should be performed for staging on this patient? Staging of the disease should include thoracic radiographs, abdominal ultrasound, and CBC and chemistry panel. Given the concern about nasal involvement in this case, a CT scan should be included in the work-up.

3 What treatment options are available and what is the prognosis? CCNU (lomustine) is currently a popular chemotherapeutic agent for this disease. Corticosteroids, l-asparaginase, dacarbazine, or combination CHOP-based protocols have also been described. In addition to chemotherapy, the use of omega-3 fatty acids, linoleic acid (in the form of Hollywood brand safflower oil), and, for diffuse cutaneous lesions, antibacterial shampoos and systemic antibiotics may be necessary to control symptoms. If staging reveals no further extension of disease beyond the nasal/oral cavity, localized radiation therapy is often helpful in controlling disease. When a solitary lesion occurs in the oral cavity, curative intent radiation therapy has resulted in long-term control and even cure.

References

Berlato D, Schrempp D, Van Den Steen N *et al.* (2011) Radiotherapy in the management of localized mucocutaneous oral lymphoma in dogs: 14 cases. *Vet Comp Oncol* **10(1):** 16–23.

deLorimier LP (2006) Updates on the management of canine epitheliotropic cutaneous T-cell lymphoma. *Vet Clin N Am Small Anim Pract* **36:**213–228.

Petersen A, Wood S, Rosser E (1999) The use of safflower oil for the treatment of mycosis fungoides in two dogs [abstract]. In: *Proceedings of the 15th Annual Meeting of the American Academy of Veterinary Dermatology.* Maui (HI), pp. 49–50.

Risbon RE, de Lorimier LP, Skorupski K *et al.* (2006) Response of canine cutaneous epitheliotropic lymphoma to lomustine (CCNU): a retrospective study of 46 cases (1999–2004). *J Vet Intern Med* **20:**1389–1397.

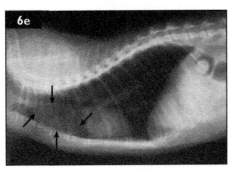

6e

CASE 6

1 What is the abnormality shown in the radiographs? On the lateral view, a soft tissue density cranial to the heart is noted (**6e**, arrows). On the VD view, the mediastinum is widened (**6f**, arrows). Interpretation: mediastinal mass.

2 **What are the most common differential diagnoses for this patient?** Differential diagnoses include lymphoma, thymoma, other less common tumor types (e.g. thyroid carcinoma, hemangiosarcoma), and benign cyst.

3 **How should the diagnosis be confirmed?** An ultrasound will help assess the character of the mass (solid, mixed echogenicity, or fluid filled) and can be followed by ultrasound-guided fine needle aspirate or biopsy.

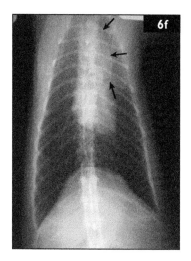

4 **The ultrasound of the mass (6c) and fluid obtained from an FNA (6d) are shown. What is the diagnosis?** The mass appears fluid filled. The FNA yielded a clear, water colored fluid, consistent with a branchial cyst. Branchial cysts are congenital, but usually asymptomatic until later in life.

5 **What therapy is indicated?** In many cases, draining the cyst with ultrasound-guided needle aspiration will help control the symptoms for prolonged periods of time. In patients whose cysts fill up more rapidly, surgical removal can be considered. This patient's cyst was drained and did not return for more than 1 year, at which time it was drained again.

References
Nelson LL, Coelho JC, Mietelka K *et al.* (2012) Pharyngeal pouch and cleft remnants in the dog and cat: a case series and review. *J Am Anim Hosp Assoc* **48**:105–112.
Zekas LJ, Adams WM (2002) Cranial mediastinal cysts in nine cats. *Vet Radiol Ultrasound* **43**:413–418.

CASE 7

1 **What are the major differential diagnoses for this patient?** The presence of a subcutaneous mass can represent neoplasia (possible vaccine-associated tumor, given the history), inflammatory lesion, trauma (swelling from an injury), or infection.

2 **What diagnostic tests can be easily performed to obtain a presumptive diagnosis?** Cytology showed predominantly segmented and degenerate neutrophils. The patient was treated with antibiotics and the abscess resolved.

3 **What considerations for future vaccination should be made for this patient?** Given the location of the abscess in an area where a vaccination had been given,

there is concern that this patient may have had a benign vaccine reaction that subsequently became infected. Cats exhibiting benign vaccine reactions may be at greater risk for subsequent tumor development. However, owing to the fact that the cat also goes outdoors, a simple cat bite abscess cannot be ruled out. Location of the vaccination could not be confirmed, and since the patient is an indoor/outdoor cat, the recommendation is to continue vaccination protocols with non-adjuvanted vaccines, but monitor closely for any post-vaccination reaction. Care should also be taken to follow the recommendation of the American Association of Feline Practitioners Advisory Panel of giving rabies vaccines below the right stifle, feline leukemia virus vaccines below the left stifle, and feline panleukopenia virus, feline herpesvirus-1, and feline calicivirus vaccines below the right elbow. A recent study showed that the immunity elicited from vaccinating in the tail was similar to other sites.

References

Hendricks CG, Levy JK, Tucker SJ (2014) Tail vaccination in cats: a pilot study. *J Feline Med Surg* **16**(4):275–280.

Macy DW, Hendrick MJ (1996) The potential role of inflammation in the development of postvaccinal sarcomas in cats. *Vet Clin N Am Small Animal Pract* **26**:103–109.

CASE 8

1 What are the differential diagnoses for this patient? Squamous cell carcinoma, fibrosarcoma, and malignant melanoma (amelanotic melanoma would be a consideration in this case owing to lack of visible pigment) are the most common malignant tumors found in the oral cavity of dogs.

2 What further staging tests should be included in the evaluation of this patient? Fine needle aspirate of the enlarged lymph node and thoracic radiographs to evaluate for metastasis should be performed first. A fine needle aspirate of the tumor may provide a presumptive diagnosis. Owing to the very caudal location of this mass, a CT scan would be helpful in providing information regarding extent of disease. A biopsy should be performed prior to or at the time of a CT scan for definitive diagnosis. Squamous cell carcinoma was diagnosed in this patient. The thoracic radiographs were normal and the lymph node was reactive.

3 What treatment options are available for this patient? Surgery (mandibulectomy) is the most effective way to achieve local control; however, tumors in the rostral portion of the oral cavity are generally more amenable to complete surgical excision. Radiation therapy is advised for those tumors with incomplete surgical excision, and this patient is likely to require postoperative radiation. The local recurrence rate following surgery is reported to be lowest with rostral tumors (~10%) and up to 50% in more caudal locations. A combination of carboplatin and piroxicam was used to treat seven dogs. Four of the seven dogs achieved complete remission. At 534 days, overall survival time had not yet been reached. Treatment with piroxicam alone can result in stable disease to measurable responses of 3–6 months' duration.

4 What is the prognosis for this patient? Squamous cell carcinoma can have a variable biologic behavior depending on the location within the oral cavity. Tumors in more caudal or tonsillar locations are extremely aggressive in comparison with rostral locations. This may, in part, be due to the inability to obtain tumor-free surgical margins in the more difficult caudal locations. A combination of surgery and radiation therapy is associated with overall median survival times of close to 3 years. However, negative prognostic indicators include the size of tumor (progression-free survival times were 8 months for dogs with tumors >4 cm in one study) and location. Tumors <2 cm in diameter had PFS times of >68 months, and tumors 2–4 cm in diameter had PFS times of 28 months.

References

deVos JP, Burm AGD, Focker AP *et al*. (2005) Piroxicam and carboplatin as a combination treatment of canine oral non-tonsillar squamous cell carcinoma: a pilot study and a literature review of a canine model of human head and neck squamous cell carcinoma. *Vet Comp Oncol* 3(1):16–24.

Kosovsky JK, Matthiesen DT, Marretta SM *et al*. (1991) Results of partial mandibulectomy for the treatment of oral tumors in 142 dogs. *Vet Surg* 20(6):397–401.

Schmidt BR, Glickman NW, DeNicola DB *et al*. (2001) Evaluation of piroxicam for the treatment of oral squamous cell carcinoma in dogs. *J Am Vet Med Assoc* 218(11): 1783–1786.

Théon AP, Rodriguez C, Madewell BR (1997) Analysis of prognostic factors and patterns of failure in dogs with malignant oral tumors treated with megavoltage irradiation. *J Am Vet Med Assoc* 210:778–784.

CASE 9

1 Based on the clinical presentation, what are the primary differential diagnoses for the cranial abdominal mass? Pancreatic or biliary carcinomas are the most likely considerations based on the dermatopathy present. A unique paraneoplastic alopecia has been observed in pancreatic carcinoma and biliary carcinoma in cats. The alopecia is symmetrical, often described as a "glistening alopecia". The face, ventrum, and medial surfaces of the limbs are most commonly affected. The hair is easily epilated and a paronychia is often seen.

2 What is the best way to make a diagnosis and potentially treat this patient? An ultrasound-guided fine needle aspirate could be attempted to obtain a cytologic diagnosis. Surgery (abdominal exploratory and attempted mass removal) is advised if cytology is not diagnostic. This patient was found to have a pancreatic mass at surgery. Several small (<3 mm) lesions found in the liver were also biopsied. Pancreatic carcinoma with metastasis to the liver was confirmed. Resolution of the paraneoplastic alopecia has been described in patients where complete excision of the pancreatic mass was achieved. Complete surgical excision, however, is usually not possible because of the presence of metastasis. The liver is the most common site for metastasis, which usually takes place very early in the course of the disease. **3 What is the prognosis for this patient?** The prognosis for pancreatic carcinoma in cats, as in other species including humans, is generally poor.

References

Linderman MJ, Brodsky EM, De Lorimier LP *et al.* (2012) Feline exocrine pancreatic carcinoma: a retrospective study of 34 cases. *Vet Comp Oncol* **11**(3):208–218.

Seaman RL (2004) Exocrine pancreatic neoplasia in the cat: a case series. *J Am Anim Hosp Assoc* **40**:238–245.

Turek MM (2003) Invited review. Cutaneous paraneoplastic syndromes in dogs and cats: a review of the literature. *Vet Dermatol* **14**:279–296.

CASE 10

1 What procedure is being performed (10)? A rostral maxillary (infraorbital) block is being performed.

2 What are the analgesic benefits? This type of block provides adjunct analgesia for painful oral surgical procedures. In the case of a rostral maxillary (infraorbital) block, the ipsilateral premolar, canine, and incisor teeth and associated soft tissues are anesthetized. The length of local anesthesia is dependent on the agent used. Lidocaine lasts 1–2 hours, mepivacaine 2–2.5 hours, and bupivacaine 2.5–6 hours. These times can be increased with the addition of epinephrine. In cats, bupivacaine given inadvertently IV can be fatal.

Reference

Beckman B, Legendre L (2002) Regional nerve blocks for oral surgery in companion animals. *Compend Contin Educ Vet* **24**:439–442.

CASE 11

1 What is the cytologic diagnosis? The cytology reveals well-granulated mast cells, indicating a mast cell tumor (MCT).

2 What are the two histologic forms of this disease? Two histologic types of MCT are recognized in cats. The most common is called the *mastocytic* form and histologically resembles canine MCTs. The mastocytic form is further divided into "compact" or "diffuse". The compact form makes up from 50 to 90% of all feline MCTs, while the diffuse form is anaplastic with a high mitotic index. The less common *histiocytic* form is characterized by histiocytic appearing mast cells, and patients often experience spontaneous regression of disease without treatment.

3 How should this patient be managed? Careful evaluation for evidence of further disease is advised. Aspiration of any enlarged lymph nodes, thoracic radiography, and abdominal ultrasound are indicated. However, the diagnostic yield of these staging tests for a cat with a solitary cutaneous MCT is expected to be low because metastasis from solitary cutaneous MCTs in cats is uncommon, as is cutaneous spread from systemic mast cell disease. Complete surgical removal of the tumor is advised. Tumors are most commonly seen on the skin of the head and neck (>50% of the time), where wide surgical excision is difficult. Marginal excision of feline MCTs appears to be more effective than in dogs. Histologic grading does not predict the behavior of cutaneous MCTs in cats as it does in dogs. Complete excision is usually curative.

4 What histologic parameter provides the most information regarding the potential for recurrence or metastasis? Histologically, anaplastic tumors or those with a high mitotic index are at the highest risk for aggressive biologic behavior.

References

Johnson TO, Schulman FY, Lipscomb TP *et al.* (2002) Histopathology and biologic behavior of pleomorphic cutaneous mast cell tumors in fifteen cats. *Vet Pathol* **39**:452–457.

Lepri E, Ricci G, Leonardi L *et al.* (2003) Diagnostic and prognostic features of feline cutaneous mast cell tumours: a retrospective analysis of 40 cases. *Vet Res Commun* **27(suppl 1)**:707–709.

Wilcock BP, Yager JA, Zink MC (1986) The morphology and behavior of feline cutaneous mastocytomas. *Vet Pathol* **23**:320–324.

CASE 12

1 What are the indications for using the pictured drug? In dogs, CCNU has activity against multicentric lymphoma, epitheliotropic lymphoma, histiocytic sarcoma, and mast cell tumors. In dogs with brain tumors, responses to CCNU have been limited, but it has been shown to be palliative. In cats, CCNU has shown benefit for use in lymphoma and mast cell tumors, and there is preliminary evidence that it may have activity against vaccine-associated sarcomas.

2 What is the mechanism of action of CCNU? CCNU is an oral alkylating agent belonging to the nitrosourea subclass. Alkylating agents destroy cancer cells by adding an alkyl group to DNA, preventing the cell's replication. CCNU is highly lipid soluble.

3 What are the side effects commonly associated with lomustine and how can they be alleviated? Myelosuppression and hepatic toxicity are the predominant side effects seen. In both dogs and cats, a potential cumulative effect of CCNU is thrombocytopenia, which can be prolonged and severe. Careful monitoring of pre- and post-treatment CBCs and using prophylactic antibiotics when neutrophil counts are significantly decreased can aid in preventing sepsis resulting from myelosuppression. If a patient experiences profound myelosuppression, reduction of subsequent CCNU dosages will be necessary. If prolonged thrombocytopenia occurs, discontinuation of therapy may be necessary. CCNU is extensively metabolized by the liver. Cumulative hepatic toxicosis can also be seen. Up to 86% of dogs treated will have liver enzyme elevations secondary to CCNU administration. Studies have shown that concurrent administration of Denamarin® (S-adenosylmethionine [SAMe] and silybin) as a liver protectant decreases the severity of hepatic enzyme elevations. In cats, the risk of clinically significant hepatic injury is considered low. Nausea and vomiting can occur secondary to CCNU but are not frequently observed in dogs or cats. In humans, taking CCNU with fluids on an empty stomach and then withholding food and water for 2 hours helps to reduce nausea.

4 What characteristic does this drug possess that is seen in very few chemotherapeutic agents? Lomustine is a highly lipid soluble drug, which allows it to cross the blood–brain barrier. One of its primary uses in human medicine is for brain tumors.

References

Heading KL, Brockley LK, Bennett PF (2011) CCNU (lomustine) toxicity in dogs: a retrospective study (2002–2007). *Aust Vet J* **89**:109–116.

Moore AS, Kitchell BE (2003) New chemotherapeutic agents in veterinary medicine. *Vet Clin N Am Small Anim Pract* **33**:629–649.

Musser ML, Quinn HT, Chretin JD (2012) Low apparent risk of CCNU (lomustine)-associated clinical hepatotoxicity in cats. *J Feline Med Surg* **14**:871–875.

Saba CF, Vail DM, Thamm DH (2012) Phase II clinical evaluation of lomustine chemotherapy for feline vaccine-associated sarcoma. *Vet Comp Oncol* **10**:283–291.

Skorupski KA, Hammond GM, Irish AM *et al.* (2011) Prospective randomized clinical trial assessing the efficacy of Denamarin for prevention of CCNU-induced hepatopathy in tumor-bearing dogs. *J Vet Intern Med* **25**:838–845.

CASE 13

1 Describe the radiographic findings. What specific structure is the arrow pointing to? Cortical lysis and loss of trabecular pattern are noted in the caudal aspect of the distal tibia. The lesion does not cross the joint space. The arrow is pointing to an area of periosteal lifting created by the lesion invading the cortical bone. There is subsequent periosteal lifting, creating what is referred to as "Codman's triangle". This radiographic finding is highly suggestive, but not pathognomonic, for a bone tumor.

2 What are the differential diagnoses? Differential diagnoses:

- *Primary bone tumor:* Owing to the location of the lesion, osteosarcoma is the most likely diagnosis, with less than a 5% chance of other primary bone tumors such as chondrosarcoma, fibrosarcoma, hemangiosarcoma, and other less common primary bone tumors such as lymphoma or solitary osseous plasmacytoma.

- *Metastatic bone tumor:* Based on the metaphyseal location of this lesion, metastatic disease from another primary tumor is less likely.
- *Osteomyelitis:* With lack of penetrating trauma, wounds, or previous surgery, bacterial osteomyelitis is highly unlikely. Fungal infection would be a consideration, especially in endemic areas and with appropriate clinical history of systemic illness.
- *Multiple myeloma:* However, other clinical findings such as monoclonal gammopathy are usually present in association.
- *Bone cyst:* Considered rare.

3 **What diagnostic tests are indicated?** An MDB to include thoracic radiographs (3 views) should be performed. Fine needle aspiration and cytology can support a tentative diagnosis, but a bone biopsy and histopathology are necessary for a definitive diagnosis. Histopathology revealed osteosarcoma in this patient.

4 **Describe both definitive and palliative treatment options for this patient.** Definitive treatment for osteosarcoma is amputation and chemotherapy (carboplatin, cis-platin, or doxorubicin reported to improve survival times). Limb sparing procedures are not recommended in the hindlimbs. Amputation alone is curative in <10% of patients and therefore is considered only palliative when chemotherapy is not used. Palliative radiation therapy, 8 Gy delivered weekly for 4 weeks, results in >90% subjective improvement and extends pain-free survival by 2–3 months. Median survival time using only this palliative radiation protocol was 5.4 months for axial sites and 10.4 months for appendicular sites. Bisphosphonates (inhibitors of osteoclast activity) provide subjective improvement for some patients with primary or metastatic bone tumors; however, RT appears to be more effective in alleviating pain.

5 **What are negative prognostic indicators for this disease?** Patients with elevations in serum alkaline phosphatase (total serum ALP >110 U/l or serum bone ALP >23 U/l) have been shown to have shorter disease-free intervals and overall survival times. Caution should be used in interpreting these values in patients that have had long standing elevations in serum ALP and/or symptoms of hyperadrenocorticism or hepatic disease.

References

Bacon NJ, Ehrhart NP, Dernell WS *et al.* (2008) Use of alternating administration of carboplatin and doxorubicin in dogs with microscopic metastases after amputation for appendicular osteosarcoma: 50 cases (1999–2006). *J Am Vet Med Assoc* **232**(10): 1504–1510.

Ehrhart N, Dernell WS, Hoffmann WE *et al.* (1998) Prognostic importance of alkaline phosphatase activity in serum from dogs with appendicular osteosarcoma: 75 cases (1990–1996). *J Am Vet Med Assoc* **213**:1002–1006.

Fan TM, deLorimier LP, O'Dell-Anderson K *et al.* (2007) Single-agent pamidronate for palliative therapy of canine appendicular osteosarcoma bone pain. *J Vet Intern Med* 21:431–439.

Garzotto CK, Berg J, Hoffman WE *et al.* (2000) Prognostic significance of serum alkaline phosphatase activity in canine appendicular osteosarcoma. *J Vet Intern Med* 14:587–592.

Green EM, Adams WM, Forrest LJ (2002) Four fraction palliative radiotherapy for osteosarcoma in 24 dogs. *J Am Anim Hosp Assoc* 38:445–451.

Phillips B, Powers BE, Dernell WS *et al.* (2009) Use of single-agent carboplatin as adjuvant or neoadjuvant therapy in conjunction with amputation for appendicular osteosarcoma in dogs. *J Am Anim Hosp Assoc* 45(1):33–38.

CASE 14

1 What procedure is being shown? A tissue core biopsy is being performed using a "tru-cut" needle core biopsy instrument.

2 What are the indications for this procedure? The indication for this procedure is to obtain a core of tissue suitable for histopathologic evaluation. Examples include:

- Larger cutaneous or subcutaneous masses that are not amenable to excisional biopsy.
- Where knowledge of the tumor type and grade will help plan a curative intent surgery.
- Intra-abdominal masses with ultrasound (US) or CT guidance.
- Intrathoracic masses with US or CT guidance.

3 What are the limitations of this procedure?

- Non-diagnostic sample due to location within the mass that is biopsied (e.g. necrotic center or cystic area of a mass).
- Diagnostic success rate is operator dependent.
- Sample size not large enough to make definitive diagnosis.

4 What are the potential complications?

- Hemorrhage (most common).
- Misplacement of needle or placement too deep, resulting in penetrating an adjoining organ.
- In cats undergoing liver biopsy, fatal hypotensive shock reactions occurred in 19% of patients in which a fully automated instrument was used. If using a semi-automatic needle core biopsy instrument, such as the one shown here, this complication did not occur.

CASE 15

1 What immunohistochemical (IHC) stains could help confirm soft tissue osteosarcoma in this patient? IHC stains such as osteonectin and osteocalcin may be helpful. This patient was positive for osteonectin and negative for osteocalcin. Positive labeling for osteonectin may be seen in some fibroblast origin soft tissue sarcomas. When combined with the overall negative labeling for osteocalcin (a more specific marker for osteogenic processes), a diagnosis of osteogenic sarcoma could not be confirmed in this case. As such, the diagnosis in this case would remain undifferentiated sarcoma, grade III.

2 In addition to an MDB, what staging tests should be performed? Given the potentially metastatic nature of a higher-grade sarcoma, abdominal ultrasound should be included in the staging process. Pre- and post-contrast CT scans could help determine the depth of invasion into the thorax.

3 What therapeutic recommendations can be made? Based on the large size of the mass, complete surgical excision is not possible. The most definitive therapy for this patient would be surgical debulking (cytoreduction) of the large volume of tumor followed postoperatively with radiation therapy. A highly skilled oncologic/soft tissue surgeon is necessary to achieve excision. Presurgical RT or chemotherapy could be attempted to cytoreduce the tumor prior to more definitive surgery. The human literature suggests that the success rate for therapy is higher if surgical debulking can be performed before RT. Recent studies have shown a benefit when using metronomic chemotherapy postoperatively when RT is not available or not elected. This patient's tumor was surgically debulked and treatment with metronomic chemotherapy chosen (**15b, c**). Despite the incomplete surgical excision, the patient remains alive and disease-free 1 year postoperatively (**15d**).

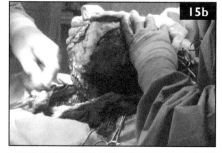

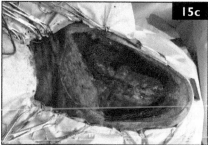

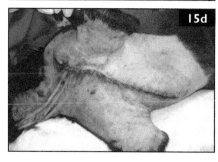

4 What is the probability of metastasis in this patient and what factors are present that indicate a poorer outcome? The metastatic rate for soft tissue sarcomas is grade dependent: <15% for grade I and II and approximately 40% for grade III tumors. Metastatic disease typically occurs late in the course of the disease. One study reported that the median time to the development of metastasis was 1 year. Unfortunately, this patient has multiple indicators for a poorer prognosis:

- Large tumor size (>5 cm).
- Histologic grade III.
- Inability to achieve microscopic tumor-free margins.

References

Elmslie RE, Glawe P, Dow SW (2008) Metronomic therapy with cyclophosphamide and piroxicam effectively delays tumor recurrence in dogs with incompletely resected soft tissue sarcomas. *J Vet Intern Med* **22**(6):1373–1379.

Kuntz CA, Dernell WS, Powers BE *et al.* (1997) Prognostic factors for surgical treatment of soft-tissue sarcomas in dogs: 75 cases (1986–1996). *J Am Vet Med Assoc* **211**:1147–1151.

Liptak JM, Forrest LJ (2013) Soft tissue sarcomas. In: Withrow SJ, Vail DM, Page RL, editors, *Small Animal Clinical Oncology*, 5th edition. St. Louis, Elsevier Saunders, pp. 356–380.

CASE 16

1 What is an appropriate diagnostic plan? An MDB, CT scan, and biopsy are recommended. The CT scan revealed extensive lysis of the hard palate created by expansion of the mass and early invasion into the nasal cavity. The mass crossed the midline and pushed against the ventral aspect of the globe. The biopsy confirmed osteosarcoma.

2 What therapeutic options can be considered? Given the location of the mass, obtaining tumor-free surgical margins is not possible. Radiation therapy and/or chemotherapy can be considered. In general, cats with axial osteosarcoma have a poor prognosis (median survival times reported to be 5–6 months), which is likely due to the location of the tumor causing problems with surgical resection. The prognosis of cats with osteosarcoma has also been associated with tumor grade and mitotic index. The metastatic rate for cats with osteosarcoma of the oral cavity is low (<10%). Cats with appendicular OSA or operable axial OSA tend to have an excellent prognosis.

References

Bitetto WV, Patnaik AK, Schrader SC *et al.* (1987) Osteosarcoma in cats: 22 cases (1974–1984). *J Am Vet Med Assoc* **190**(1):91–93.

Heldmann E, Anderson MA, Wagner-Mann C (2000) Feline osteosarcoma: 145 cases (1990–1995). *J Am Anim Hosp Assoc* **36**:518–521.

CASE 17

1 What therapeutic options offer the best chance of long-term control? Although in a difficult location, complete surgical excision should be attempted. If histologically tumor-free margins cannot be obtained, radiation therapy should follow. Evaluation of histologic grade, mitotic index, PCR for *c-KIT* mutation, and immunohistochemistry (Ki-67, AgNOR, and c-KIT staining) may also be performed on the biopsy specimen to provide additional information to predict the biologic behavior of this patient's tumor. Chemotherapy may be considered if aggressive behavior is suspected on the basis of histopathology and/or additional tests.

2 How does the location of this tumor impact the prognosis? In general, mast cell tumors located on the muzzle in dogs have been shown to have a more aggressive clinical course than similarly graded mast cell tumors in other locations. Prognostic factors affecting survival time of dogs with muzzle MCT included tumor grade and presence of metastasis at diagnosis. The overall median survival time in this group of patients was 30 months, regardless of treatment type.

Surgery was performed on this patient, and 10 mm microscopic lateral tissue margins and one fascial plane below the tumor were accomplished. However, the skin margin nearest the nares was close at 2 mm (**17b**). The tumor was histologically grade II (Patnaik system) and low grade (Kiupel *et al.*) with a mitotic index of 2. The PCR for the *c-KIT* mutation was negative, and the remainder of the values low grade. No further treatment was pursued and this patient was alive and disease-free 4 years post surgery, after which time he was lost to follow-up.

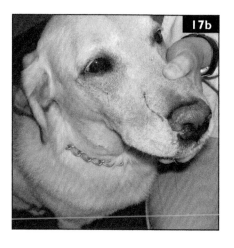

References

Gieger TL, Théon AP, Werner JA *et al.* (2003) Biologic behavior and prognostic factors for mast cell tumors of the canine muzzle: 24 cases (1990–2001). *J Vet Intern Med* 17(5):687–692.

Kiupel M, Webster JD, Bailey KL *et al.* (2011) Proposal of a 2-tier histologic grading system for canine cutaneous mast cell tumors to more accurately predict biological behavior. *Vet Pathol* 48:147–155.

Webster JD, Yuzbasiyan-Gurken V, Miller RA *et al.* (2007) Cellular proliferation in canine cutaneous mast cell tumors: association with c-KIT and its role in prognostication. *Vet Pathol* 44:298–308.

Answers

CASE 18

1 Describe the CT findings. What structure is the arrow pointing to? There is a soft tissue mass on the ventral midline of the neck. There are calcified areas within and throughout the tumor. The mass is abutting the trachea and has a broad based attachment to the underlying tissues. The arrow is pointing to the endotracheal tube.

2 In addition to the MDB, what further staging tests should be performed? Careful evaluation of regional lymph nodes is important and, if they are enlarged, FNA and cytology should be performed. Because thyroid tumors tend to be very vascular, FNA or incisional biopsies of the tumors can be difficult owing to bleeding. If an incisional biopsy is to be performed, a ventral midline approach is advised to avoid seeding of tissue along the jugular furrow. CT (as performed in this case) or MRI for surgical planning is advised in cases where tumors are not freely moveable. A thyroid hormone panel to include a T3, T4, TSH, and thyroglobulin autoantibodies should be run. Although the majority of thyroid tumors in dogs are non-functional, a small percentage of patients will exhibit symptoms of

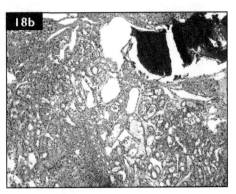

hyperthyroidism. In this patient, lymph nodes were not palpable, the thyroid panel was normal, and an incisional biopsy revealed a follicular epithelial cell thyroid carcinoma (18b). The slides (H & E stain) from the biopsy of this patient showed that sections of the mass were composed of a poorly defined, infiltrative, unencapsulated neoplasm composed of acini, packets, and trabeculae of neoplastic epithelial cells. Infiltration into associated connective tissue was

a prominent feature. Mitoses were rare to absent. There were irregular fragments of metaplastic bone within the tumor. (Courtesy of M. Kiupel, MSU.)

3 What therapies can be considered for this patient? Surgery is the treatment of choice for freely moveable thyroid tumors. If masses are small and freely moveable, surgery may be all that is necessary. Postoperative RT may be needed if tumor-free margins are not achieved. For larger fixed tumors, RT can be used as the primary therapy or to attempt to shrink tumors to a more operable size. Preoperative RT may reduce the size of the tumor and result in the formation of a fibrous capsule, making the tumor more amenable to surgical excision. In one study, dogs treated with definitive radiation showed stabilization or a decrease in tumor size. In some patients, maximal tumor reduction was reached at up to 22 months after treatment. Progression-free survival rates were 80% at 1 year and 72% at 3 years. Radioactive 131I has been shown to be effective in dogs regardless of their thyroid hormone functional status (e.g. hypothyroid, euthyroid, hyperthyroid). Patients with incomplete surgical margins, advanced unresectable, or metastatic thyroid tumors were treated with 131I and median survival times exceeding 2 years were reported for non-metastatic thyroid tumors and 1 year for metastatic thyroid tumors. In this patient, because of the clinical and histologic evidence of disease infiltrating into the surrounding tissue, RT, 131I, and chemotherapy were provided as options to make the tumor more amenable to surgery. The owner declined further therapy, but the patient lived 2 years beyond biopsy with thyroid supplementation alone. The supplementation of thyroid hormone was used to decrease TSH production through negative feedback. TSH is believed to influence tumor cell growth, even in non-functional tumors. This has been documented in humans, but is only anecdotal to date in dogs. The role of chemotherapy in the treatment of canine thyroid tumors has not been well defined, although doxorubicin, cis-platin, actinomycin-D, and mitoxantrone have been reported to be effective and may be considered in patients with non-resectable or metastatic tumors. In one study, postoperative chemotherapy did not improve survival in patients with or without metastasis. In this patient, the tumor slowly progressed in size and she was ultimately euthanized because of weight loss and upper airway obstruction.

References
Barber LG (2007) Thyroid tumors in dogs. *Vet Clin N Am Small Anim Pract* 37:755–773.
Hammer AS, Couto CG, Ayl RD *et al.* (1994) Treatment of tumor-bearing dogs with actinomycin D. *J Vet Intern Med* 8(3):236–239.
Jeglum KA, Whereat A (1983) Chemotherapy of canine thyroid carcinoma. *Compend Contin Educ Vet* 5:96–98.
Nadeau ME, Kitchell BE (2011) Evaluation of the use of chemotherapy and other prognostic variables for surgically excised canine thyroid carcinoma with and without metastasis. *Can Vet J* 52:994–998.
Ogilvie GK, Obradovich JE, Elmslie RE *et al.* (1991) Efficacy of mitoxantrone against various neoplasms in dogs. *J Am Vet Med Assoc* 198:1618–1621.
Théon AP, Marks SL, Feldman ES *et al.* (2000) Prognostic factors and patterns of treatment failure in dogs with unresectable differentiated thyroid carcinomas treated with megavoltage irradiation. *J Am Vet Med Assoc* 216:1775–1779.
Turrel JM, McEntee MC, Burke BP *et al.* (2006) Sodium iodide I 131 treatment of dogs with nonresectable thyroid tumors: 39 cases (1990–2003). *J Am Vet Med Assoc* 229:542–548.

CASE 19
1 Describe the CT scan. There are two intensely contrast-enhancing masses in the region of the thyroid glands. Based on the degree of contrast enhancement, the tumors are very vascular. The jugular and carotid vessels are closely associated with the masses bilaterally. Although the masses appeared well circumscribed on CT, the physical examination supported that they were firmly attached to the tissues of the jugular furrows. The masses were also noted to be very close to or attached to the carotid arteries and jugular veins.

2 What other therapy could be offered for this patient? Radioactive 131I could be used. However, in this patient, an alternating course of doxorubicin and carboplatin chemotherapy was used. Following chemotherapy, the masses were smaller (by approximately 25%) and became freely moveable. Bilateral thyroidectomies were performed.

3 How common are bilateral thyroid tumors? Approximately 25–47% of canine thyroid carcinomas will develop bilaterally.

4 What is the rate of metastasis seen in bilateral thyroid carcinoma? Dogs with bilateral thyroid carcinomas were 16 times more likely to have metastases than dogs with unilateral tumors in one study. In a more recent study of 15 cases of bilateral thyroid gland carcinoma, outcomes were more favorable and metastatic rate much lower; median survival time was 38.3 months.

5 What potential complications exist for bilateral thyroidectomy? Complications of thyroid surgery include intraoperative hemorrhage, laryngeal paralysis due to damage to the recurrent laryngeal nerves, and hypoparathyroidism. It is usually not possible to preserve the parathyroid glands when bilateral thyroidectomy is performed. Given this concern, vitamin D (in the form of calcitriol) and calcium were started 3 days prior to surgery. Ionized calcium levels were measured preoperatively and carefully monitored postoperatively (daily initially, then weekly).

References

Théon AP, Marks SL, Feldman ES *et al.* (2000) Prognostic factors and patterns of treatment failure in dogs with unresectable differentiated thyroid carcinomas treated with megavoltage irradiation. *J Am Vet Med Assoc* **216**:1775–1779.

Tuohy JL, Worley DR, Withrow SJ (2012) Outcome following simultaneous bilateral thyroid lobectomy for treatment of thyroid gland carcinoma in dogs: 15 cases (1994–2010). *J Am Vet Med Assoc* **241**:95–103.

CASE 20

1 Based on the appearance of the mass, what are the differential diagnoses? The large, relatively circumscribed appearance of this mass is highly suggestive of a granular cell tumor (or granular cell myoblastoma). Other differential diagnoses to consider are melanoma, squamous cell carcinoma, and mast cell tumor, although plasmacytoma, epitheliotropic T cell lymphoma (or other round cell tumors), sarcomas, and other more rare types of tumors are possible.

2 Is surgery an option? Given the location and size of the tumor, glossectomy was not considered a reasonable option for this patient. However, because of the circumscribed appearance of this tumor, local surgical excision was advised.

3 What is the likely outcome for this patient? The tumor was well circumscribed and was removed preserving tongue function (20b). The histologic diagnosis was granular cell myoblastoma (GCMB). GCMB carries an excellent prognosis with long-term permanent local control of disease achieved in >80% of patients treated surgically. If tumor-free margins are not possible, re-excision of any regrowth is usually successful. Despite tumor cells extending to the margins in this patient, no recurrence was seen at 2 years postoperatively.

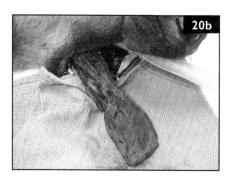

References

Beck ER, Withrow SJ, McChesne AE *et al.* (1986) Canine tongue tumors: a retrospective review of 57 cases. *J Am Anim Hosp Assoc* **22**:525–532.

Liptak JM, Withrow SJ (2013) Cancer of the gastrointestinal tract. In: Withrow SJ, Vail DM, Page RL, editors, *Small Animal Clinical Oncology*, 5th edition. St. Louis, Saunders Elsevier, p. 392.

Turk MAM, Johnson GC, Gallina AM *et al.* (1983) Canine granular cell tumor (myoblastoma): a report of four cases and review of the literature. *J Small Anim Pract* **24**:637–645.

Rallis TS, Tontis DK, Soubasis NH *et al.* (2001) Immunohistochemical study of a granular cell tumor on the tongue of a dog. *Vet Clin Pathol* **30**:62–66.

CASE 21

1 Describe the CT scan. The scan shows a large mineralized mass dorsal to the calvarium. The mass is abutting the bone but does not appear to be invading into the bone. This tumor is often described as having a "popcorn ball" appearance radiographically and on CT.

2 What therapeutic options exist for this patient? Surgery is considered the treatment of choice for these patients. Multilobular tumors of bone commonly occur on the calvarium, maxilla, and mandible. Mandibular tumors appear to have a better prognosis, most likely because the location is more amenable to surgery. Given the fact that this mass does not appear to be invading into the bone, surgical debulking could be considered in this case. Appearance of the well-circumscribed tumor is shown in **21c**. Based on the size and location of the mass, obtaining histologically tumor-free margins would be difficult and

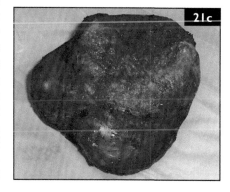

therefore postoperative radiation therapy would be recommended. Chemotherapy (MTD or metronomic) has not been sufficiently evaluated for multilobular tumors of bone.

3 What are the most important prognostic factors for this type of tumor? Histologic grade and ability to achieve a complete surgical excision are the most important prognostic indicators. Overall, recurrence is noted postoperatively in <58%, with a median time to recurrence of 26 months. Grade III tumors had a 78% recurrence rate, whereas grade I tumors had 30% and grade II 47% recurrence rates. With histologically tumor-free margins, recurrence rates were reported to be approximately 25% vs. incomplete surgical excision resulting in 75% recurrence. Overall median survival times are approximately 21 months, with grade I >29 to >50 months, grade II 17–22 months, and grade III 11–13 months, depending on the study reported. Even in patients where surgery is not likely to achieve a complete excision, recurrence tends to be slow. This patient's tumor remained a grade I and despite microscopically incomplete surgical margins, he was still disease-free at 18 months post surgery (**21d, e**).

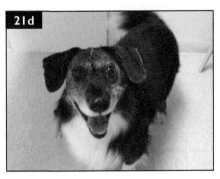 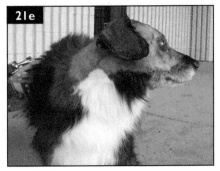

References

Dernell WS, Straw RC, Cooper MR *et al.* (1998) Multilobular osteochondrosarcoma in 39 dogs: 1979–1993. *J Am Anim Hosp Assoc* **34**:11–18.

Hathcock JT, Newton JC (2000) Computed tomographic characteristics of multilobular tumor of bone involving the cranium in 7 dogs and zygomatic arch in 2 dogs. *Vet Radiol Ultrasound* **41**:214–217.

Straw RC, LaCouteur RA, Powers BE *et al.* (1989) Multilobular osteochondrosarcoma of the canine skull: 16 cases (1978–1988). *J Am Vet Med Assoc* **195**:1764–1769.

CASE 22

1 What is the most common tumor type observed in the canine tongue? Squamous cell carcinoma (SCC) accounts for approximately 50% of tongue tumors in dogs. SCC tends to have an ulcerated appearance, making it most likely in this patient.

Although tongue tumors in general are rare in dogs, the next most common tongue tumors are granular cell myoblastoma and malignant melanoma. A variety of other tumor types have been rarely reported such as mast cell tumor, fibrosarcoma, adenocarcinoma, hemangiosarcoma, leiomyosarcoma, myxoma, lymphoma, and lipoma, to name a few. Cytology from a fine needle aspirate was consistent with squamous cell carcinoma.

2 What are the criteria for surgical resection of tongue tumors? Up to 60% of the tongue can be removed for unilateral tumors not crossing the midline or tumors confined to the rostral portion of the tongue. Up to 100% resection of the tongue has been reported in five dogs, with minimal postoperative complications. Feeding tubes were necessary in the postoperative period but, in the long term, function was only mildly affected.

3 Is this patient a candidate for surgery? This patient's tumor crosses the midline and is located too far caudally to remove surgically and preserve any of the tongue. The owner did not want to pursue more aggressive glossectomy.

4 What is the prognosis for this patient? This patient's prognosis is extremely poor owing to the tumor's location and extent of local disease. In patients with inoperable tumors, radiation therapy can be considered. However, this patient's tumor has already eroded through the tongue and his quality of life has been significantly affected. Humane euthanasia was advised. For patients whose tumors are operable, the prognosis is further determined by histologic grade. Grade I tumors have median survival times of 16 months post surgery, grade II 4 months, and grade III 3 months. The overall 1-year survival time is 50%, but approaches 80% for grade I SCC removed with histologically tumor-free margins.

References

Carpenter LG, Withrow SJ, Powers BE *et al.* (1993) Squamous cell carcinoma of the tongue in 10 dogs. *J Am Anim Hosp Assoc* **29**:17–24.

Dennis MM, Ehrhart N, Duncan CG *et al.* (2006) Frequency of and risk factors associated with lingual lesions in dogs: 1,196 cases (1995–2004). *J Am Vet Med Assoc* **228**:1533–1537.

Dvorak LD, Beaver DP, Ellison GW *et al.* (2004) Major glossectomy in dogs: a case series and proposed classification system. *J Am Anim Hosp Assoc* **40**:331–337.

CASE 23

1 Describe the ultrasound findings. What is the likely diagnosis? The image has been obtained from the ventral abdominal wall, therefore the top of the image represents the ventral aspect of the bladder. There is a soft tissue mass in the trigone area of the bladder. Given the patient's age, breed, and the location of the mass, transitional cell carcinoma is likely.

2 What staging tests should be performed and how should the diagnosis be confirmed? An MDB should be performed, but the urinalysis should be obtained by free catch or catheterization rather than cystocentesis. A complete abdominal ultrasound should be performed with special attention to evaluating the bladder, prostate, kidneys, ureters, and sublumbar lymph nodes. Traumatic catheterization can be used to obtain a cytologic specimen. If available, cystoscopy can be used to obtain a biopsy sample.

3 What procedures should be avoided when attempting to obtain a diagnosis? A diagnosis should be attempted through non-surgical means if possible. Ultrasound-guided FNA or cystocentesis should be avoided. The incidence of transplantation of tumor cells causing abdominal wall seeding has been reported to be as high as 10% of cases undergoing cystotomy and is also described in patients undergoing FNA or cystocentesis. Recent reports suggest that abdominal wall seeding of TCC was more likely to occur when dogs underwent cystotomy than FNA or cystocentesis. In fact, the incidence rate for development of body wall TCC was only 1.6% in patients not undergoing cystotomy. The use of FNA for tumors should be reserved for those patients in whom a diagnosis could not be obtained through non-surgical means.

4 How should this patient be treated? TCC of the bladder is commonly treated with a combination of mitoxantrone chemotherapy and piroxicam. Surgical treatment is usually reserved for patients whose tumors are not suspected to be TCC on the basis of their radiographic and ultrasound appearance and location within the bladder (i.e. not located in the trigone region). Even when tumors appear to be small and circumscribed, it is uncommon to achieve a complete tumor-free margin because of the infiltrative nature of TCC. Total cystectomy procedures (e.g. ureterocolonic anastomosis) have been described, but they are technically difficult and metastasis tends to occur early with survival times rarely exceeding 5 months. More recently, total cystectomy with implantation of the ureters into the proximal aspect of the vagina was performed on one dog, with a favorable outcome (survival of 447 days). For the majority of TCC patients, medical management is advised. The combination of mitoxantrone chemotherapy and piroxicam, or carboplatin and piroxicam, has yielded favorable response and survival times. MST for patients treated with piroxicam alone is approximately 6 months. When mitoxantrone is added, MST is 291 days. Progression-free intervals were 109 days with mitoxantrone/piroxicam compared with 73.5 days for carboplatin/piroxicam (these were not statistically different). When mitoxantrone was the first-line treatment, MST was 247.5 days, vs. 263 days when carboplatin was used as the first-line treatment; however, rescue treatment was allowed in this study. Metronomic chlorambucil was reported to be effective in patients that had failed other chemotherapy treatment. A 70% response rate (PR and SD – no CR) was seen, with a PFS of 119 days and overall MST of 221 days. Vinblastine has also been shown to have antitumor activity against TCC in dogs. The median PFI was 122 days with MST of 147 days. Metronomic chlorambucil has not been fully evaluated as a first-line therapy, but has shown efficacy in patients with TCC who had failed other therapies. The median PFI after starting metronomic chlorambucil was 119 days, with the MST from the start of chlorambucil 221 days. Intensity-modulated and image-guided radiation therapy was well tolerated and resulted in an excellent MST of 654 days in one study.

References

Allstadt SD, Rodriguez CO, Boostrom B *et al.* (2015) Randomized phase III trial of piroxicam in combination with mitoxantrone or carboplatin for first-line treatment of urogenital tract transitional cell carcinoma in dogs. *J Vet Intern Med* **29**:261–267.
Boston S, Singh A (2014) Total cystectomy for treatment of transitional cell carcinoma of the urethra and bladder trigone in a dog. *Vet Surg* **43**:294–300.
Henry CJ, McDaw DL, Turnquist SE *et al.* (2003) Clinical evaluation of mitoxantrone and piroxicam in a canine model of human invasive bladder cancer. *Clin Cancer Res* **9**:906–911.
Higuchi T, Burcham CN, Childress MO *et al.* (2013) Characterization and treatment of transitional cell carcinoma of the abdominal wall in dogs: 24 cases (1985–2010). *J Am Vet Med Assoc* **242**:499–506.
Nolan MW, Kogan L, Griffin LR *et al.* (2012) Intensity-modulated and image-guided radiation therapy for treatment of genitourinary carcinomas in dogs. *J Vet Intern Med* **26**:987–995.

CASE 24

1 What diagnostic and staging tests should be performed on this patient prior to treatment recommendations? An MDB is advised. FNA of the regional lymph node should also be performed. An FNA of the tumor can be attempted, but because of the probable secondary inflammation and infection, it may not yield a definitive diagnosis. A tissue biopsy is necessary to determine tumor type more accurately.

2 What is the most common digital tumor seen in dogs? What are the other differential diagnoses? Squamous cell carcinoma is the most common digital tumor seen in dogs. In one large retrospective study, SCC accounted for 51.6% of digital tumors. Other tumor types included malignant melanoma (15.6%), osteosarcoma (6.3%), hemangiopericytoma (4.7%), benign soft tissue tumors (7.8%), and malignant soft tissue tumors (14%). Pododermatitis can be difficult to distinguish from malignancy on radiographs alone, but seemed less likely in this patient given the progression while on antibiotics and the severe lysis noted on the radiographs.

3 What therapy is advised and what is the prognosis for this patient? Amputation of the digit is advised. In this patient, the FNA was consistent with SCC, so amputation was pursued (**24c**). Histopathology confirmed SCC and the margins of the surgery were tumor-free. One- and two-year survival rates following digital amputation for

Answers

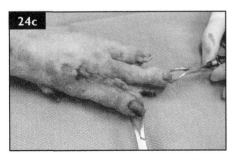

SCC have ranged from 50 to 95% and 18 to 74%, respectively, depending on the study quoted. When looking at specific sites of the digit, subungual SCC had more favorable survival times (survival rates of 95% at 1 year and 74% at 2 years) compared with other sites in the digit (60% at 1 year, 40% at 2 years).

References

Henry CJ, Brewer WG, Whitley EM *et al.* (2005) Canine digital tumors: a Veterinary Cooperative Oncology Group retrospective study of 64 dogs. *J Vet Intern Med* **19**: 720–724.

Marino DJ, Matthiesen DT, Stefanacci JD *et al.* (1995) Evaluation of dogs with digit masses: 117 cases (1981–1991). *J Am Vet Med Assoc* **207**:726–728.

Voges AK, Neuwirth L, Thompson JP *et al.* (1996) Radiographic changes associated with digital, metacarpal and metatarsal tumors, and pododermatitis in the dog. *Vet Radiol Ultrasound* **37**:327–335.

Wobeser BK, Kidney BA, Powers BE *et al.* (2007) Diagnosis and clinical outcomes associated with surgically amputated canine digits submitted to multiple veterinary diagnostic laboratories. *Vet Pathol* **44**:355–461.

CASE 25

1 Describe the radiograph and list the differential diagnoses. There is a proliferative and lytic lesion of the right ilium, extending into the soft tissues surrounding the

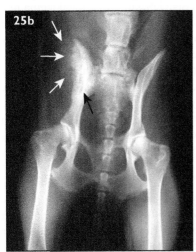

ilium (**25b**). The lesion is consistent with a primary tumor of the ilium. Osteosarcoma and chondrosarcoma are the most common tumors seen in this location. A tumor arising in the soft tissue and invading the bone is a less likely consideration.

2 What further diagnostic tests should be performed? An MDB to include thoracic radiographs, 3 views, is advised. A bone biopsy and CT for surgical planning are advised. Histopathology for this case confirmed OSA.

3 What therapeutic options are available for this patient and what is the prognosis? Surgical removal of the tumor would require hemipelvectomy. Osteosarcoma of the axial skeleton represents approximately 20–25% of all OSA in the dog. Pelvic OSA is the least common of the axial sites, therefore information regarding prognosis with various types of treatments is limited. Pelvic OSA appears to behave similarly to appendicular OSA, therefore surgical excision followed by chemotherapy is advised. With axial OSAs the ability to achieve a tumor-free surgical margin is the most important prognostic indicator. The use of CT or MRI to assist in surgical planning improves the chances of achieving a complete excision and in avoiding surgery in cases where disease is found to be too extensive. In several studies, smaller dogs appeared to do better than larger dogs. Serum ALP level as a predictor of outcome has not been fully evaluated for axial OSA.

References
Ehrhart NP, Ryan SD, Fan TM (2013) Osteosarcoma in dogs. In: Withrow SJ, Vail DM, Page RL, editors, *Small Animal Clinical Oncology*, 5th edition. St. Louis, Elsevier Saunders, pp. 463–503.
Heyman SJ, Diefenderfer DL, Goldschmidt MH *et al.* (1992) Canine axial skeletal osteosarcoma. A retrospective study of 116 cases (1986–1989). *Vet Surg* **21**:304–310.
Kramer A, Walsh PJ, Seguin B (2008) Hemipelvectomy in dogs and cats: technique overview, variations, and description. *Vet Surg* **37**:413–419.

CASE 26
1 What further diagnostic tests are necessary in this patient? An MDB and careful evaluation of the regional lymph nodes are advised. The MDB was within normal limits. Regional lymph nodes were not palpable.
2 Assuming localized disease only, what is the best way to control disease or cure this patient? The best chance for a cure is complete surgical excision with wide tumor-free margins. This represents a challenge in this patient given the location of the tumor, because removal of the metatarsal pad could cause significant postoperative problems.
3 What are the primary concerns with removal of the metatarsal pad in dogs? Removal of the metatarsal pad causes severe problems for dogs because the wear, especially on rougher surfaces, usually results in an open non-healing area and extreme discomfort when walking. In cats, removal of the metatarsal pad is better tolerated. The best way to treat this patient surgically is to remove the pad in the hope of obtaining a wider and deeper tumor-free margin and to perform a digital pad advancement flap for reconstruction of the metatarsal pad.
4 What non-surgical treatment could be considered? Radiation therapy prior to surgery could be considered as a primary treatment, to attempt to shrink the mass to a more easily operable size, or as post-surgical treatment in the event that tumor-free margins are not obtained. Chemotherapy (either MTD or metronomic) would

be more effective in treating microscopic disease than in treating macroscopic disease.

5 If tumor-free margins are not achieved, what further therapy could be considered? For intermediate-grade (grade II) soft tissue sarcomas, recurrence and metastatic rates are highly dependent on the tumor's mitotic index. Postoperative RT or metronomic chemotherapy could be considered to delay recurrence. The risk of metastasis is low for this patient (<15%).

Follow up/discussion

Following routine preparation and draping, an elliptical skin incision was made around the metatarsal pad to include the previous surgical scar and open pad wound (**26b**). The pad and scar were dissected out and removed, the deep dissection plane being at the level of the flexor tendons. The distal edge of the pad was left, to allow attachment of the transplanted pad.

A plantar phalangeal fillet of the 5th digit was then performed (**26c**). A section of skin on the plantar aspect between the digital pad and metatarsal wound was resected to allow the pad to be advanced into the wound. The pad was then sutured to the remnants of the metatarsal pad (**26d**). The postoperative appearance of the surgical resection is shown (**26e**). Histopathology from this surgery revealed wide, clean margins. No further treatment was advised. The patient remains clinically normal and disease-free 18 months following the surgery.

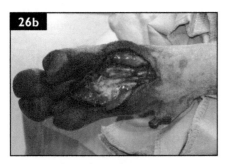

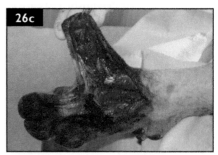

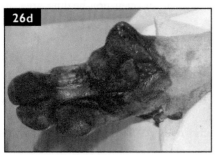

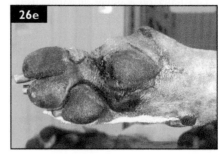

References

Cantatore M, Renwick MG, Yool DA (2013) Combined Z-plasty and phalangeal fillet for reconstruction of a large carpal defect following ablative oncologic surgery. *Vet Comp Orthop Traumatol* **26**:510–514.

Elmslie RE, Glawe P, Dow SW (2008) Metronomic therapy with cyclophosphamide and piroxicam effectively delays tumor recurrence in dogs with incompletely resected soft tissue sarcomas. *J Vet Intern Med* **22**:1373–1379.

Forrest LJ, Chun R, Adams WM *et al.* (2000) Postoperative radiotherapy for canine soft tissue sarcoma. *J Vet Intern Med* **14**:578–582.

Kuntz CA, Dernell WS, Powers BE *et al.* (1997) Prognostic factors for surgical treatment of soft-tissue sarcomas in dogs: 75 cases (1986–1996). *J Am Vet Med Assoc* **21**:1147–1151.

CASE 27

1 What are the differential diagnoses for this lesion? SCC, cutaneous lymphosarcoma, folliculitis (feline demodecosis or dermatophytosis), eosinophilic dermatitis, feline progressive histiocytosis (FPH), and solar dermatitis are considerations.

2 A biopsy was performed and the histopathologic diagnosis was feline progressive histiocytosis (FPH). What is the expected clinical course of this disease? FPH is a rare histiocytic proliferative disorder that is considered a reactive or neoplastic proliferation of dendritic cells (DCs) or macrophages. It is most typically seen as solitary or multiple plaques, papules, or nodules with a predilection for the feet, legs, and face. Early in the course of the disease, there may be minimal to slow progression of the lesion(s), which can remain limited to the skin for prolonged periods of time (reported up to 3 years). As the disease progresses, the microscopic appearance of the cells becomes more aggressive and eventually can be difficult to distinguish from histiocytic sarcoma. In advanced stages, lymph node involvement and internal organ metastasis can be seen.

3 What treatment should be recommended? Unfortunately, FPH is poorly responsive to steroids or chemotherapy. Lack of response to interferon-γ, retinoids, cyclosporine A, leflunomide, vincristine, vinblastine, nitrogen mustard, and l-asparaginase is reported. Surgical excision can be considered for solitary smaller lesions. Approximately 50% of patients treated surgically suffered local recurrences. Radiation therapy has not been described but may be palliative. There are anecdotal transient responses reported to CCNU.

References

Affolter VK, Moore PF (2006) Feline progressive histiocytosis. *Vet Pathol* **43**:646–655.

Moore PF (2014) A review of histiocytic diseases of dogs and cats. *Vet Pathol* **5**:167–184.

CASE 28

1 Describe the cytology. What is the diagnosis? There is an abnormal population of round cells exhibiting anisocytosis, anisokaryosis, and anisonucleoleosis (variation in size of nucleoli). There are also dark blue/black pigment granules seen in the cytoplasm of the cells. This cytology is most consistent with melanoma. The diagnosis is oral malignant melanoma (OMM).

2 What further staging tests are important? An MDB to include 3-view thoracic radiographs is indicated. Evaluation of the regional lymph nodes should include fine needle aspiration and cytology. Cytology is usually reliable if melanoma cells are identified; however, a negative cytology does not completely rule out metastatic disease. In patients with normally palpating lymph nodes, 40% were found to be positive for melanoma on histopathology. Therefore, removal of the draining lymph nodes is a more accurate way to determine whether metastasis has occurred, and should be considered. Some authors have recommended removal of the ipsilateral and contralateral lymph nodes. Sentinel node mapping and removal is of diagnostic, prognostic, and clinical benefit in humans, but studies in dogs are lacking.

3 Describe treatment options. Therapy would be aimed at controlling local disease and attempting to prevent metastasis. Unfortunately, OMM in dogs carries a very poor prognosis. Surgical removal is not possible in this patient without creating a large oronasal fistula. Therefore radiation therapy to control local disease could be considered. Additional systemic therapies such as chemotherapy or the Oncept® canine melanoma vaccine have yielded inconsistent results. Recently, a large retrospective study failed to show a survival advantage with any form of postoperative treatment vs. surgery alone. However, this patient does not have operable disease, so additional systemic therapy could be palliative. When RT alone was compared with RT with adjuvant carboplatin therapy, there was no difference in MST. However, using carboplatin following local treatment for OMM resulted in a survival advantage in another report.

References

Bergman PJ, Kent MS, Farese JP (2013) Melanoma. In: Withrow SJ, Vail DM, Page RL, editors, *Small Animal Clinical Oncology*, 5th edition. St. Louis, Elsevier Saunders, pp. 321–334.

Boston SE, Lu X, Culp WTN *et al.* (2014) Efficacy of systemic adjuvant therapies administered to dogs after excision of oral malignant melanomas: 151 cases (2001–2012). *J Am Vet Med Assoc* 245:401–407.

Dank G, Rassnick KM, Sokolovsky Y *et al.* (2012) Use of adjuvant carboplatin for treatment of dogs with oral malignant melanoma following surgical excision. *Vet Comp Oncol* 12:78–84.

Murphy S, Hayes AM, Blackwood L *et al.* (2005) Oral malignant melanoma – the effect of coarse fractionation radiotherapy alone or with adjuvant carboplatin therapy. *Vet Comp Oncol* 3:222–229.

Williams LE, Packer RA (2003) Association between lymph node size and metastasis in dogs with oral malignant melanoma: 100 cases (1987–2001). *J Am Vet Med Assoc* 222(9):1234–1236.

CASE 29

1 Describe the ultrasound findings. There is a crescent shaped hypoechoic subcapsular thickening noted in the kidney (red arrow). There is increased cortical echogenicity with some irregularity to the renal margins. These ultrasound findings are highly suggestive of renal lymphoma in cats. In one study, >80% of cats with these ultrasound findings were diagnosed with renal lymphoma.

2 An ultrasound-guided FNA of the kidney was performed and cytology is shown (29b). What is the clinical diagnosis? Cytology was most suggestive of lymphoma. There is moderate blood contamination in the cytology specimen, but there is an obvious population of larger lymphocytes. A mitotic figure is present (arrow). Immunocytochemistry was subsequently performed that confirmed B cell lymphoma.

3 Based on the degree of renal failure present, is this patient a reasonable candidate for treatment? For patients that respond to chemotherapy, reversal of even severe azotemia may be observed.

4 What are the possible causes of this patient's ataxia? Weakness and dehydration are most likely contributing to the suspected appearance of ataxia. However, renal lymphoma has a high incidence of CNS involvement. Chemotherapy protocols that include drugs that cross the blood–brain barrier (such as cytosine arabinoside or CCNU) may be helpful when treating renal lymphoma, although this has not been substantiated.

References
Taylor SS, Goodfellow MR, Browne WJ *et al.* (2009) Feline extranodal lymphoma: response to chemotherapy and survival in 110 cats. *J Small Anim Pract* 50:584–592.
Valdes-Martinez A, Cianciolo R, Mai W (2007) Association between renal hypoechoic subcapsular thickening and lymphosarcoma in cats. *Vet Radiol Ultrasound* 48:357–360.

CASE 30

1 Describe the lesion seen on CT. There is a contrast-enhancing lesion, measuring approximately 2.1 × 2 cm, in the pituitary fossa. This patient's lesion is most suggestive of a pituitary macroadenoma.

2 What is the cause of the oculomotor dysfunction? Pressure from the tumor on the optic chiasm is most likely.

3 **What therapy is recommended and what is the prognosis for this patient?**
Radiation therapy is the treatment of choice for pituitary macroadenomas. While
pituitary macroadenomas are relatively uncommon in dogs, overall survival of
patients is increased with RT. In one study, the MST of patients with functional
pituitary macroadenomas and macrocarcinomas treated with radiation therapy
was 743 days. The best prognosis is for dogs without clinical signs whose tumors
are less than 1.5 cm. In a separate study, the prognostic factors that independently
affected overall survival time negatively were larger tumor size and severity of
neurologic signs.

References

deFornel P, Delisle F, Devauchelle P *et al.* (2007) Effects of radiotherapy on pituitary
corticotroph macrotumors in dogs: a retrospective study of 12 cases. *Can Vet J* **48:**
481–486.

Dow SW, LeCouteur RA, Rosychuk RAW *et al.* (1990) Response of dogs with functional
pituitary macroadenomas and macrocarcinomas to radiation. *J Small Anim Pract*
31:287–294.

Theon AP, Feldman EC (1998) Megavoltage irradiation of pituitary macrotumors in dogs
with neurologic signs. *J Am Vet Med Assoc* **213:**225–231.

CASE 31

1 **What therapeutic options should be considered for this patient?** Unfortunately,
there are no good alternatives to amputation in this case. Owing to the fact that
the tumor encompasses 360° of the leg, curative intent radiation therapy would
be difficult. Unless it is possible to spare normal tissue from the radiation field,
there is concern that lymphatic and vascular supply to the distal limb would be
compromised. Chemotherapy is likely to be of minimal benefit, especially given
that the tumor is low grade. Therefore, despite the owner's aversion to amputation,
it would be the best treatment for this pet in terms of both a cure and palliation of
pain.

2 **What is the long-term prognosis for this patient with treatment?** With
amputation, the prognosis for this patient is excellent for long-term tumor control.
The leg was ultimately amputated and the owners were very pleased with cosmetic
and functional result. Preoperative tumor size and tumor type were the most
significant predictors of the outcome of cats with soft tissue sarcomas in one study.
Postoperative median survival times were 643 days if tumors were <2 cm, 558 days
if 2–5 cm, and 394 days for tumors >5 cm. Of the soft tissue sarcomas evaluated,
fibrosarcomas and nerve sheath tumors had the best prognosis (MSTs 640 days
and 645 days respectively).

Answers

Reference
Dillon JD, Mauldin GN, Baer KE (2005) Outcome following surgical removal of nonvisceral soft tissue sarcomas in cats: 42 cases (1992–2000). *J Am Vet Med Assoc* **12**:1955–1957.

CASE 32

1 Describe the radiographic findings. The radiograph shows a compression fracture of the distal radius and ulna. There is a large lytic lesion in the distal radius at the level of the metaphysis. Diagnosis: pathologic fracture.

2 What further diagnostic tests are recommended for this patient? In a 10-year-old Rottweiler with a lytic distal radial lesion and pathologic fracture, osteosarcoma is the primary rule out. Therefore, an MDB should be performed. Survey radiographs of the appendicular skeleton or nuclear bone scan to rule out further metastasis can also be considered. A bone biopsy is needed to obtain a definitive diagnosis.

3 What is the appropriate treatment plan? Repair of pathologic fractures has been described. In one study, using a bone plate and interlocking nails for repair, limb use was immediate after surgery and provided palliation for patients. A median survival time of 166 days following repair was noted, but adjunctive therapy with chemotherapy, radiation, or pamidronate was used in some patients. Definitive treatment would involve amputation and chemotherapy. Various chemotherapy agents and protocols have been described in the literature. The platinum compounds (carboplatin, cis-platin, lobaplatin) used singly or in combinatin with doxorubicin have been studied. Doxorubicin as a single agent has also been reported. The ease of administration of carboplatin has made it a more popular choice than cis-platin, which is nephrotoxic and requires aggressive pre- and post-treatment diuresis. A recent study comparing the use of carboplatin alone and alternating carboplatin and doxorubicin post-amputation showed superior results with carboplatin as a single agent. Dogs receiving carboplatin (six total dosages) alone had significantly longer DFI (425 vs. 135 days) than dogs treated with alternating dosages of carboplatin and doxorubicin (three dosages of each). The MST for the carboplatin alone group was 479 days; that for the carboplatin/doxorubicin group was 287 days. These results are the most favorable to date for patients undergoing amputation and chemotherapy. Overall MSTs with various chemotherapeutic protocols approach 1 year, with 2-year survival rates of <28%. Palliative protocols using RT are not likely to be helpful in this patient unless the fracture is repaired. When considering pain control, amputation would be the preferred option.

References
Boston SE, Bacon NJ, Culp WTN *et al.* (2011) Outcome after repair of a sarcoma-related pathologic fracture in dogs: a Veterinary Society of Surgical Oncology retrospective study. *Vet Surg* **40**(4):431–437.

Selmic LE, Burton JH, Thamm DH *et al.* (2014) Comparison of carboplatin- and doxorubicin-based chemotherapy protocols in 470 dogs after amputation for treatment of appendicular osteosarcoma. *J Vet Intern Med* 28:554–563.

Skorupski KA, Uhl JM, Szivek A *et al.* (2016) Carboplatin versus alternating carboplatin and doxorubicin for the adjuvant treatment of canine appendicular osteosarcoma: a randomized, phase III trial. *Vet Comp Oncol* 14(1):81–87, doi:10.1111/vco.12069.

Szewczyk M, Lechowski R, Zabielska K (2015) What do we know about canine osteosarcoma treatment? – Review. *Vet Res Commun* 39:61–67.

CASE 33

1 What diagnostic tests are recommended for this patient? The status of the patient's remission should be assessed with CBC, chemistry panel, thoracic radiographs, abdominal ultrasound, and FNA of the new lesions.

- Blood work was normal. Physical examination, thoracic radiographs, and abdominal ultrasound confirmed complete remission. The FNAs were inconclusive, revealing only normal epithelial cells.
- A biopsy of the skin lesions revealed canine cutaneous viral squamous papillomas, which are benign growths caused by infection with canine papillomavirus. These masses are most commonly seen in young dogs and older immunosuppressed dogs, but can be seen in dogs of any age. They often regress spontaneously.

2 What therapy is indicated? The immune suppression is most likely secondary to chemotherapy, although this is uncommon in dogs. This patient was weaned off prednisone and chemotherapy was delayed until the lesions regressed. Chemotherapy was started again, but a more conservative treatment interval of every 2–3 weeks was initiated rather than weekly induction therapy.

Reference
Lange CE, Favrot C (2011) Canine papillomaviruses. *Vet Clin N Am Small Anim Pract* 41:1183–1195.

CASE 34

1 What are the differential diagnoses for this patient? When a splenic mass is noted, approximately one-third are benign (hematoma, extramedullary hematopoiesis, abscess) and two-thirds are malignant. Of those tumors that are malignant, approximately two-thirds are diagnosed as hemangiosarcoma (HSA) and the remaining one-third have other types of malignancy (fibrosarcoma, undifferentiated sarcoma, etc.). Therefore, almost 50% of splenic masses detected are ultimately diagnosed as hemangiosarcoma.

2 Does the patient's breed play a role in determining the most likely diagnosis? German Shepherd Dogs are at higher risk for the development of splenic hemangiosarcoma. However, they are also at higher risk for development of splenic hematoma. Although this dog's breed raises suspicion for hemangiosarcoma, histopathology is necessary to make a definitive diagnosis.

3 What further diagnostic tests should be performed? MDB, coagulation panel (~75% of patients with HSA have clinical or subclinical DIC), and abdominal ultrasound are advised. Blood work and thoracic radiographs were normal in this patient. The ultrasound revealed a large, mostly fluid-filled mass associated with the spleen. There was no evidence of free fluid or other lesions in the abdomen.

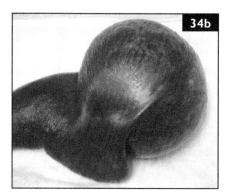

4 What is the recommended treatment and the expected prognosis for this patient? Surgical exploratory is the recommendation for this patient. Although breed and age would raise concern for neoplasia, the only way to obtain a definitive diagnosis and provide therapy is through surgery. The patient's tumor is shown (**34b**). The diagnosis was a benign hematoma.

References
Hammer AS, Couto CG (1992) Diagnosing and treating canine hemangiosarcoma. *Vet Med* 3:188–201.
Hammer AS, Couto CG, Swardson C *et al.* (1991) Hemostatic abnormalities in dogs with hemangiosarcoma. *J Vet Intern Med* 5:11–14.
Johnson KA, Powers BE, Withrow SJ *et al.* (1989) Splenomegaly in dogs: predictors of neoplasia and survival after splenectomy. *J Vet Intern Med* 3:160–166.
Srebrenik N, Appleby RC (1991) Breed prevalence and sites of hemangioma and hemangiosarcoma in dogs. *Vet Rec* 129:408–409.

CASE 35

1 What additional diagnostic tests are indicated for this patient? Diagnostic tests indicated include:

- To complete the MDB, thoracic radiographs should be performed. There was no evidence of thoracic metastasis seen in this patient.
- Ultrasound-guided fine needle aspirates of the liver can be useful in obtaining a preliminary diagnosis. In this case, they were performed, and revealed hepatocytes with mild anisocytosis and cellular atypia.

Answers

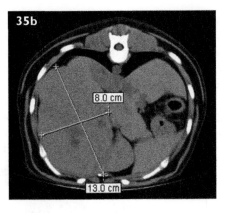

- CT scanning is a useful tool to determine extent of disease and to help with surgical planning – the CT scan from this patient is shown (35b). There was no further evidence of disease beyond the primary tumor site.

2 What is the significance of the mass being on the left side? Masses arising in the left side of the liver appear to be more amenable to surgical resection and, as a result, carry a more favorable prognosis than those on the right.

3 What are the primary rule outs for this mass? Hepatoma and hepatocellular carcinoma are the most likely considerations. If it is hepatocellular carcinoma, "massive" hepatocellular carcinoma is probable given the large size and solitary nature of the mass.

4 Is this patient a poor candidate for surgery because of the large size of the mass? Both hepatoma and massive hepatocellular carcinoma carry an excellent prognosis with surgical excision. Despite their large size, most can be surgically removed. Even if microscopic disease remains following surgery, regrowth is typically very slow and quality of life significantly improves with surgery. At surgery, this

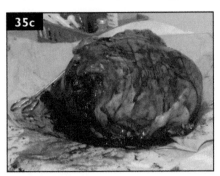

patient's tumor was removed from the left lateral liver lobe (35c). Complete excision of the mass was possible. Histopathology documented a well-differentiated hepatocellular carcinoma. Median survival times for dogs with massive hepatocellular carcinoma are >1,460 days (median not reached) for dogs undergoing surgery, compared with only 270 days for patients treated medically.

Reference

Liptak JM, Dernell WS, Monnet E et al. (2004) Massive hepatocellular carcinoma in dogs: 48 cases (1992–2002). J Am Vet Med Assoc 225:1225–1230.

CASE 36

1 What are the likely causes of the lymphadenopathy? Lymphoma is the most likely consideration. With a normal body temperature, normal CBC, and no other abnormalities noted, the peripheral lymphadenopathy and cranial organomegaly are not likely to be caused by any infectious process. The degree of node enlargement and the clinically normal status of this patient are most consistent with lymphoma.

2 What further tests should be performed prior to instituting treatment? An MDB is advised. However, thoracic radiographs need only include 2 views (lateral and VD) as lymphoma is more likely to effect sternal, mediastinal, or hilar nodes, which can be adequately assessed on 2 views. In addition, if lymphoma were to spread to the lungs, it tends to do so diffusely as an interstitial infiltrate rather than as solitary or a limited number of lung masses. Fine needle aspiration and cytology are advised for a presumptive diagnosis. IHC or ICC is advised to differentiate between T and B cell lymphoma. In addition to routine staging tests and cytology/biopsy, an echocardiogram is advised for this patient. Although there is no current evidence of cardiac abnormalities, Boxers are predisposed to cardiomyopathy, which may in initial phases be occult. With the potential use of cardiotoxic chemotherapy (doxorubicin), an echocardiogram is advised as a baseline for any breed, such as the Boxer, which is at increased risk for cardiac abnormalities.

3 What is the likelihood that this patient has T cell lymphoma? Approximately 70% of Boxers diagnosed with lymphoma will have T cell lymphoma. Although patients with T cell lymphoma have been shown to carry a poorer prognosis than those with B cell lymphoma in some studies, there appears to be a subset of T cell lymphoma patients whose disease behaves in more of a chronic low-grade fashion.

References

Lurie DM, Lucroy SM, Griffey SM et al. (2004) T-cell-derived malignant lymphoma in the boxer breed. *Vet Comp Oncol* 2:171–175.

Lurie DM, Milner RJ, Suter SE et al. (2008) Immunophenotypic and cytomorphologic subclassification of T-cell lymphoma in the boxer breed. *Vet Immunol Immunopathol* 125:102–110.

Valli VE, Kass PH, San Myint M et al. (2013) Canine lymphomas: association of classification type, disease stage, tumor subtype, mitotic rate, and treatment with survival. *Vet Pathol* 50:738–748.

CASE 37

1 What device is being placed in this patient and what is it used for? A subcutaneous vascular access port (SVAP) is being placed into the jugular vein of a Shar Pei with lymphoma. SVAPs provide open access to a vessel without having to place catheters repeatedly for chronic treatments such as chemotherapy. In patients whose veins are too small to access repeatedly or in breeds, such as Shar Peis, who have very difficult veins to work with, SVAP may be the only reasonable method to deliver IV chemotherapy. These ports have also been used in patients undergoing radiation therapy for induction of anesthesia, because multiple anesthetic episodes are required during a radiation protocol. Fortunately, most complications are minor and self-limiting, but there is a low risk of serious complications.

2 **What are the advantages of this device?**
- Immediate and easy access to a vein without having to place a catheter repeatedly.
- Less stress to patient.
- Avoids damage to peripheral veins from repeated catheter placement.
- No activity restrictions for patients once ports are placed.

3 **What are the disadvantages that can be seen?**
- Bacterial infection/abscess formation.
- Seroma.
- Breakage of port–catheter junction.
- Port migration.
- Requires surgical procedure to put in place.

Reference

Culp WTN, Mayhew PD, Reese MS *et al.* (2010) Complications associated with use of subcutaneous vascular access ports in cats and dogs undergoing fractionated radiotherapy: 172 cases (1996–2007). *J Am Vet Med Assoc* **236**:1322–1327.

CASE 38

1 **What risk factor(s) would exist for increased toxicity to chemotherapy in this patient (38)?** Because this patient is a Collie, there is a 70% chance that he has a mutation in the multi-drug resistance gene *ABCB1* (*MDR1*). This gene encodes a protein, P-glycoprotein (P-gp), an adenosine triphosphate (ATP)-driven pump that transports substrate drugs across cell membranes. P-gp is expressed in a variety of mammalian tissues including the intestinal tract, kidney, liver, and endothelial cells of brain capillaries. At the blood–brain barrier, for example, P-gp is expressed at the luminal membrane of endothelial cells of the brain capillaries and restricts the entry of drugs into the central nervous system. Mutations in *MDR1* can result in reduced ability to pump some drugs out of the brain, resulting in neurologic symptoms. Likewise, mutations in *MDR1* can also affect excretion of these drugs from other tissues, causing increased toxicity. In some cases, reactions to certain drugs can be life threatening. Other breeds affected by the *MDR1* mutation include (but are not limited to) Shetland Sheepdogs (15% frequency), Long-haired Whippets (65% frequency), McNab Shepherds (30% frequency), English Shepherds (15% frequency), and German Shepherds (10% frequency).

2 What additional tests should be run before planning a chemotherapy protocol? Identification of the mutant *MDR1* (*ABCB1-1Δ*) gene can be done through DNA testing currently performed at Washington State University. Test results will indicate whether the dog has the *MDR1* mutation and whether it has one copy or two copies of the mutant gene: *Normal/Normal* (these dogs do not carry the mutation and will not pass on the mutation to their offspring); *Mutant/Mutant* (homozygous for the mutant allele – these dogs would be expected to experience toxicity to certain drugs); *Mutant/Normal* (heterozygous for the mutant allele – these dogs carry the mutation and *may* pass on the mutant gene to their offspring; they may also experience toxicity to certain drugs).

3 What drugs should be avoided in this patient? A mutation in the gene encoding P-gp can render patients extremely susceptible to toxicity resulting from the administration of many drugs that use P-gp as a substrate, including chemotherapeutic agents. Drugs known to cause problems in dogs with the *MDR1* mutation include acepromazine, butorphanol, erythromycin, ivermectin, loperamide, and certain antineoplastic agents (e.g. vincristine, vinblastine, actinomycin-D, etoposide, docetaxel, and doxorubicin) and these should probably be avoided completely in Mutant/Mutant dogs. These drugs should be used with caution, and probably at reduced doses, in Mutant/Normal dogs.

References

Mealey KL (2006) Adverse drug reactions in herding-breed dogs: the role of p-glycoprotein. *Compend Contin Educ Vet* **28**:23–33.

Mealey KL (2013) Adverse drug reactions in veterinary patients associated with drug transporters. *Vet Clin N Am Small Anim Pract* **43**:1067–1078.

Mizukami K, Chang HS, Yabuki A *et al.* (2012) Rapid genotyping assays for the 4-base pair deletion of canine *MDR1/ABCB1* gene and low frequency of the mutant allele in Border Collie dogs. *J Vet Diag Invest* **24**:127–134.

CASE 39

1 Describe the pretreatment (39b) and post-treatment (39c) radiographs. The proximal aspect of the third metacarpal bone in **39b** has a well-defined lytic lesion. In the post-treatment radiograph (**39c**), there has been bone remodeling which has decreased the amount of lysis visible.

2 What curative-intent therapeutic options can be offered to this patient? Given the location of the lesion, surgical removal of the affected metacarpal bone is not possible without amputation of the leg. Owing to the metastatic nature of osteosarcoma, chemotherapy should be used postoperatively (e.g. carboplatin). Non-surgical limb-sparing stereotactic radiotherapy (SRT) in combination with chemotherapy (e.g. carboplatin alone or with doxorubicin) has yielded results similar to those of amputation and chemotherapy. Generally, smaller more blastic lesions are better candidates for SRT than larger lytic ones, because pathologic fracture is a frequent complication of SRT used for OSA.

3 Describe options for palliative therapy. Palliative options include RT (e.g. four 8–10 Gy dosages). In addition to palliative RT, chemotherapy can be considered in order to delay the progression of local disease and onset of metastasis. At the end of four 8 Gy fractions of RT and four carboplatin chemotherapy treatments, the lesion was markedly improved radiographically (**32c**) and the patient was no longer lame.

References

Coomer A, Farese J, Milner R *et al.* (2009) Radiation therapy for canine appendicular osteosarcoma. *Vet Comp Oncol* 7:15–27.

Farese JP, Milner R, Thompson MS *et al.* (2004) Stereotactic radiosurgery for treatment of osteosarcomas involving the distal portions of the limbs in dogs. *J Am Vet Med Assoc* 225:1567–1572.

CASE 40

1 Describe the abnormality observed. There are multiple darkly pigmented spots on the iris of the left eye (OS). Anisocoria (mydriasis OS) is also noted, which could be a result of decreased mobility of the iris or adhesions. This condition is called iris melanosis. Iris melanosis in cats refers to dark pigmentation changes within the iris. It can be diffuse and progressive. The proliferating melanocytes are entirely limited to the anterior surface of the iris. Benign lesions tend to be flat and should not protrude above the surface of the iris. It typically starts as a benign condition. In some patients, it remains benign. In others, progression to malignancy can be seen. Without histology from enucleation, the diagnosis of malignancy can be difficult.

2 What are the recommendations for this patient? Because transition to malignancy can take months to years, careful monitoring of the eye is generally recommended. A thorough ophthalmic examination is necessary. Melanotic changes can interfere with the drainage angle and result in glaucoma. Transition from a smooth to fuzzy appearance of the iris, increased thickness or irregularities, pigment dispersion into the aqueous humor, distortion or decreased mobility of the iris, increased intraocular pressure, and extension into the posterior surface of the iris are all changes that raise concern. In this patient, there is evidence of possible decreased mobility of the iris. If no further abnormalities are present, careful monitoring is advised. However, if additional abnormalities such as increased intraocular pressure are present, enucleation should be considered. A more rapid progression can occur in younger cats.

Reference
Finn M, Krohne S, Stiles J (2008) Ocular melanocytic neoplasia. *Compend Contin Educ Vet* 30:19–25.

CASE 41

1 Describe the cytologic findings and give a diagnosis. The sample is very cellular with the predominant population being round cells. The nuclei are eccentric in location and there is a perinuclear clear zone which represents the Golgi apparatus. There is moderate anisocytosis and anisokaryosis present. The findings are most consistent with a plasma cell tumor.

2 What staging tests should be performed? Cutaneous plasmacytomas are usually benign in their behavior. Less than 1% of cutaneous plasmacytomas were determined to be part of systemic multiple myeloma. Nodal metastasis was seen in only 2% of cases in one large study. Patients with extramedullary plasmacytomas in the intestinal tract or solitary osseous plasmacytomas should be staged with bone marrow aspirates, serum electrophoresis, and skeletal survey radiographs because the probability of metastasis is somewhat greater. However, those that exist as solitary tumors in the skin are typically benign. Careful evaluation for regional lymph node enlargement is warranted, but more aggressive staging is likely to be unrewarding.

3 What are the treatment recommendations for this patient? Given the size of this mass, complete surgical excision would be difficult. Radiation therapy or chemotherapy could reduce the size of the mass and make it more amenable to surgery. This patient was treated with prednisone. The mass decreased by approximately 50% in size and was then removed surgically. Marginal surgical excision is usually adequate. Three years following surgery, the mass had not recurred.

References
Clark GN, Berg J, Engler SJ et al. (1992) Extramedullary plasmacytoas in dogs: results of surgical excision in 131 cases. *J Am Anim Hosp Assoc* 28:105–111.
Gupta A, Fry JL, Meindel M et al. (2014) Pathology in practice. *J Am Vet Med Assoc* 244:163–165.

CASE 42

1 Are these lesions consistent with progression of lymphoma? This would be a very unusual presentation for progression of lymphoma and appears more clinically consistent with calcinosis circumscripta, given the location and appearance of the lesions. Calcinosis circumscripta is an uncommon syndrome of ectopic deposition of calcium salts in soft tissue. It most often occurs in young large breed dogs and is generally idiopathic, although disorders of calcium are also incriminated in some patients. It can be seen in patients with renal disease, vitamin D excess, nutritional imbalance (disordered calcium:phosphorus ratio in foods), parathyroid tumors, Cushing's disease, or any other disorder where calcium balance is abnormal.

2 How could these lesions be a result of therapy? Excessive exogenous steroids are also implicated. This patient was on 2 mg/kg daily of prednisone as part of her chemotherapy protocol.

3 What other diagnostic tests should be done on this patient? Approximately 85% of Boxers diagnosed with lymphoma will have T cell lymphoma. T cell lymphomas are commonly associated with hypercalcemia. A serum chemistry panel including a calcium level should be obtained. This patient's calcium level was normal.

4 What is the recommended therapy for these lesions? Surgical excision is usually curative. Because there were no other findings to explain the calcium dysregulation in this patient, the calcinosis circumscripta was considered to be either idiopathic or iatrogenic secondary to steroid administration. Following discontinuation of the steroids, the lesions did partially regress.

References
Lurie DM, Milner RJ, Suter SE *et al.* (2008) Immunophenotypic and cytomorphologic subclassification of T-cell lymphoma in the boxer breed. *Vet Immunol Immunopathol* **125**:102–110.
Tafti AK, Hanna P, Bourque AC (2005) Calcinosis circumscripta in the dog: a retrospective pathological study. *J Vet Med* **52**:13–17.

CASE 43

1 Describe the radiographic findings (43b). There is a lytic expansile bone lesion of the left third metatarsal bone. The lesion occupies at least 75% of the length of the bone. The cortex is almost completely destroyed and there is periosteal new bone evident.

2 An MDB and a fine needle aspirate of the lesion were performed. The MDB was normal and the cytology slide is shown (43c). What is the presumptive diagnosis? The radiographic and cytologic findings are most consistent with neoplasia. The cytology is consistent with sarcoma, but the type of sarcoma cannot be definitively diagnosed without histopathology. A primary bone tumor is most likely. A biopsy confirmed osteosarcoma.

3 What is the recommended treatment and expected outcome? Hindlimb amputation offers the best chance for a cure. Osteosarcoma in cats differs greatly from the same disease in dogs. Feline OSA has a far lower incidence of metastasis (80–90% in dogs vs. 5–10% in cats). Wide surgical excision, in this case amputation, has a high probability of resulting in long-term control. Post-amputation chemotherapy has not been shown to improve survival times in cats. Histologically, the appearance of feline OSA is similar to that of canine OSA, although feline OSA tends to have a lower mitotic index. In one study, mitotic index was the only specific histologic variable that significantly affected survival statistics for cats. The most important clinical variable influencing survival time is the ability to obtain tumor-free margins with surgery. The MST for feline OSA has been reported to range from 24 to 44 months.

References
Dimopoulou M, Kirpensteijn J, Moens H *et al.* (2008) Histologic prognosticators in feline osteosarcoma: a comparison with phenotypically similar canine osteosarcoma. *Vet Surg* 37:466–471.

Ehrhart ND, Ryan SD, Fan TM (2013) Tumors of the skeletal system. Primary bone tumors of cats. In: Withrow SJ, Vail DM, Page RL, editors, *Small Animal Clinical Oncology*, 5th edition. St. Louis, Elsevier Saunders, pp. 494–495.

Heldmann E, Anderson MA, Wagner-Mann C (2000) Feline osteosarcoma: 145 cases (1990–1995). *J Am Anim Hosp Assoc* 36:518–521.

CASE 44

1 What are the primary differential diagnoses for this mass? Amelanotic melanoma, squamous cell carcinoma, and fibrosarcoma are the most likely considerations.

2 The owners only wished to pursue palliative therapy. What would be advised and what diagnostic tests would be necessary prior to instituting palliative therapy? The biologic behavior and expectations for disease progression and metastatic behavior can vary considerably for these three tumor types. Thoracic radiographs and cytology or histopathology of the primary tumor and lymph node should be considered. Thoracic radiographs were normal and the biopsy revealed an amelanotic melanoma. There was evidence of metastatic disease in the ipsilateral submandibular lymph node.

3 What palliative therapy would most likely have the greatest impact on improving this patient's quality of life? The primary causes of the patient's poor quality of life are the secondary infection present, the physical obstruction to eating created by the mass, and pain due to likely bone involvement of the tumor. Antibiotics should be used to decrease secondary infection. Radiation therapy offers the best chance to provide control of bone pain and to reduce the size of the tumor to improve his ability to eat. Palliative RT is effective for local control of oral malignant melanoma in >70% of patients treated. Unfortunately, despite adequate local control of disease, metastatic disease remains the primary challenge.

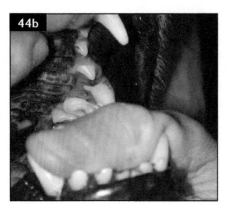

44b

Follow up/discussion
The post-RT photograph (**44b**) shows almost complete resolution of the oral tumor. However, the patient died 4 months later, due to pulmonary metastasis.

References
Bateman KE, Catton PA, Pennock PW *et al*. (1994) 0-7-21 radiation therapy for the treatment of canine oral melanoma. *J Vet Intern Med* **8**:267–272.
Cancedda S, Bley CR, Aresu L *et al*. (2014) Efficacy and side effects of radiation therapy in comparison with radiation therapy and temozolomide in the treatment of measurable canine malignant melanoma. *Vet Comp Oncol*, doi:10.1111/vco.12122: 1-12.
Khan N, Khan MK, Almasan A *et al*. (2011) The evolving role of radiation therapy in the management of malignant melanoma. *Int J Radiation Oncology Biol Phys* **80**:645–654.
Murphy S, Hayes AM, Blackwood L *et al*. (2005) Oral malignant melanoma – the effect of coarse fractionation radiotherapy alone or with adjuvant carboplatin therapy. *Vet Comp Oncol* **3**:222–229.
Proulx DR, Ruslander DM, Dodge RK *et al*. (2003) A retrospective analysis of 140 dogs with oral melanoma treated with external beam radiation. *Vet Radiol Ultrasound* **44**:352–359.

CASE 45
1 Describe the abnormality seen on this radiograph (45) of a 12-year-old Labrador Retriever presented for an acute onset of forelimb lameness. There is a lesion of the mid-shaft humerus. The lesion is predominantly lytic but areas of bone production are also noted. The location of this lesion is more suggestive of a metastatic tumor than a primary tumor because the lesion has developed at the site where the blood supply enters the bone.

2 What staging tests would be required before further prognostic information can be given? Given the possibility that this could represent a metastatic site, a work-up to include a thorough physical examination, thoracic radiographs, and abdominal ultrasound should initially be performed. If there is no other evidence of cancer on these tests, biopsy of the bone lesion would be indicated. In the event that a diagnosis of osteosarcoma, chondrosarcoma, or other type of sarcoma that can be primary in the bone is identified, a nuclear bone scan could be considered to look for another primary bone tumor site. A biopsy of the bone lesion would be required to determine histologic type. If histopathology reveals a type of tumor not expected to be primary in the bone (e.g. carcinoma), then further investigation to identify a primary site is indicated.

3 What therapeutic options would be recommended in this case? Therapeutic options would depend on the histologic diagnosis. If the biopsy results suggest a primary bone tumor with no other evidence of metastasis or another primary site, then amputation plus chemotherapy (depending on histology) is advised. If the lesion is considered to be metastatic from another site, palliative therapy such as radiation therapy, bisphosphonate therapy, or even amputation for pain control is recommended.

4 What tumors are most commonly associated with bone metastasis? Mammary gland adenocarcinoma, prostatic carcinoma, transitional cell carcinoma, head and neck squamous cell carcinoma, pulmonary carcinoma, and multiple myeloma can metastasize to bones. Primary OSA can spread to other bone sites and HSA has been reported to metastasize to bone.

Reference
Simmons JK, Hildreth III BE, Supsavhad W *et al*. (2015) Animal models of bone metastasis. *Vet Pathol* **52**:827–841.

CASE 46

1 Describe the CT findings. There is a 6.8 × 5.3 cm mass in the right side of the neck that is abutting the trachea and appears to be destroying or displacing a portion of the vertebrae. The mass appears multilobulated in nature. The origin of the mass could not be determined with certainty. Although the tonsils were normal on the CT scan, metastasis from a tonsillar or salivary gland origin cannot be excluded.

2 Is this a surgical case? Given the close proximity to the trachea and muscles/transverse processes of the vertebrae, complete surgical excision is not possible and marginal excision would be difficult.

3 What therapy is advised? Chemotherapy and/or palliative radiation therapy could be considered. A PFS of 12–18 months was seen in patients with non-tonsillar oral SCC treated with RT, although intraoral disease was not seen in this patient. When patients with non-tonsillar oral SCC were treated with piroxicam and carboplatin in another study, the median follow up was 543 days, with time to recurrence and progression not yet reached. Toceranib phosphate (Palladia®) appears to have biologic activity against head and neck carcinomas in dogs. The response rate was 75% (one CR, five PR) with a median duration of response of almost 20 weeks (range 4–48 weeks). However, given the size and invasiveness of this patient's tumor, a guarded prognosis for response to therapy must be given.

References

deVos JP, Burm AGD, Focker AP *et al.* (2005) Piroxicam and carboplatin as a combination treatment of canine oral non-tonsillar squamous cell carcinoma: a pilot study and a literature review of a canine model of human head and neck squamous cell carcinoma. *Vet Comp Oncol* 3:16–24.

London C, Mathie T, Stingle N *et al.* (2012) Preliminary evidence for biologic activity of toceranib phosphate (Palladia®) in solid tumours. *Vet Comp Oncol* 10:194–205.

CASE 47

1 Describe the clinical appearance and likely diagnosis for this patient. The clinical appearance of this patient is highly suggestive of inflammatory mammary carcinoma (IMC).

2 What additional diagnostic tests should be performed? IMC has a high rate of metastasis, which can occur through vascular or lymphatic routes; therefore, in addition to the MDB, abdominal ultrasound is advised. At the time of diagnosis, >80% of patients have evidence of distant metastasis. Coagulopathies (DIC) are seen in approximately 20% of patients with IMC, therefore a coagulation panel is also advised. Fine needle aspiration is usually not helpful owing to the extensive inflammation associated with the tumor. Definitive diagnosis is best made on a biopsy. Dermal lymphatic involvement is the hallmark for the pathologic diagnosis of IMC.

3 Given the clinical appearance of the lesions and histopathology results, what treatment can be considered and what is the prognosis for this patient? IMC typically carries a very poor prognosis. Median survival times are approximately 60 days. Patients with coagulopathies have the shortest survival times. Patients receiving some sort of medical therapy have slightly improved survival times. Surgical excision is not possible in this patient because the disease is extending down the hindlimbs. Chemotherapy is mostly ineffective for IMC. High intra-tumor levels of COX-2 are seen in IMC and have been associated with increased recurrence, metastasis, and decreased disease-free survival and overall survival. Therefore, COX-2 inhibitors such as piroxicam are recommended for IMC to provide pain relief and potentially anti-cancer benefit. The MST reported for IMC patients treated with piroxicam was 185 days in one study.

References

de M Souza CH, Toledo-Piza E, Amorin R *et al.* (2009) Inflammatory mammary carcinoma in 12 dogs: clinical features, cyclooxygenase-2 expression, and response to piroxicam treatment. *Can Vet J* 50:506–510.

Marcanato L, Romanelli G, Stefanello D *et al.* (2009) Prognostic factors for dogs with mammary inflammatory carcinoma: 43 cases (2003–2008). *J Am Vet Med Assoc* 235:967–972.

CASE 48

1 Name the disorder noted on the radiograph (48a) of this 10-year-old Golden Retriever that presented for lameness and swelling of the distal limbs. The extensive periosteal reaction is most consistent with paraneoplastic hypertrophic osteopathy (HO). The palisading periosteal reaction in the absence of bone lysis is the hallmark of HO. The pathology of HO is poorly understood. It may be secondary to vagal nerve stimulation from a primary lesion or from some substance secreted from the primary lesion itself. Ligation of the vagal nerve has resulted in resolution of HO in humans.

2 What is the next diagnostic step for this patient? Thoracic radiographs should be performed. The most common cause of HO is a space-occupying lesion in the lungs. A mass in the lungs leads to a paraneoplastic syndrome causing periosteal new bone proliferation of the distal limbs that ascends over time. Although lung lesions are the most common cause, HO can be associated with intra-abdominal neoplasia (e.g. urinary tract neoplasia: botryoid rhabdomyosarcoma of the bladder). A large intrathoracic mass was found in this patient.

3 How is this disorder treated? Removal of the intrathoracic mass should allow resolution of the HO. Non-steroidal anti-inflammatory drugs may be helpful for the pain and discomfort associated with HO. The author has noted clinical improvement with piroxicam. Although anecdotal in dogs, bisphosphonate therapy has been described in humans for the treatment of hypertrophic osteopathy.

References

Jayaker BA, Abelson AG, Yao Q (2011) Treatment of hypertrophic osteoarthropathy with zoledronic acid: case report and review of the literature. *Semin Arthritis Rheum* **41**: 291–296.

Withers SS, Johnson EG, Culp WTN *et al.* (2015) Paraneoplastic hypertrophic osteopathy in 30 dogs. *Vet Comp Oncol* **13**:157–165.

CASE 49

1 What is the most likely diagnosis, based on the physical examination? Based on the erosive nature of the lesion and the abnormal proliferative tissue seen protruding from the rostral portion of the nasal cavity on brief otoscopic examination, squamous cell carcinoma is most likely.

2 What diagnostic tests should be performed? A deep wedge biopsy of the abnormal tissue should be performed. In this case, the diagnosis was confirmed as SCC. Although this cancer has a low rate of metastasis, thoracic radiographs should be obtained as part of the MDB.

3 What therapeutic options should be considered? Nasal planum resection ("nosectomy") offers the best chance of a cure for earlier, localized lesions (**49b**, intraoperative picture of nosectomy). Nasal planum SCC can fall into one of two main categories: superficial minimally invasive and deeply infiltrative. More advanced,

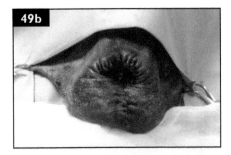

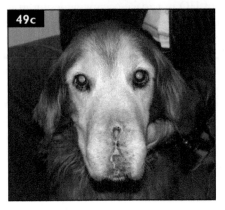

infiltrative lesions may be difficult to cure surgically. CT or MRI can help with surgical planning on more infiltrative lesions. Postsurgical radiation therapy would be advised if clean margins are not attainable. If adequate clean margins can be obtained, the rate of recurrence would be considered low. Pet owners adequately prepared for the cosmetic changes of this type of surgery through postoperative photographs are usually satisfied with the outcome. While cosmetics are altered, functional changes are uncommon. SCC of the nasal planum in dogs can be locally invasive and stubborn. Other therapies described, such as cryosurgery, lasers, photodynamic therapy, intralesional carboplatin therapy, and RT as a single modality, offer poor local control rates in dogs. Delayed node metastasis (>1 year after successful nasal planum resection with clean margins) has been reported and treated successfully with node removal.

Figure **49c** shows the postoperative appearance of a patient that had undergone nasal planum resection for a very large, invasive SCC.

References
Gallegos J, Schmiedt CW, McAnulty JF (2007) Cosmetic rostral nasal reconstruction after nasal planum and premaxilla resection: technique and results in two dogs. *Vet Surg* **36**:669–674.
Withrow SJ (2013) Tumors of the respiratory system. In: Withrow SJ, Vail DM, Page RL, editors, *Small Animal Clinical Oncology*, 5th edition. St. Louis, Elsevier Saunders, pp. 432–435.

CASE 50

1 What are the primary differential diagnoses for this mass? Approximately one-third of splenic masses are benign (hematoma, extramedullary hematopoiesis, abscess), approximately two-thirds are malignant. Of the malignant tumors, approximately two-thirds are hemangiosarcoma and the remainder are other cancers, including members of the soft tissue sarcoma group (fibrosarcoma, myxosarcoma, malignant histiocytosis, etc.).

2 What further diagnostic tests should be performed prior to surgical removal of the mass? Thoracic radiographs to rule out metastasis, CBC, and chemistry panel would be advised in addition to the abdominal radiographs and ultrasound already performed.

Approximately 75% of patients with hemangiosarcoma are in DIC (most subclinical), therefore the presurgical blood work should also include a coagulation panel. Because of the heart murmur heard and the concern for hemangiosarcoma, an echocardiogram would also be advised for this patient to rule out atrial masses.

3 What prognosis can be given to this pet's owner prior to surgery? Without the histopathology results, it is difficult to give a prognosis. In the event of a hematoma or a low-grade malignancy, splenectomy could be curative. With the diagnosis of hemangiosarcoma, a median survival time of 2 months can be expected with no further therapy. Postoperative chemotherapy (doxorubicin +/– cyclophosphamide [Cytoxan] or metronomic chemotherapy) extends median survival expectations to 8–10 months. The metastatic potential for other types of sarcoma tends to increase with tumor grade. This patient's tumor was confirmed to be an intermediate-grade fibrosarcoma. Given the high mitotic index (MI) noted on histopathology, postoperative chemotherapy was advised. Survival times of patients with non-lymphomatous, non-angiomatous sarcomas of the spleen have been shown to be closely linked to the tumor's MI. Patients with tumors with an MI of <9 have MSTs of approximately 7–8 months, whereas those with MIs of >9 have 1–2-month MSTs.

References

Hammer AS, Cuoto CG, Swardson C et al. (1991) Hemostatic abnormalities in dogs with hemangiosarcoma. *J Vet Intern Med* **5**:11–14.

Lana S, U'Ren L, Plaza S et al. (2007) Continuous low-dose oral chemotherapy for adjuvant therapy of splenic hemangiosarcoma in dogs. *J Vet Intern Med* **21**:764–769.

Ogilvie GK, Powers BE, Mallinckrodt CH et al. (1996) Surgery and doxorubicin in dogs with hemangiosarcoma. *J Vet Intern Med* **10**:379–384.

Spangler WL, Culbertson MR, Kass PH (1994) Primary mesenchymal (nonangiomatous/nonlymphomatous) neoplasms occurring in the canine spleen: anatomic classification, immunohistochemistry, and mitotic activity correlated with patient survival. *Vet Pathol* **31**:37–47.

CASE 51

1 Is this patient a good candidate for radiation therapy? The mass appears to be involving the entire circumference of the hock and tibia. When tumors involve the entire circumference of the limb, RT cannot be used because there is no normal skin to "spare" from the treatment field. Treating the entire circumference of the limb would result in possible death of vessels and lymphatics to the distal limb. A portion of the limb needs to be pulled out of the radiation field for this purpose.

2 What further staging tests are indicated? Although the metastatic potential for HPC is low, the tumor has been growing for close to 2 years. Thoracic radiographs and abdominal ultrasound are advised to rule out potential spread.

3 What treatment is most appropriate for this patient? If all tests are negative, amputation would provide the best chance for long-term control and potentially cure for this patient.

Answers

CASE 52

1 Describe the radiographic and cytologic findings and give the diagnosis. The lateral radiograph of the thorax shows a large soft tissue cranial thoracic mass causing dorsal elevation of the trachea. The cranial aspect of the heart shadow is obliterated by the mass. The cytology reveals large lymphocytes, with the majority of the lymphocytes at least 2–3 times larger than the size of the red blood cells. Lymphocytes contain prominent, multiple nucleoli of varying shapes and sizes. There is scant basophilic cytoplasm. The diagnosis is lymphoma.

2 What staging tests and further diagnostic tests should be considered? A feline MDB including retroviral testing should be performed. In addition to the MDB, an abdominal ultrasound for staging and immunocytochemistry for confirmation and typing of the lymphoma is recommended.

3 Is this disease unusual for this age and breed of cat? What is the likely result of retroviral testing in this patient? Younger (median of 3 years of age) Siamese and Oriental breed cats are over-represented with mediastinal lymphoma. Males also appear to be over-represented. Prior to the common practice of vaccinating against FeLV, mediastinal lymphoma was most often seen in young FeLV-positive cats. Now, the majority of cats presenting with mediastinal lymphoma are FeLV negative.

4 What treatment is recommended and what are the survival expectations? Chemotherapy is the treatment of choice. Responses are often rapid. In severely compromised patients, radiation therapy can also be used for a rapid induction of remission. The radiograph shown (**52c**) was taken 48 hours after starting chemotherapy (vincristine). The best prognostic indicator for cats with mediastinal lymphoma is the

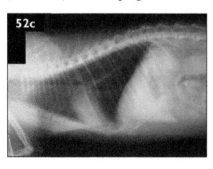

ability to achieve a complete remission. Cats achieving CR survived longer (median of 980 days vs. 42 days for cats only achieving PR). Age, breed, sex, presence of other sites, retroviral status, and pretreatment with steroids did not affect the response to treatment. In addition, there was no statistical difference in survival times based on the chemotherapy protocol chosen (CHOP, University of Winsconsin, etc.).

References

Fabrizio F, Calam AE, Dobson JM *et al.* (2014) Feline mediastinal lymphoma: a retrospective study of signalment, retroviral status, response to chemotherapy and prognostic indicators. *J Feline Med Surg* **16**:637–644.

Guzera M, Cian F, Leo C *et al.* (2014) The use of flow cytometry for immunophenotyping lymphoproliferative disorders in cats: a retrospective study of 19 cases. *Vet Comp Oncol* doi:10.1111/vco.12098.

Louwerens M, London CA, Pedersen NC *et al.* (2005) Feline lymphoma in the post-feline leukemia virus era. *J Vet Intern Med* **19**:329–335.

CASE 53

1 Based on the clinical appearance, what is the most likely diagnosis? The appearance is highly suggestive of a dermal melanoma/melanocytoma; however, basal cell carcinoma (BCC) can also be pigmented.

2 An excisional biopsy was performed, which confirmed a dermal melanoma. What features of the histopathology report are necessary to determine further treatment and outcome for this patient? It is important to know whether the melanoma is considered benign or malignant, whether the margins are free of tumor, and to evaluate the mitotic index. In this case, the patient's biopsy revealed a benign dermal melanoma with no mitotic figures seen. The margins were free of tumor. Close monitoring for recurrence was recommended; however, it is likely that the patient was cured. Mitotic index ≥3 per 10 hpf is associated with a more guarded prognosis. Less than 10% of more benign appearing dermal melanomas ever metastasize, but recurrence is common if complete margins are not achieved. One report suggested that histologic type (benign vs. malignant) does not provide prognostic information, so caution is advised when managing feline patients with dermal melanomas.

References

Luna LD, Higginbotham ML, Henry CJ (2000) Feline non-ocular melanoma: a retrospective study of 23 cases (1991–1999). *J Feline Med Surg* 2(4):173–181.

Smedley RC, Spangler WL, Esplin DG *et al.* (2011) Prognostic markers for canine melanocytic neoplasms: a comparative review of the literature and goals for future investigation. *Vet Pathol* 48(1):54–72.

CASE 54

1 Describe the tumor tissue and likely diagnosis. This is a large, well-circumscribed, cystic mass. The appearance is suggestive of a benign cystadenoma.

2 Approximately what percentage of hepatobiliary tumors in cats are benign? Bile duct adenomas (biliary cystadenomas) are the most common benign liver tumors in cats and represent approximately 50% of hepatobiliary tumors.

3 What further treatment beyond surgery is recommended? Surgical excision is the treatment of choice and can be curative, with no further therapy indicated postoperatively. These tumors are often well circumscribed, as shown here; they are usually cystic, usually only cause clinical signs when they become large, and do not metastasize. In patients with multiple or inoperable cystadenomas, quality of life can be negatively impacted as they grow. In patients that are experiencing pain or compromise of liver function due to pressure exerted by the masses, ultrasound-guided aspiration and drainage of the larger cysts can provide relief.

References

Adler R, Wilson DW (1995) Biliary cystadenoma of cats. *Vet Pathol* 32:415–418.

Lawrence HJ, Hollis N, Harvey HJ (1994) Nonlymphomatous hepatobiliary masses in cats: 41 cases (1972–1991). *Vet Surg* 23:365–368.

CASE 55

1 Describe the abnormalities on this ultrasound image. The prostate is enlarged with areas of calcification. The urethra is widened and there is suspicious tissue infiltrating into the neck of the bladder.

2 Why is prostatic neoplasia the primary differential? This patient was castrated at a young age. How does this affect your diagnostic considerations? The fact that this patient was castrated at a young age decreases the likelihood of benign prostatic disease such as hypertrophy or infection. Prostatic enlargement with secondary calcification is more likely to be a result of neoplasia.

3 How should the diagnosis be confirmed? Castration does not prevent the development of prostatic cancer in dogs. Earlier studies showed that castration did not have a sparing effect on the risk of the development of prostatic carcinoma in dogs. Subsequently, it was shown in epidemiologic studies that castration actually increases the risk of cancer development. Neutered males have a significantly increased risk for bladder TCC, prostate TCC, prostatic adenocarcinoma, and prostatic carcinoma.

References

Nyland TG, Wallack ST, Wisner ER (2000) Needle-tract implantation following us-guided fine-needle aspiration biopsy of transitional cell carcinoma of the bladder, urethra, and prostate. *Vet Radiol Ultrasound* **43**(1):50–53.

Obradovich JE, Walshaw R, Goullaud E (1987) The influence of castration on the development of prostate carcinoma in the dog: 43 cases (1978–1985). *J Vet Intern Med* **1**:183–187.

Teske E, Naan ED, Kijk EM *et al.* (2002) Canine prostate carcinoma: epidemiological evidence of an increased risk in castrated dogs. *Mol Cell Endocrinol* **197**:251–255.

CASE 56

1 Describe the cytology. There are clusters of cohesive epithelial cells with minimal anisocytosis, although cellular borders are poorly defined. The nuclei appear fairly uniform. There are minimal criteria for malignancy observed. Despite the relatively benign appearance of the cytology, the probability that this tumor is benign is fairly low. For this reason, histopathology is necessary to make a definitive diagnosis.

2 What are the primary diagnostic considerations? Primary rule outs for an anal gland mass are anal sac gland adenocarcinoma (ASGAC) and anal gland infection. However, based on the finding of an atypical epithelial cell population on aspiration, an anal gland tumor is more likely.

3 What specific abnormality on a serum chemistry panel has prognostic significance? An elevated calcium level is commonly associated with AGSAC, with 25–50% of patients presenting with hypercalcemia. The finding of hypercalcemia has been associated with a more guarded prognosis; however, this has been an inconsistent finding. Therefore, the presence of hypercalcemia should not discourage treatment.

4 In addition to the MDB, what further testing should be done to make a definitive diagnosis and stage this patient? An abdominal ultrasound should be performed, paying careful attention to the sublumbar lymph nodes. These nodes are frequently enlarged, even when primary tumors are very small. An incisional or tru-cut biopsy (needle core biopsy) of the anal gland mass can give a definitive diagnosis. In patients with smaller tumors that have no evidence of lymphadenopathy, an excisional biopsy (removal of the abnormal anal gland) may be diagnostic and therapeutic.

References
Bennett PF, DeNicola DB, Bonney P *et al.* (2002) Canine anal sac adenocarcinomas: clinical presentation and response to therapy. *J Vet Intern Med* **16**:100–104.

Gauthier M, Barber LG, Burgess KE (2009) Identifying and treating anal sac adenocarcinoma in dogs. *Vet Med* **104**:74–81.

Potanas CP, Padgett S, Gamblin RM (2015) Surgical excision of anal sac apocrine gland adenocarcinomas with and without adjunctive chemotherapy in dogs: 42 cases (2005–2011). *J Am Vet Med Assoc* **246**:877–884.

Williams LE, Gliatto JM, Dodge RK *et al.* (2003) Carcinoma of the apocrine glands of the anal sac in dogs: 113 cases (1985–1995). *J Am Vet Med Assoc* **223**(6):825–831.

CASE 57

1 What instructions should be provided for owners regarding handling of these medications? Owners should be provided with latex chemotherapy gloves to handle and administer the oral chemotherapy. Gloves should be disposed of in a plastic chemotherapy bag and brought back to the hospital for appropriate disposal. Local authorities need to be consulted regarding appropriate disposal. Powder-free latex gloves approved for chemotherapy (**57b**, red arrow) should be sent home with the owner to handle any chemotherapy to be dispensed at home. A chemotherapy transport bag (**57c**) should also be provided. Any used latex gloves, pill bottles, etc. should be placed in the bag and returned to the clinic for proper disposal.

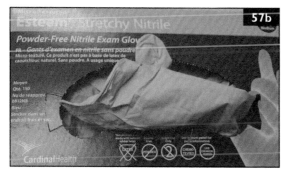

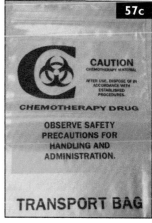

2 Is it safe to cut/split tablets? NO. Splitting of chemotherapy tablets of all types is discouraged. Cytotoxic drug particles have been found up to 12 inches away from where a pill was split or crushed. Given the small dosages used, especially for smaller pets, compounding into the appropriate sizes may be necessary.

Reference
Gustafson DL, Page RL (2013) Cancer chemotherapy. In: Withrow SJ, Vail DM, Page RL, editors, *Small Animal Clinical Oncology*, 5th edition. St. Louis, Elsevier Saunders, pp. 157–179.

CASE 58

1 In considering cancer as an underlying cause for this patient's hypercalcemia, what must a physical examination include? The tumors most likely to be associated with paraneoplastic hypercalcemia include anal sac gland adenocarcinoma, lymphoma, multiple myeloma, and mammary gland tumors, although other malignancies can potentially cause hypercalcemia. Careful evaluation for lymphadenopathy and mammary masses, and a digital rectal examination should be performed.

2 A 1.0 cm mass is detected on digital rectal examination that appears to be within the right anal gland. Cytology from a fine needle aspirate is suggestive of anal sac gland adenocarcinoma (ASGAC). What is the suspected cause of the hypercalcemia? Paraneoplastic hypercalcemia is most commonly associated with the tumor's release of a parathyroid hormone-related peptide (PTHrP) by the tumor cells that mimics parathyroid hormone, causing excessive release of calcium from the bone when the body does not require the additional calcium. Not all cases of paraneoplastic hypercalcemia are caused by PTHrP. Inflammatory cytokines such as interleukin-1 beta, tumor necrosis factor alpha, and transforming growth factor beta may stimulate osteoclast bone resorption alone or in conjunction with PTHrP. Hypercalcemia is reported to occur in 25–50% of patients with ASGAC at diagnosis.

3 How should this patient be managed? Hypercalcemia of this degree is considered a medical emergency. An ionized calcium will provide a more accurate determination of calcium levels and should be used to monitor response to therapy. Thoracic radiographs and an abdominal ultrasound should be performed to complete staging. Saline diuresis should be instituted and tumor removal performed as soon as the patient is considered medically stable. If the calcium does not decrease substantially with saline diuresis and the patient is not yet medically stable enough for surgery, the addition of prednisone, furosemide, and, in extreme cases, bisphosphonate therapy may be necessary.

4 Despite the small size of the primary mass, an ultrasound examination (58) revealed significantly enlarged sublumbar lymph nodes (4.48 × 5.54 cm). How does this affect the treatment approach and the prognosis? A CT scan may aid in determining whether the lymph nodes are operable. If amenable to surgical resection, removal of the primary mass and sublumbar nodes is recommended. However, based on the regional metastasis and hypercalcemia, this patient's prognosis is guarded. Chemotherapy is advised postoperatively. Radiation therapy is considered in the event that clean surgical margins are not achieved. In patients with ASGAC, multi-modality therapy appears superior to surgery, chemotherapy, or RT alone. Responses have been reported to carboplatin, cis-platin, actinomycin-D, mitoxantrone, and melphalan chemotherapy and tyrosine kinase inhibitors (TKIs, e.g. toceranib). The combination of surgery (including lymph node removal), RT, and chemotherapy has been associated with prolonged survival times (MST ranging from 17 to 31 months). In one case series, toceranib was given to patients that had failed other forms of therapy. The median duration of partial response was 22 weeks, and a median duration of treatment of 25 weeks was reported, indicating its efficacy in this disease.

5 What factors are considered negative prognostic indicators? The following factors have been associated with a more guarded prognosis:

- Size of tumor: significant survival advantage noted for smaller tumors (stage 1, primary tumor <2.5 cm diameter, no metastasis) associated with MST of 1,205 days in one study.
- Lymph node metastasis: removal of lymph nodes is associated with significant improvement in survival times. The size of the lymph nodes was prognostic in one study: <4.5 cm, MST of 492 days vs. >4.5 cm, MST 335 days.
- Distant metastasis beyond regional nodes (MST approximately 70 days).
- Not performing surgery.
- Single modality therapy.
- Hypercalcemia: some studies suggest a poorer survival time with hypercalcemia while others do not.

References
Bergman PH (2013) Paraneoplastic syndromes. In: Withrow SJ, Vail DM, Page RL, editors, *Small Animal Clinical Oncology*, 5th edition. St. Louis, Elsevier Saunders, pp. 83–97.
London C, Mathie T, Stingle N *et al.* (2012) Preliminary evidence for biologic activity of toceranib phosphate (Palladia®) in solid tumors. *Vet Comp Oncol* 10(3):194–205.
Polton GA, Brearley MJ (2007) Clinical stage, therapy, and prognosis in canine anal sac gland carcinoma. *J Vet Intern Med* 21:274–280.
Turek MM, Forrest LJ, Adams WM *et al.* (2003) Postoperative radiotherapy and mitoxantrone for anal sac adenocarcinoma in the dog: 15 cases (1991–2001). *Vet Comp Oncol* 1:94–104.
Williams LE, Gliatto JM, Dodge RK *et al.* (2003) Carcinoma of the apocrine glands of the anal sac in dogs: 113 cases (1985–1995) *J Am Vet Med Assoc* 223(6):825–831.

CASE 59

1 What is the biologic behavior of this tumor in dogs? Solitary plasma cell tumors are most typically seen in older dogs (average 9–10 years) and are most common in larger-breed dogs. Solitary plasma tumors are usually described as extramedullary plasmacytomas (EMP) or solitary osseous plasmacytomas (SOP). These tumors can occur on the trunk, head, or limbs, and in the oral cavity, including the gingiva and tongue. In the case of SOP, underlying bone involvement is seen. They are usually benign tumors which carry an excellent prognosis with complete surgical excision. In one large series of over 300 cases reported, only 1% were accompanied by systemic multiple myeloma. Less than 4% recurred after surgery, most commonly when margins were incomplete, and less than 2% developed distant disease at other sites. Solitary EMPs do not arise from bone. They are locally aggressive but rarely metastasize. Surgical excision is usually curative.

2 What further diagnostic tests should be performed? Despite the low reported incidence of systemic disease being associated with EMP or SOP, an MDB is advised. Radiographs of the jaw are also advised to rule out underlying bone involvement.

3 Is any further treatment necessary? In order to achieve a cure, more aggressive surgery or RT can be considered. However, based on the low incidence of recurrence even after conservative surgery, close monitoring of the local site is also an option for this patient. If recurrence is noted, more aggressive surgery to include underlying bone may be required.

References

Smithson CW, Smith MM, Tappe J *et al.* (2012) Multicentric oral plasmacytomas in 3 dogs. *J Vet Dent* **29**:96–110.

Wright ZM, Rogers KS, Marshall JH (2008) Survival data for canine extramedullary plasmacytomas: a retrospective analysis (1996–2006). *J Am Anim Hosp Assoc* **44**: 75–81.

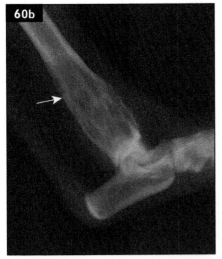

60b

CASE 60

1 Describe the radiographic lesion. There is a lytic lesion of the distal tibia (metaphyseal region). The lesion is multilocular, sharply defined, and primarily lytic. The cortical bone is thin owing to the expansile nature of the lesion and there appears to be a possible pathologic fracture on the caudal aspect of the lesion (**60b,** arrow).

2 What in this dog's signalment and the radiographic appearance of this lesion would indicate that the lesion is less likely to be osteosarcoma? Although osteosarcoma can occur in smaller dogs, the majority of dogs with OSA are of

larger breeds. The multilocular appearance of this lesion is most consistent with a benign bone cyst. However, this diagnosis cannot be made based on radiographs alone.
3 List the differential diagnoses for this patient and diagnostic recommendations. Other considerations include a primary bone tumor: a very lytic osteosarcoma, hemangiosarcoma, myeloma, or other sarcoma is possible. A bone biopsy is required to make a definitive diagnosis. Given the possibility of a primary bone tumor, an MDB to include thoracic radiographs is advised before a bone biopsy is performed. Because the lesion is extremely lytic, hemangiosarcoma is high on the differential list among the primary bone tumors mentioned. For this reason, abdominal ultrasound and echocardiography can be considered prior to biopsy. The histologic diagnosis in this patient was a simple bone cyst. There are two types of bone cyst recognized: a simple bone cyst (SBC), which is a true cyst of primary intraosseous origin, and an aneurysmal bone cyst (ABC), which is a spongy, multiloculated mass filled with free-flowing blood. The SBC is characterized histologically by thin fibrous walls lined by mesothelial or endothelial cells, whereas ABCs are rarely lined by epithelium and most likely represent an arteriovenous malformation. Often, curettage and packing the space with autogenous bone graft can be used for treatment. However, given the early pathologic fracture and extremely thin cortical bone in this case, the owner elected amputation.

Reference
Stickle R, Flo G, Render J (1999) Radiographic diagnosis – benign bone cyst. *Vet Radiol Ultrasound* 40(4):365–366.

CASE 61
1 What are the primary differential diagnoses for this mass? Hemangiosarcoma, splenic sarcoma (non-angiomatous, non-lymphomatous), lymphoma, and mast cell tumor are the primary differential diagnoses for malignant tumors. Hematomas, abscesses, regenerative nodules, and extramedullary hematopoiesis are examples of benign splenic masses. Approximately 80% of masses associated with acute non-traumatic hemoabdomen are malignant.
2 What further tests should be performed to complete the preoperative staging? Screening for metastasis is required prior to surgery. HSA has a high metastatic rate. The liver, omentum, mesentery, and lungs are the most common sites of metastasis. Older studies report right atrial involvement in approximately 25% of dogs with HSA, while a more recent study reports a rate of 8.7%. Metastasis can, however, occur in virtually any area of the body. In addition to the MDB with thoracic radiographs, complete staging for suspected HSA should include:
- *Coagulation testing:* ~75% of patients with HSA have coagulopathies at the time of diagnosis, with up to 50% meeting the criteria for DIC.

- *Electrocardiography*: Evidence of changes suggestive of pericardial effusion should be followed by echocardiography.
- *Echocardiography*: This is useful to detect pericardial effusion and a right atrial mass.
- *Abdominal ultrasound*: Careful evaluation of the spleen and liver for evidence of potential metastatic lesions. If lesions are present in the liver that could be representative of regenerative or benign nodules and not cancer, surgery should still be performed but biopsies of any suspicious areas also be performed.

3 **Histopathology revealed hemangiosarcoma (HSA). What treatment should be considered postoperatively and what are the survival expectations?** With splenectomy alone, reported median survival times range from 19 to 86 days, with less than 10% of patients alive at 1 year. Even with the addition of chemotherapy, 1-year survival expectations are <10%, but MSTs improve to 141–179 days. MSTs of 277 days were observed with immunotherapy with L-MTP-PE (liposomal muramyl tripeptide phosphatidylethanolamine) when used in conjunction with surgery and chemotherapy. Metronomic chemotherapy (continuous low-dose oral administration of chemotherapy) has been used postoperatively in patients undergoing splenectomy for HSA. A combination of cyclophosphamide, etoposide, and piroxicam used in this setting yielded an MST of 178 days, which compares with those seen with conventional chemotherapy.

References

Aronsohn MG, Dubiel B, Roberts B *et al.* (2009) Prognosis for acute nontraumatic hemoperitoneum in the dog: a retrospective analysis of 60 cases (2003–2006). *J Am Anim Hosp Assoc* 45(2):72–77.

Boston SE, Higginson G, Monteith G (2011) Concurrent splenic and right atrial mass at presentation in dogs with HSA: a retrospective study. *J Am Anim Hosp Assoc* 47(5): 336–341.

Hammer AS, Couto CG, Swardson C *et al.* (1991) Hemostatic abnormalities in dogs with hemangiosarcoma. *J Vet Intern Med* 5:11–14.

Lana S, U'Ren L, Plaza S *et al.* (2007) Continuous low-dose oral chemotherapy for adjuvant therapy of splenic hemangiosarcoma in dogs. *J Vet Intern Med* 21:764–769.

Ogilvie GK, Powers BE, Mallinckrodt CH *et al.* (1996) Surgery and doxorubicin in dogs with hemangiosarcoma. *J Vet Intern Med* 10:379–384.

Pintar J, Breitschwerdt EB, Hardie EM *et al.* (2003) Acute nontraumatic hemoabdomen in the dog: a retrospective analysis of 39 cases (1987–2001). *J Am Anim Hosp Assoc* 39(6):518–522.

Vail DM, MacEwen EF, Kurzman ID *et al.* (1995) Liposome-encapsulated muramyl tripeptide phosphatidylethanolamine adjuvant immunotherapy for splenic hemangiosarcoma in the dog: a randomized multi-institutional clinical trial. *Clin Cancer Res* 1(10):1165–1170.

CASE 62

1 What is the cytologic diagnosis? This appears to be a round cell tumor with minimal cytoplasmic granules noted. The predominant cells appear to be coalescing, suggestive of an epithelial malignancy; therefore, histopathology is necessary to confirm the diagnosis.

2 A splenectomy was performed. Histopathology confirmed the diagnosis of poorly differentiated mast cell tumor. What further information can be gained from the tissue sample that will help in making treatment recommendations for this patient? Further evaluation of the tissue sample should include the following immunohistochemical stains: AgNOR, Ki67, and cKIT staining. In addition, PCR to determine whether there is a mutation on exon 8 or 11 should be included. This patient's mast cell tumor prognostic panel is shown here:

Microscopic description:
Immunohistochemical labeling for KIT showed perimembrane labeling consistent with a KIT pattern **2**. Labeling for Ki67 showed strong nuclear labeling in an average of **24** cells per grid. Labeling for AgNOR showed an average of **4** positive AgNORs per nucleus in neoplastic cells.

Diagnosis(es):
KIT pattern: 2; Ki67: 24; AgNORs/cell: 3; AgNOR × Ki67: 72
PCRs for mutations in exons 8 and 11 of the *c-KIT* gene were negative

Comments:
Correlation between expression of the KIT receptor and the histologic grade of canine mast cell tumors has been made based on the expression pattern of the KIT protein. The expression pattern of the neoplastic cells in this tumor was consistent with a KIT pattern 2. Dogs with KIT patterns 2 and 3 may have a lower disease-free survival and overall survival time compared with those with expression 1. In one study 30% of dogs with KIT pattern 3 were dead within 6 months and 20% of dogs with pattern 2 were dead within 10 months. Mast cell tumors that have a high proliferation activity, characterized by large numbers of neoplastic cells being positive for Ki67 (>23/grid) and that have a high AgNOR count (AgNOR × Ki67 >54) have been associated with a significantly worse prognosis and decreased survival times.

3 What is the prognosis for this patient? Visceral mast cell tumors in dogs are rare and carry a very poor prognosis. It would seem unlikely that the disease in the spleen represents metastasis from a primary low-grade mast cell tumor removed 3 years prior. Based on the aggressive nature of this cancer, systemic therapy is advised. Patients that are positive for mutations of the *c-KIT* gene could be candidates for tyrosine kinase inhibitor therapy (e.g. toceranib, masitinib). Therapeutic outcome for either chemotherapy or TKI therapy has not been fully evaluated in canine visceral mast cell tumors.

References
O'Keefe DA, Couto CG, Burke-Schwartz C *et al.* (1987) Systemic mastocytosis in 16 dogs. *J Vet Intern Med* **1**:75–80.
Takahashi T, Kadosawa T, Negase M *et al.* (2000) Visceral mast cell tumors in dogs: 10 cases (1982–1997). *J Am Vet Med* Assoc **216**(2):222–226.

CASE 63

1 Describe the photograph. There are multiple coalescing nodules throughout the abdomen affecting the peritoneal serosal surfaces.

2 What is the probable diagnosis? This probably represents carcinomatosis, a condition in which multiple carcinomas develop simultaneously after dissemination of cancer from a primary source. A biopsy confirmed carcinomatosis. Dissemination occurs with the direct seeding of tumor cells on serosal membranes. Peritoneal, pleural, and leptomeningial carcinomatosis can occur. In addition to carcinomas, similar spreading patterns may be seen with sarcomas (sarcomatosis) and mesothelioma.

3 What treatments can be considered and what is the prognosis for this patient with or without treatment? The most successful treatment outcomes reported have been with the use of intracavitary (IC) chemotherapy. The direct delivery of chemotherapy into a body cavity is usually safe and can be effective. Mitoxantrone, carboplatin, and cis-platin are the chemotherapeutic agents that have been evaluated in veterinary medicine. The procedure is performed following thoracocentesis or abdominocentesis. The chemotherapy agents are diluted in saline and then injected through an administration set into the peritoneal or pleural cavity as a slow IV bolus. The MST for dogs not receiving any treatment is generally <30 days. With IC chemotherapy, MSTs are closer to 1 year, with some dogs experiencing prolonged survival times of close to 3 years. However, patients that have extensive advanced metastasis throughout abdominal organs as well as the peritoneal surfaces generally have a very poor prognosis.

References
Charney SC, Bergman PJ, McKnight JA *et al.* (2005) Evaluation of intracavitary mitoxantrone and carboplatin for treatment of carcinomatosis, sarcomatosis and mesothelioma, with or without malignant effusions: a retrospective analysis of 12 cases (1997–2002). *Vet Comp Oncol* **3**(4):171–181.
Moore AS, Kirk C, Cardona A (1991) Intracavitary cisplatin chemotherapy experience with six dogs. *J Vet Intern Med* **5**:227–231.

CASE 64

1 What further tests would help in determining a treatment plan? The mass appears minimally pigmented, but a biopsy should be performed to determine tumor type. Although this patient had a history of OMM, tonsillar spread is not common so other types of neoplasia such as SCC should be ruled out. A CT scan would help in determining extent of disease for surgical planning. If this is not available, an excisional biopsy should be performed if possible.

2 An excisional biopsy revealed an undifferentiated round cell tumor with cells seen at the margins of the surgical sample. What further information from the biopsy can help in determining a more definitive diagnosis and the biologic behavior of this tumor? Immunohistochemistry (Melan-A, PNL-2, TRP-1, TRP-2 – Diagnostic melanoma panel*) can be useful in determining whether this is a melanoma. In this case, IHC confirmed malignant melanoma. Although all oral malignant melanomas are considered aggressive, the mitotic index and Ki67 levels can provide information regarding the biologic behavior of the patient's tumor. Therefore, a melanoma prognostic panel* was also performed in this case, revealing a high Ki67 level (28) and mitotic index of 10 per hpf, indicating a poor prognosis. Ki67 (MIB-1) is expressed in all proliferating cells, but increased expression is associated with a poorer prognosis for many tumor types, including canine oral melanoma. Ki67 levels >19.5 are associated with a very poor prognosis.

3 What treatment options can be considered? Treatment options include surgical removal of the tonsil followed by radiation therapy, or RT alone if the tumor is determined to be too invasive on the basis of CT scanning. It is not clear whether the melanoma vaccine provided any additional benefit over surgery alone in this patient. Tumors with a mitotic index of <4/10 hpf have >80% 3-year survival rates and the MST for patients with stage II oral melanoma was reported to be 818 days.

WHO Staging Scheme for Dogs With Oral Melanoma

T: Primary tumor
T_1: Tumor ≤2 cm in diameter
T_2: Tumor 2–4 cm in diameter
T_3: Tumor >4 cm in diameter

N: Regional lymph nodes
N_0: No evidence of regional lymph node involvement
N_1: Histologic/cytologic evidence of lymph node involvement
N_2: Fixed nodes

M: Distant metastasis
M_0: No evidence of distant metastasis
M_1: Evidence of distant metastasis

Stage grouping			
Stage I	T_1	N_0	M_0
Stage II	T_2	N_0	M_0
Stage III	T_2	N_1	M_0 or T_3 N_0 M_0
Stage IV	Any T, any N, and M_1		

TNM = tumor, nodes, metastasis.

---

* Melanoma diagnostic panel and prognostic panel were developed and performed at Michigan State University, Diagnostic Center for Population and Animal Health.

Answers

References

Bergin IL, Smedley RC, Esplin DG et al. (2011) Prognostic evaluation of Ki67 threshold value I canine oral melanoma. *Vet Pathol* **48**(1):41–53.

Hoinghaus R, Mischke R, Hewicker-Trautwein M (2002) Use of immunocytochemical techniques in canine melanoma. *J Vet Med A Physiol Pathol Clin Med* **48**(4):198–202.

Ramos-Vara JA, Miller MA (2011) Immunohistochemical identification of canine melanocytic neoplasms with antibodies to melanocytic antigen PNL2 and tyrosinase: comparison with Melan A. *Vet Pathol* **48**(2):443–450.

Ramos-Vara JA, Beissenherz ME, Miller MA et al. (2000) Retrospective study of 338 canine oral melanomas with clinical, histologic and immunohistochemical review of 129 cases. *Vet Pathol* **37**(6):597–608.

Tuohy JL, Selmic LE, Worley DR et al. (2014) Outcome following curative-intent surgery for oral melanoma in dogs: 70 cases (1998–2011). *J Am Vet Med Assoc* **245**:1266–1273.

CASE 65

1 Describe the cells seen on cytology. There is a mixed population of epithelial cells exhibiting anisocytosis, anisokaryosis, and anisonucleoleosis. However, owing to the possibility of dysplastic epithelial cells, a biopsy is needed to confirm the diagnosis.

2 What are the differential diagnoses for this patient? Transitional cell carcinoma (TCC) is the most common urethral cancer. Other urethral tumors reported in the dog include squamous cell carcinoma, leiomyoma, leiomyosarcoma, plasma cell tumor, lymphoma, and chondrosarcoma. Non-neoplastic causes of a thickened urethra include proliferative urethritis (also referred to as lymphoplasmacytic urethritis or granulomatous urethritis), inflammation secondary to urethral calculi, and chronic infection.

3 What further diagnostic tests should be performed on this patient? An MDB and full abdominal ultrasound are indicated; however, cystocentesis is not advised to obtain a sample for UA – a free-catch or catheterized urine sample is advised instead. Although not visible on ultrasound, infiltrative disease along the bladder wall cannot be ruled out, so the risk of peritoneal seeding of tumor cells still exists. In addition, there is clinical evidence that the patient has at the very least a partial urethral obstruction, and therefore a cystocentesis would be contraindicated. With ultrasound, it is difficult to see more than the proximal portion of the urethra. Contrast urethrography or transrectal ultrasound will provide better images. Cystoscopy or surgery is usually required to obtain a tissue biopsy. In some cases, catheterization can result in obtaining pieces of tissue. In this case, tumor tissue was visualized at the urethral opening, making a biopsy easier to obtain. Histopathology confirmed transitional cell carcinoma.

4 What treatment should be offered? Based on the degree of disease present in the urethra and the partial obstruction likely present, a urinary catheter needs to be placed. Unfortunately, maintaining a urinary catheter can be difficult and, if available, a urethral stent or tube cystostomy should be considered. Piroxicam alone or in combination with chemotherapy has been shown to increase median survival times in patients with TCC. Chemotherapeutic agents with activity against TCC include mitoxantrone, vinblastine, carboplatin, and metronomic chlorambucil. The addition of weekly coarse fraction radiation therapy with mitoxantrone and piroxicam did not offer a survival advantage over chemotherapy alone. RT as part of multi-modality therapy for bladder and/or urethral TCC has been described. Photodynamic therapy has been sporadically described with some significant prolongation of survival times noted in urethral TCC.

References
Allstadt SD, Rodriguez Jr. CO, Boostrom B *et al.* (2015) Randomized phase III trial of piroxicam in combination with mitoxantrone or carboplatin for first-line treatment of urogenital tract transitional cell carcinoma in dogs. *J Vet Intern Med* 29:261–267.
Arnold EJ, Childress MO, Fourez LM *et al.* (2011) Clinical trial of vinblastine in dogs with transitional cell carcinoma of the urinary bladder. *J Vet Intern Med* 25:1385–1390.
Fulkerson CM, Knapp DW (2015) Management of transitional cell carcinoma of the urinary bladder in dogs: a review. *Vet J* 205:217–225
Knapp DW, Richardson RCX, Chan TCK *et al.* (1994) Piroxicam therapy in 34 dogs with transitional cell carcinoma of the urinary bladder. *J Vet Intern Med* 8:273–278.
McMillan SK, Knapp DW, Ramos-Vara JA *et al.* (2012) Outcome of urethral stent placement for management of urethral obstruction secondary to transitional cell carcinoma in dogs: 19 cases (2007–2010). *J Am Vet Med Assoc* 241:1627–1632.
Nolan MW, Kogan L, Griffin LR *et al.* (2012) Intensity-modulated and image-guided radiation therapy for treatment of genitourinary carcinomas in dogs. *J Vet Intern Med* 26:987–995.

CASE 66

1 Should this recurrent mass be biopsied? A new biopsy is indicated to be certain that the cancer has not changed in its biologic behavior (grade and aggressiveness). A needle core biopsy was performed. The mass remained a grade II soft tissue sarcoma believed to be of peripheral nerve sheath origin.

2 What treatment recommendations can be made for this patient? Based on the close association of the tumor with the sacrum, it would be difficult to obtain clean surgical margins even with hemipelvectomy. Therefore, this patient was treated with radiation therapy in order to reduce the size of the tumor and sterilize the peripheral margins. Following RT, a hemipelvectomy was performed. Clean margins were obtained and the patient lived 18 months before several metastatic lesions were noted on thoracic radiographs. Based on previous reports of metronomic chemotherapy delaying the recurrence of incompletely excised soft tissue sarcomas, cyclophosphamide and piroxicam were instituted to delay progression of the metastatic disease. The patient lived an additional 8 months following detection of lung metastasis, for an overall survival time of 26 months.

Answers

References

Bray JP (2014) Hemipelvectomy: modified surgical technique and clinical experiences from a retrospective study. *Vet Surg* 43(1):19–26.

Bray JP, Worley DR, Henderson RA *et al.* (2014) Hemipelvectomy: outcome in 84 dogs and 16 cats. A Veterinary Society of Surgical Oncology retrospective study. *Vet Surg* 43(1):27–37.

Elmslie RE, Glawe P, Dow SW (2008) Metronomic therapy with cyclophosphamide and piroxicam effectively delays tumor recurrence in dogs with incompletely resected soft tissue sarcomas. *J Vet Intern Med* 22(6):1373–1379.

Case 67

1 What are the differential diagnoses for this lesion? Differentials for this lesion can include melanoma (amelanotic, based on appearance), squamous cell carcinoma, epitheliotropic lymphoma, fibrosarcoma (although typically FSA has intact epithelium covering the mass), plasma cell tumor, and mast cell tumor. Granuloma or infection secondary to a foreign body is possible, but less likely. Considerations for the lymph node enlargement include regional neoplastic metastasis or a reactive lymph node due to obvious secondary infection within the mass.

2 What is the diagnostic approach to this lesion? Fine needle aspirates of the primary oral lesion and the prominent lymph node can give a presumptive diagnosis. In this case, a malignant round cell tumor was seen cytologically. The lymph node showed no obvious malignant cells and appeared reactive. Histopathology would be necessary to differentiate further the type of round cell tumor and to assess the lymph node. Following an MDB, surgical excision of the oral lesion and removal of the prominent ipsilateral lymph node for histopathology was advised. A full-thickness lip resection is required to obtain tumor-free margins. Once a histologic diagnosis is confirmed, additional therapy may be required.

Follow-up/discussion

The initial surgical approach is shown (**67b**) and the postoperative appearance of the lip resection (**67c**; the incision from submandibular node removal can also be seen). The diagnosis was amelanotic melanoma and tumor-free margins

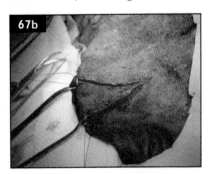

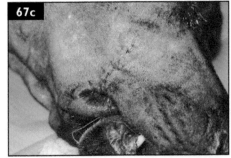

were obtained. The mitotic index was 15 per 10 hpf. The lymph node showed no evidence of metastatic neoplasia. The Oncept® canine melanoma vaccine was used postoperatively.

References
Grosenbaugh DA, Leard AT, Bergman PJ *et al.* (2011) Safety and efficacy of a xenogeneic DNA vaccine encoding for human tyrosinase as adjunctive treatment for oral malignant melanoma in dogs following surgical excision of the primary tumor. *Am J Vet Res* 72:1631–1638.

Smedley RC, Spangler WL, Esplin DG *et al.* (2011) Prognostic markers for canine melanocytic neoplasms: a comparative review of the literature and goals for future investigation. *Vet Pathol* 48:54–72.

CASE 68

1 What is the clinical diagnosis? The cytology supports a soft tissue sarcoma. The prominent regional lymph node suggests possible metastasis or may represent a reactive node.

2 What diagnostic tests are indicated? Thoracic radiographs, a regional radiograph of the affected foot, and fine needle aspirate of the popliteal lymph node are advised. A tissue biopsy is indicated to determine type of sarcoma and grade. Removal of the popliteal lymph node for biopsy is also indicated.

3 What is the expected biologic behavior of this cancer? The biologic behavior depends on the histologic grade. Soft tissue sarcomas tend to be locally invasive with a low metastatic rate. However, with grade III tumors, the metastatic rate approaches 50%.

4 Based on the location and size of this mass, complete surgical excision would only be possible with limb amputation. The owners have declined amputation. Describe a treatment plan that does not include amputation. For grade I or II soft tissue sarcomas, radiation therapy can be considered in an attempt to cytoreduce the tumor and facilitate subsequent limb-preserving excision. If the tumor is a grade III and/or there is metastasis to the regional lymph node, chemotherapy should be considered in addition to RT, although there are no data demonstrating improvements in outcome for patients with high-risk soft tissue sarcomas receiving postoperative chemotherapy. Even with significant reduction in tumor volume, it still may be difficult to obtain clean surgical margins following RT.

References
Kuntz CA, Dernell WS, Powers BE *et al.* (1997) Prognostic factors for surgical treatment of soft-tissue sarcomas in dogs: 75 cases (1986–1996). *J Am Vet Med Assoc* 21:1147–1151.

Selting KA, Powers BA, Thompson LJ *et al.* (2005) Outcome of dogs with high-grade soft tissue sarcomas treated with and without adjuvant doxorubicin chemotherapy: 39 cases (1996–2004). *J Am Vet Med Assoc* 227:1442–1448.

CASE 69

1 List the differential diagnoses for this lesion. The majority of vaginal tumors are of smooth muscle or fibrous tissue origin. In the intact patient, polyps or leiomyoma are most common. Other benign tumors possible are fibroma and fibroleiomyoma. Malignant vaginal tumors are far less common in the intact female. Other less common tumors that can occur in the vaginal area include lipomas, soft tissue sarcomas, myxoma, adenocarcinoma, hemangiosarcoma, transmissible venereal tumor (TVT), osteosarcoma, or carcinomas arising from the bladder or urethra that present with masses near the urethral papilla. Histopathology confirmed leiomyoma in this patient.

2 What additional therapy is recommended? Leiomyomas are usually estrogen responsive tumors and can regress with ovariohysterectomy. While tumors will regress, they often will not regress completely, so surgical removal of the mass is still advised.

References

Saba CF, Lawrence JA (2013) Tumors of the female reproductive system. In: Withrow SJ, Vail DM, Page RL, editors, *Small Animal Clinical Oncology*, 5th edition. St. Louis, Elsevier Saunders, pp. 535–537.
Thacher C, Bradley RL (1983) Vulvar and vaginal tumors in the dog: a retrospective study. *J Am Vet Med Assoc* 183:690–692.

CASE 70

1 Describe the cytology. What is the most common exocrine pancreatic neoplasia in the cat? There is a cluster of epithelial cells exhibiting moderate anisocytosis and anisokaryosis consistent with carcinoma. Pancreatic adenocarcinoma is the most common cancer diagnosed. Neoplastic disorders of the pancreas may be primary (adenoma, adenocarcinoma) or secondary (metastasis from another primary tumor) and either benign or malignant. Histopathology is necessary to obtain a definitive diagnosis.

2 If cancer is confirmed histologically, what is the likelihood of finding further metastasis in the abdominal cavity? At the time of diagnosis of pancreatic adenocarcinoma in cats, >50% of patients have evidence of regional or distant metastasis. This cancer is highly malignant and widespread metastasis can result; however, the most common sites for metastasis are the liver, regional lymph nodes, duodenal wall, and peritoneum. Metastasis to the lungs, spleen, and kidneys can also occur.

3 What treatment options are available for this cat? Unfortunately, the prognosis for pancreatic adenocarcinoma is poor to grave. Stabilization and palliation of disease can be attempted with MTD chemotherapy (e.g. doxorubicin, carboplatin, mitoxantrone, gemcitabine), metronomic chemotherapy, or TKIs. However, no effective medical treatments have been reported. Gastrointestinal bypass (gastrojejunostomy) can provide short-term relief if bowel obstruction has occurred or is imminent.

References

Seaman RL (2004) Exocrine pancreatic neoplasia in the cat: a case series. *J Am Anim Hosp Assoc* 40:238–245.
Withrow SJ (2013) Exocrine pancreatic cancer. In: Withrow SJ, Vail DM, Page RL, editors, *Small Animal Clinical Oncology* 5th edition. St. Louis, Elsevier, pp. 401–402.

CASE 71

1 What are the most common skin tumors in the cat? Basal cell tumors, mast cell tumors, fibrosarcoma, squamous cell carcinoma, and sebaceous adenomas are most common, in descending order of incidence.

2 Based on its appearance, what is the most likely diagnosis? The most common pigmented skin tumor in the cat is a basal cell tumor. The term basal cell tumor (BCT), however, has been used in the past to describe collectively various epithelial tumors such as basal cell carcinoma (BCC), trichoblastoma, and solid–cystic ductular sweat gland adenomas and adenocarcinomas. BCCs are considered rare in cats, and many tumors previously diagnosed as BCTs are now actually put into separate categories of solid–cystic apocrine ductular adenoma and trichoblastoma.

3 What diagnostic tests are indicated? Evaluation of regional lymph nodes and thoracic radiographs are indicated. A fine needle aspirate should first be performed if the mass is large enough to obtain a diagnostic sample. An excisional biopsy is usually needed to make a more definitive diagnosis. In this case, a benign BCT was diagnosed and margins were clean but narrow.

4 What treatment is indicated? Surgical removal through excisional biopsy is usually curative for benign BCTs. Although less common, malignant BCTs are seen. In the case of a malignant BCT, wider margins are preferred. If it is not possible to obtain clean surgical margins, radiation therapy is advised postoperatively for malignant BCTs. Chemotherapy has been suggested, but its role is not widely known.

References

Diters RW, Walsh KM (1984) Feline basal cell tumors: a review of 124 cases. *Vet Pathol* 21:51–56.
Hauck ML (2013) Tumors of the skin and subcutaneous tissues. In: Withrow SJ, Vail DM, Page RL, editors, *Small Animal Clinical Oncology*, 5th edition. St. Louis, Elsevier Saunders, pp. 305–320.

Answers

CASE 72

1 Describe the lesion seen on the CT scans. There is a large lytic and productive expansile lesion that appears to be arising from the rib. It extends dorsally to the rib heads and is adjacent to the vertebral body. At least 25% of the volume of the mass is extending into the pulmonary parenchyma.

2 What are the two most common tumors seen arising from the ribs? Osteosarcoma (OSA) is the most common primary rib tumor, accounting for approximately 65% of cases previously reported. Chondrosarcoma (CSA) is the second most common, accounting for 28–35% of cases. Other tumors are possible, including fibrosarcoma and hemangiosarcoma, but are uncommon.

3 From the rostral to caudal direction, the mass appeared to be affecting at least three ribs. Is curative intent surgical resection likely in this patient? The treatment of choice for primary rib OSA is surgical resection followed by chemotherapy (carboplatin or cis-platin and/or doxorubicin are reported). However, based on the local extent of disease in this patient, surgical excision would be unlikely to result in tumor-free margins. It is possible to resect multiple ribs and reconstruct the thoracic wall with various techniques, but the dorsal extent of disease affecting the vertebral body is what makes this patient a poor candidate for curative-intent surgery. Radiation therapy and/or chemotherapy would be palliative.

4 Histopathology confirmed OSA in this patient. What is the prognosis for this patient? Describe the prognostic significance of the elevated ALP. The MST for patients with primary rib OSA that undergo curative-intent surgery and chemotherapy is 240–290 days. Increased total ALP was associated with significantly decreased survival in dogs with primary rib OSA (210 days vs. 675 days in one study).

References
Liptak JM, Dernell WS, Rizzo SA *et al.* (2008) Reconstruction of chest wall defect after rib tumor resection: a comparison of autogenous, prosthetic, and composite techniques in 44 dogs. *Vet Surg* **37**:479–487.

Liptak JM, Kamstock DA, Dernell WS *et al.* (2008) Oncologic outcome after curative-intent treatment in 39 dogs with primary chest wall tumors (1992–2005). *Vet Surg* **37**:488–496.

Pirkey-Ehrhart N, Withrow SJ, Straw RC *et al.* (1995) Primary rib tumors in 54 dogs. *J Am Anim Hosp Assoc* **31**:65–69.

CASE 73

1 What are the two most common tumors seen in the oral cavity of cats? Squamous cell carcinoma is the most common oral tumor in cats, accounting for 70–80% of all oral tumors. Fibrosarcoma is the second most common, making up 13–17%. The remaining tumors noted are rare and individually make up less than 3% of feline oral tumors.

2 What non-malignant lesions could be present in this cat? Odontogenic tumors (such as calcifying epithelial odontogenic tumor (CEOT), ameloblastic fibroma, keratinizing ameloblastoma, complex odontoma, etc. have been described). There is a syndrome of benign mandibular swelling reported in cats which can mimic oral neoplasia.

3 Assuming this is a malignant tumor, what diagnostic and therapeutic options are available for this patient? An incisional biopsy is recommended to classify the lesion further prior to aggressive surgery or other therapy. In this case, the diagnosis was fibrosarcoma. Aggressive surgical resection (hemimandibulectomy) is generally recommended for oral FSA in cats. The large size of this tumor, and the fact that it was crossing the midline, made obtaining tumor-free surgical margins extremely difficult. Full course or palliative radiation therapy could be considered. Stereotactic radiotherapy would allow more precise delivery of RT with fewer side effects and fewer fractions (dosages) of radiation. The placement of an esophageal or gastric feeding tube could be considered to maintain a good plane of nutrition and hydration.

References

Liptak JM, Withrow SJ (2013) Cancer of the gastrointestinal tract, oral tumors. In: Withrow SJ, Vail DM, Page RL, editors, *Small Animal Clinical Oncology*, 5th edition. St. Louis, Elsevier Saunders, pp. 381–398.

Northrup NC, Selting KA, Rassnick KM *et al.* (2006) Outcomes of cats with oral tumors treated with mandibulectomy: 42 cases. *J Am Anim Hosp Assoc* **42**:350–360.

Stebbins KE, Morse CC, Goldschmidt MH (1989) Feline oral neoplasia: a ten-year survey. *Vet Pathol* **26**:121–128.

CASE 74

1 What is the clinical diagnosis? Based on the pedunculated appearance and texture of this mass, the most likely diagnosis is sebaceous adenoma.

2 What recommendations should be made? Cytology of the lesion is indicated and in this case was consistent with a benign adenoma. Removal of the lesion is suggested if it is causing any discomfort for the patient. In certain anatomic locations, sebaceous adenomas will be at risk of bleeding if rubbed or bumped.

CASE 75

1 Describe the CT findings and suggest differential diagnoses. There is a 3.5 × 4.0 cm mass with non-uniform enhancement and well-defined margins. The mass is located adjacent to the descending aorta and medial to the left kidney. The location of the mass is most consistent with a left adrenal tumor. In cats, adrenal tumors are uncommon. Approximately 50% of adrenal cortical tumors in cats are carcinomas, but metastasis is uncommon. When seen, cortisol and aldosterone are the most common hormones produced. Pheochromocytomas are extremely rare in cats.

2 What further diagnostic testing is indicated for this patient? Typically, endocrine testing is recommended in cats with adrenal masses. For example, if cortisol excess is suspected, a low-dose dexamethasone suppression test is recommended. This patient has evidence of hypertension and hypokalemia that could be consistent with an aldosterone secreting tumor. Plasma aldosterone levels were 1,760 pmol/l (reference range, 194–388). The presumptive diagnosis is an aldosterone secreting adrenal tumor. The diagnosis is based primarily on imaging and histopathology.

3 What treatment is recommended? Adrenalectomy is the treatment of choice. Medical management/stabilization is recommended prior to surgery, including potassium supplementation to correct hypokalemia, spironolactone (aldosterone antagonist), and amlodipine besylate (to decrease blood pressure). Surgical removal and histopathology of this patient's mass revealed an adrenocortical adenoma. Plasma aldosterone levels normalized after surgery.

4 What are survival expectations with treatment? With surgical excision, the prognosis for cats surviving the immediate postoperative period is good, with median survival times of 1,297 days most recently reported. The only significant factor affecting survival time was an increased length of anesthesia (>4 hours). With medical management alone (listed above), survival times of 1–3 years are reported.

References

Ash RA, Harvey AM, Tasker S (2005) Primary hyperaldosteronism in the cat: a series of 13 cases. *J Fel Med Surg* 7:173–182.

Lo AJ, Holt DE, Brown DC *et al.* (2014) Treatment of aldosterone-secreting adrenocortical tumors in cats by unilateral adrenalectomy: 10 cases (2002–2012). *J Vet Intern Med* 28:137–143.

CASE 76

1 What is the prognosis and the expected metastatic rate of this cancer? The prognosis for SCC in the oral cavity of cats is unfortunately very poor. Fewer than 10% of cats undergoing therapy survive 1 year. SCC tends to be a locally invasive tumor with a low metastatic potential. When spread occurs, it usually involves the local lymph nodes or, rarely, the lungs.

2 Are there any environmental or lifestyle factors that increase the risk of this cancer in cats? Several studies evaluating lifestyle and environmental factors have suggested that environmental tobacco smoke, flea products, and diet may be associated with an increased risk of oral SCC development.

3 What therapies are described for this disease? The combination of surgery, RT, and chemotherapy generally offers the best chance for control of oral SCC. Patients receiving no treatment have an average survival time of 2–3 months. Any single treatment used alone (surgery, RT, or chemotherapy) provides no significant survival advantage, but may provide pain relief. Inhibition of COX-2 activity alone or in combination with RT and/or chemotherapy may improve response rates and survival times, although <10% of cats will have tumors that express COX-2. Regardless of treatment type, however, less than 10% of patients survive to 1 year. Unfortunately, most patients presenting with advanced tongue involvement are not good surgical candidates owing to extensive local disease and location. Marconato *et al.* reported encouraging results using a multi-modality approach. Neoadjuvant bleomycin, piroxicam, and thalidomide followed by surgery and RT yielded positive results in three cats with sublingual SCC. The three cats were alive at 759, 458, and 362 days.

4 Develop a palliative therapeutic plan for this cat. The most significant morbidity associated with tongue SCC is inability to eat and drink. Weight loss, inability to groom, and regional pain contribute to an overall declining quality of life. Palliative intervention should include:

- Pharmacologic pain management (e.g. piroxicam or meloxicam, buprenorphine or tramadol, etc.).
- Sustainable nutritional support (PEG tube, or pharyngostomy tube).
- Attention to patient's comfort (keeping patient brushed and clean, removing any saliva or blood from the hair coat and oral cavity area).
- Controlling secondary infection with antibiotics.
- A palliative radiation course (total radiation doses of 24–40 Gy administered in 3–4 fractions once weekly for 4–5 weeks has been described) +/– chemotherapy can be considered, but nutritional support is critical in treated patients.
- Careful assessment of quality of life issues and euthanasia once pain is no longer able to be alleviated.

References

Bertone ER, Snyder LA, Moore AS (2003) Environmental and lifestyle risk factors for oral squamous cell carcinoma in domestic cats. *J Vet Intern Med* **17**:557–562.

Marconato L, Buchholz J, Keller M *et al.* (2012) Multimodality therapeutic approach and interdisciplinary challenge for the treatment of unresectable head and neck squamous cell carcinoma in six cats: a pilot study. *Vet Comp Oncol* **11**:101–112.

Sabhlok A, Ayl R (2014) Palliative radiation therapy outcomes for cats with oral squamous cell carcinoma (1999–2005). *Vet Radiol Ultrasound* **55**:565–570.

CASE 77

1 The mass measured 2 cm. The surgical scar measured 3.1 cm. Is this adequate surgical planning? Assuming that 2–3 cm lateral margins and one fascial plane below the tumor are considered standard, the surgical scar should be at least 6–8 cm. In this case, it is unlikely that a wide excision was obtained. The surgical margins were documented histologically to have tumor cells present at all margins.

2 Interpret the prognostic panel. Mast cell tumors that have a high proliferation activity are associated with a poorer prognosis. Studies have supported that Ki67 of >23/grid and an AgNOR × Ki67 of >54 are associated with a significantly worse prognosis and decreased survival times. Likewise, a significantly shorter survival time is associated with the presence of a *c-KIT* mutation in exon 8 or exon 11, or KIT pattern 2 or 3. Therefore, this patient's prognosis is considered to be favorable.

3 Does the subcutaneous location of the tumor provide any additional prognostic information? Recent studies have shown that patients with subcutaneous tumors have a favorable prognosis. In a case series of 306 dogs with subcutaneous MCTs, metastasis occurred in only 13 dogs (4%) and only 24 dogs had local recurrence (8%), even though 171 dogs (56%) had incomplete surgical margins. The tumor recurrence rate for patients with incomplete surgical margins was only 12%. Median survival times were not reached in the study, but 5-year survival rates were 86%. High mitotic index (>4), infiltrative growth pattern, and presence of multinucleated cells were linked to a less favorable prognosis. In another report of dogs with subcutaneous MCT, no dogs possessed mutations in exon 11 of *c-KIT*.

4 What are the treatment options for this patient? The subcutaneous location, low mitotic index, and low-grade classification of this tumor are all favorable. Recurrence rates, even with incomplete excision, tend to be very low. If no further treatment is pursued in this patient, the recurrence rate is <12%. Wider surgical excisions to obtain tumor-free margins or cautious monitoring are reasonable options.

References

Thompson JJ, Pearl DL, Yager JA *et al.* (2011) Canine subcutaneous mast cell tumor: characterization and prognostic indices. *Vet Pathol* 48:156–168.

Thompson JJ, Yager JA, Best SJ *et al.* (2011) Canine subcutaneous mast cell tumors: cellular proliferation and KIT expression as prognostic indices. *Vet Pathol* 48:169–181.

Webster JD, Yuzbasiyan-Gurkan V, Miller RA *et al.* (2007) Cellular proliferation in canine cutaneous mast cell tumors: association with c-KIT and its role in prognostication. *Vet Pathol* 44:298–308.

CASE 78

1 What type of radiograph is being illustrated? This is a "port film", which is a radiographic image taken by the linear accelerator to confirm the position of the patient and the geometry of the treatment beam.

2 What is the purpose of this radiograph? Portal imaging is done to ensure that the patient's desired treatment field is exactly aligned with the beam that the machine is delivering. Accuracy in reproducing the treatment field over the course of multiple fractions of radiation is crucial. In addition to port films, "radiation tattoos" or ink marks (78b) are used to mark the treatment field on the patient to help in consistency and reproducibility of radiation delivery.

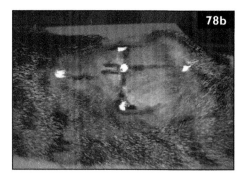

CASE 79

1 What is the most likely diagnosis? The primary differential diagnosis for this lesion is squamous cell carcinoma (SCC). Early lesions often appear to be scratches or trauma related.

2 What are possible causes or predisposing factors for development of this lesion? Cutaneous SCC is a sunlight (actinically) induced tumor of older cats thought to be related to chronic exposure to UVB radiation. It occurs more commonly in white or partly white cats, which appear to be 5 times more likely to develop cutaneous SCC than cats of any other color. Long-haired breeds may be more protected against sun exposure owing to better hair cover. Siamese cats appear to be protected by the distribution of their markings. Sunlight may induce *p53* mutations, allowing development of SCC; 7–20% of cats with SCC are FIV-positive.

3 What are the most important criteria when considering surgery of the nasal planum? The size of the tumor and the depth of invasion dictate the ability to remove tumors in this location surgically. Tumors typically begin as pre-invasive carcinoma (in situ) and eventually progress to larger sizes with invasion of fascia, cartilage, muscle, or bone. More superficial tumors that have not invaded the subcutaneous or fascial layers are more amenable to surgical resection. Surgical removal of the nasal planum offers long-term control when tumors are not deeply invasive (i.e. tumors limited to the most superficial cutaneous layers). T_1 and T_2 tumors may be surgically treatable without nasal planum resection, but for T_3 and T_4 tumors, nasal planum resection may be the only surgical option.

Answers

4 Describe a non-surgical option for the treatment of this patient. Various non-surgical treatments have been described including RT, cryosurgery, strontium-90 plesiotherapy, retinoids, and photodynamic therapy. RT results in a median disease-free interval of approximately 1 year and appears to be effective for earlier stage disease. Cryosurgery (T_1 or T_2) was associated with median remissions of 26.7 months in one study of 102 cats. For superficial SCC (≤3 mm depth) strontium-90 plesiotherapy was effective with median remission times of 692 days and 1,071 days in two separate studies. Photodynamic therapy refers to the use of systemic or topically applied photosensitizing agents that can be activated by visible light. Several studies have reported the response rate to various types of photosensitizers. A 100% complete remission rate was achieved using a liposomal photosensitizing agent with 1-year control rates of 75%. Unfortunately, photodynamic therapy is not widely available. Intralesional carboplatin has been described and resulted in a complete remission rate of 76%, with 55% 1-year progression-free survival.

Follow-up/discussion
The postoperative appearance of a patient that underwent nasal planum resection ("nosectomy") is shown (**79b**). This procedure is generally well tolerated. There was a crusty discharge which lasted approximately 1 month postoperatively in this patient and then resolved.

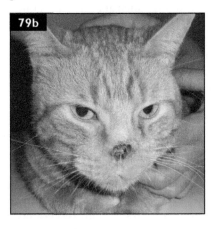

79b

WHO Staging System

Stage	Description
T_{is}	Pre-invasive carcinoma (carcinoma in situ) not breaching the basement membrane
T_1	Tumor <2 cm diameter, superficial or exophytic
T_2	Tumor 2–5 cm diameter, or with minimal invasion irrespective of size
T_3	Tumor >5 cm diameter, or with invasion of the subcutis irrespective of size
T_4	Tumor invading other structures such as fascia, muscle, bone or cartilage

References
Bexfield NH, Stell AJ, Gear RN *et al.* (2008) Photodynamic therapy of superficial nasal planum squamous cell carcinoma in cats: 55 cases. *J Vet Intern Med* **22**:1385–1389.
Buchholz J, Wergin M, Walt H *et al.* (2007) Photodynamic therapy of feline cutaneous squamous cell carcinoma using a newly developed liposomal photosensitizer: preliminary results concerning drug safety and efficacy. *J Vet Intern Med* **21**:770–775.

Clarke RE (1991) Cryosurgical treatment of feline cutaneous squamous cell carcinoma. *Aust Vet Pract* **21**:148–153.

Goodfellow M, Hayes A, Murphy S *et al.* (2006) A retrospective study of ^{90}strontium plesiotherapy for feline squamous cell carcinoma of the nasal planum. *J Fel Med Surg* **8**:169–176.

Hammond GM, Gordon IK, Theon AP *et al.* Evaluation of strontium Sr 90 for the treatment of superficial squamous cell carcinoma of the nasal planum in cats: 49 cases (1990–2006). *J Am Vet Med Assoc* **231**:736–741.

Murphy S (2013) Cutaneous squamous cell carcinoma in the cat. *J Fel Med Surg* **15**:401–407.

deVos JP, Burm AGO, Focker BP (2004) Results from the treatment of advanced stage squamous cell carcinoma of the nasal planum in cats, using a combination of intralesional carboplatin and superficial radiotherapy: a pilot study. *Vet Comp Oncol* **2**:75–81.

CASE 80

1 Describe the thoracic radiograph. Based on the radiograph and physical examination, what is the presumptive diagnosis? There is significant lymphadenopathy involving the hilar, sternal, and mediastinal lymph nodes. Clinically, lymphoma would be a likely diagnosis. However, the presence of the vacuolated cells raises suspicion for histiocytic sarcoma (HS).

2 What is the interpretation of the ICC and what is the diagnosis? When trying to differentiate between lymphoma and HS, CD3, CD79a, and CD18 should be run. Macrophages and granulocytes express 10 times more CD18 than lymphocytes, and lymphoma usually expresses either CD3 or CD79a, allowing differentiation between the two tumor types. Therefore, the diagnosis in this case is HS. CD204 is a more recently described useful immunohistochemical marker of canine HS.

3 What is the prognosis for this patient? Histiocytic sarcoma carries a very poor prognosis, especially when widespread disease is identified. Untreated, the clinical course is rapid and fatal. CCNU (lomustine) appears to be the most effective chemotherapeutic agent used to date, but the overall response rate tends to be just under 50%, with a median survival time of 172 days in patients that achieve a CR or PR. For patients with localized disease treated aggressively (surgery and/or RT) and adjunct CCNU, MSTs were 568 days in one study. Periarticular HS, without evidence of metastatic disease and treated aggressively with combination therapy (surgery, radiation, CCNU), has been associated with a favorable prognosis (980 days).

4 What is the significance of the normal blood work? There is a more aggressive form of this disease called hemophagocytic HS. In this form, approximately 95% of patients present with a regenerative anemia, 90% with thrombocytopenia, and 95% with hypoproteinemia. In hemophagocytic HS, grossly visible mass lesions are generally lacking. The lack of any of these changes and presence of obvious masses makes hemophagocytic HS less likely. The prognosis for this form of HS is grave.

Answers

References

Kato Y, Murakami M, Hoshino Y et al. (2013) The class A macrophage scavenger receptor CD204 is a useful immunohistochemical marker of canine histiocytic sarcoma. *J Comp Pathol* 148:188–196.

Klahn SL, Kitchell BE, Dervisis NG (2011) Evaluation and comparison of outcomes in dogs with periarticular and nonperiarticular histiocytic sarcoma. *J Am Vet Med Assoc* 239: 90–96.

Moore PF (2014) A review of histiocytic disease of dogs and cats. *Vet Pathol* 51:167–184.

CASE 81

1 **Describe the abnormality pictured here.** The temporal side of the right pupil is paralyzed. This is often referred to as a "reverse D" shaped pupil.

2 **What are the differential diagnoses?** "D" or "reverse D" shaped pupils, also called spastic pupil syndrome, is most commonly related to FeLV infection, especially when the papillary changes are intermittent. Other disorders such as posterior synechia, iris coloboma or malformation (congenital), developmental or acquired iris/lens abnormalities, or trauma are possible, but all of these changes are typically not intermittent.

3 **What is unique about the feline pupil that allows this abnormality to occur?** The innervation of the feline pupil is unique. The temporal half and the nasal half of the pupil are innervated separately. Therefore, localized nerve damage can result in a hemi-dilated pupil.

Reference

Aroch I, Ofri R, Sutton G (2007) Ocular manifestations of systemic disease. In: Gelatt KN, editor, *Veterinary Ophthalmology*, 4th edition. Ames, Wiley-Blackwell, pp. 1406–1469.

CASE 82

1 **What is the significance of the fluid being bloody throughout the thoracocentesis procedure?** If blood were only seen at the beginning of the procedure, then iatrogenic bleeding from the procedure itself is possible. When the character of the fluid is bloody throughout the tap, the fluid is representative of the underlying disease process.

2 **What diagnostic tests are indicated once the fluid has been removed?** Fluid analysis to include cytology, PCV, and biochemical analysis is advised. It can be very difficult cytologically to differentiate between reactive mesothelial cells and malignancy (mesothelioma, carcinoma, and adenocarcinoma). With no history of trauma, malignancy is a common cause of hemorrhagic effusions. Effusions associated with malignancy are commonly exudative, with normal or increased pH (>7.4), glucose >10 but <80 mg/dl, <30% neutrophils, and increased cell counts.

Pathologic hemorrhage (as opposed to iatrogenic hemorrhage) is supported by the presence of hemosiderin, low platelets, and erythrophagocytosis. The presence of platelets usually indicates ongoing iatrogenic hemorrhage. Post-thoracocentesis radiographs of the thorax should be taken to evaluate for masses or other abnormalities that the fluid may have been obscuring in the initial radiographs. An echocardiogram is used to rule out pericardial effusion and/or cardiac tumors. An abdominal ultrasound should be performed to determine whether another primary tumor site is present. Blood work should include coagulation analysis.

3 List the differential diagnoses for a hemorrhagic pleural effusion. Non-neoplastic causes of hemorrhagic effusions include trauma, lung lobe torsion, and pancreatitis. Neoplastic causes include mesothelioma, carcinomatosis, and sarcomatosis. Patients with pericardial effusion secondary to neoplasia (e.g. atrial hemangiosarcoma and heart base tumors) can also present with pleural effusion that can be bloody. This patient was diagnosed at necropsy with carcinomatosis.

Reference
Rizzi TE, Cowell RL, Tyler RD *et al.* (2008) Effusions: abdominal, thoracic, and pericardial. In: Cowell RL, Tyler RD, Meinkoth JH *et al.*, editors, *Diagnostic Cytology and Hematology of the Dog and Cat*, 3rd edition. St. Louis, Mosby, pp. 235–255.

CASE 83

1 What are the differential diagnoses for this lesion? Squamous cell carcinoma is the most common oral tumor in cats; however, this is not a typical location for SCC. Fibrosarcoma (FSA) is the second most common feline oral tumor, which is the primary rule out given the appearance of the lesion. Eosinophilic granuloma (EG) is a consideration; however, this lesion appears more smooth and circumscribed than the typical EG. An odontogenic tumor is also possible. FSA was the histologic diagnosis.

2 What is the likelihood of metastasis? The majority of oral tumors in cats are locally invasive and late to metastasize. This is true for FSA. Lymph node and lung metastasis are uncommon.

3 What diagnostic tests should be performed? An MDB plus oral radiographs or, preferably, CT scanning are indicated. A CT was performed on this patient and a significant amount of bone destruction was noted.

4 The tumor extends too far back on the hard palate to be operable. What therapeutic options are available? Radiation therapy is the best treatment option, although oral FSAs are traditionally poorly responsive. However, in this case RT would at least provide palliation of the bone pain. At the end of a full course of RT, the patient showed significant clinical improvement (better appetite, no longer bleeding), but the tumor appeared relatively unchanged in size. Following

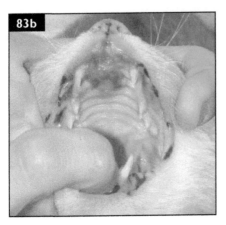

radiation, the mass continued to regress and is shown 4 months later (83b). This patient was euthanized 2 years after treatment because of recurrence of disease. A second course of RT could have been performed, but other age-related health issues precluded further therapy.

References

Burk RL (1996) Radiation therapy in the treatment of oral neoplasia. *Vet Clin N Am Small Anim Pract* 26:155–163.

Liptak JM, Withrow SJ (2013) Cancer of the gastrointestinal tract. Oral tumors. In: Withrow SJ, Vail DM, Page RL, editors, *Small Animal Clinical Oncology*, 5th edition. St. Louis, Elsevier Saunders, pp. 381–398.

CASE 84

1 What clinical diagnosis does this represent? Based on the aggressive recurrence and histologically benign diagnosis, this represents a histologically low-grade but biologically high-grade fibrosarcoma. This is a syndrome that tends to occur in large breed dogs, with younger Golden and Labrador Retrievers appearing to be predisposed. These tumors commonly arise on the hard palate and maxillary arcade.

2 What was the mistake made in the clinical interpretation of this patient's disease? Based on the younger age of the patient, the breed, and the low-grade fibrosarcoma diagnosis, it should have been recognized that this could be a histologically low-grade but biologically high-grade fibrosarcoma and more aggressive treatment recommended.

3 Based on the current clinical presentation, what further diagnostic evaluation and treatment options are available? Given the maxillary location of this tumor, a CT scan is advised for surgical planning. If the tumor crosses the midline of the hard palate or is deemed inoperable, radiation therapy should be pursued in hopes of cytoreduction for a more effective surgery. Thoracic radiography and careful evaluation of regional lymph nodes should be performed prior to surgery. Although the metastatic rate at diagnosis tends to be very low, <20% of patients will ultimately develop either lymph node or lung metastasis. The

Answers

prognosis for this patient has to be considered guarded owing to the problematic issue of local recurrence. A median survival time of 1 year has been suggested with surgery alone. When RT is used postoperatively, MSTs increased to 18–26 months.

4 What features of this patient's tumor can help predict outcome? The T_3 clinical stage (T_1: <2 cm diameter; T_2: 2–4 cm diameter; T_3: >4 cm diameter) is associated with a higher local recurrence rate due to difficulty in obtaining a clean surgical margin. Patients with tumors in the rostral location tend to have better outcomes because of the greater ability to achieve local surgical control. Completeness of excision is important. In cases where the margins are free of tumor but are <5 mm, completeness of excision is in question and RT is recommended.

Reference

Ciekot PA, Powers BE, Withrow SJ *et al.* (1994) Histologically low-grade, yet biologically high-grade, fibrosarcomas of the mandible and maxilla in dogs: 25 cases (1982–1991). *J Am Vet Med Assoc* **204**:610–615.

CASE 85

1 Describe the radiographs and list the differential diagnoses. There is a well-circumscribed soft tissue density in the right caudal lung field. Differential diagnoses include:

- Primary lung tumor.
- Metastatic lung tumor.
- Abscess.
- Granuloma.

2 Describe the cytology. The sample is very cellular with the predominant population being epithelial cells. There is minimal anisocytosis and anisokaryosis. The cells at the top of the slide appear to be forming acini. Presumptive diagnosis: pulmonary adenocarcinoma.

3 What additional diagnostic tests should be performed? An abdominal ultrasound to rule out another primary source is indicated. Owing to the fact that the mass is solitary, metastasis from another primary site is less likely. A CT scan of the lungs should be performed to help confirm that the mass is truly solitary.

4 What treatment is indicated and what are the most important prognostic indicators for this patient? The treatment of choice for primary lung neoplasia is surgery. Adjunct therapy (such as chemotherapy) would be determined on the basis of histopathology. Histologic grade was the single most important predictor of prognosis in one study, with an MST of 2.5 months postoperatively for cats with poorly differentiated tumors and an MST of 23 months for cats with

201

Answers

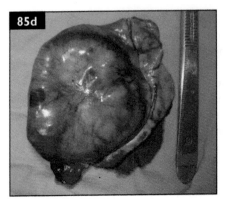

85d

well-differentiated tumors. This patient's tumor was removed surgically (85d). The histologic diagnosis was well-differentiated adenocarcinoma.

References
Hahn KA, McEntee MF (1997) Primary lung tumors in cats: 86 cases (1979–1994). *J Am Vet Med Assoc* 211:1257–1260.
Hahn KA, McEntee MF (1998) Prognosis factors for survival in cats after removal of a primary lung tumor: 21 cases (1979–1994). *Vet Surg* 27:307–311.

CASE 86

1 **Describe the radiograph.** The bladder wall appears thickened with a soft tissue density filling the majority of the bladder. There appears to be air/emphysema within or near the bladder wall. The soft tissue density appears to be separated from the bladder wall.

2 **Explain the interpretation of the BTA test in this patient.** The bladder tumor antigen test is not accurate when there is hematuria present. Red blood cells in the urine result in false positives.

3 **What are the differential diagnoses for this patient?** The radiographic findings are more consistent with a blood clot. Emphysematous cystitis is another consideration (usually secondary to diabetes). Underlying causes of a blood clot (or clots) in the bladder include trauma, bleeding disorders, neoplasia, and cystitis. Because this patient had been missing, trauma was suspected.

References
Billet JHG, Moore AH, Holt PE (2002) Evaluation of a bladder tumor antigen test for the diagnosis of lower urinary tract malignancies in dogs. *Am J Vet Res* 63:370–373.
Henry CJ, Tyler JW, McEntee MC *et al.* (2003) Evaluation of a bladder tumor antigen test as a screening test for transitional cell carcinoma of the lower urinary tract in dogs. *Am J Vet Res* 64:1017–1020.

CASE 87

1 **Describe the radiograph and give the differential diagnoses.** There is a diffuse nodular pattern within the lung parenchyma. There is no obvious evidence of pneumonia or lymphadenopathy. The primary differential is diffuse metastatic lung disease (from an extrapulmonary primary source or a primary pulmonary

neoplasia that has metastasized within the lungs). Fungal disease such as blastomycosis is also a consideration – a diffuse interstitial military pattern with hilar lymphadenopathy tends to be more common with fungal pneumonia.

2 In addition to the MDB, an abdominal ultrasound was performed and was normal. What further testing is indicated in order to differentiate between malignancy and a non-neoplastic cause? Given that the physical examination and an abdominal ultrasound failed to identify a primary source of cancer, a lung aspirate should be considered. Lung aspirates are usually an inexpensive, safe, and effective way to obtain a diagnosis. Seeding of tumor cells along needle tracts has been reported, but this is the quickest way to identify cancer or fungal disease.

References

Rossi F, Aresu L, Vignoli M *et al.* (2015) Metastatic cancer of unknown primary in 21 dogs. *Vet Comp Oncol* **13**:11–19.

Warren-Smith CMR, Roe K, DeLa Puerta B *et al.* (2011) Pulmonary adenocarcinoma seeding along a fine needle aspiration tract in a dog. *Vet Rec* **169**:181.

Wood EF, O'Brien RT, Young KM (1998) Ultrasound-guided fine-needle aspiration of focal parenchymal lesions of the lung in dogs and cats. *J Vet Intern Med* **12**:338–342.

CASE 88

1 Describe the lesion. There is a mass immediately behind the arytenoid cartilages. The mass has a smooth surface and is mildly erythematous. The mass is almost completely obstructing the airway. Tonsillar involvement could not be appreciated.

2 List the differential diagnoses. Abscess, granuloma, and neoplasia are the primary considerations. Among the neoplastic diseases reported in this location are benign tumors (osteochondroma) and malignant tumors (adenocarcinoma, chondrosarcoma, lymphoma, osteosarcoma, plasmacytoma, and squamous cell carcinomas).

3 Surgical debulking was performed because of the severe clinical symptoms. A biopsy revealed squamous cell carcinoma. What is the recommended treatment? Debulking surgery (removing visible disease) followed by RT and/or chemotherapy would be advised, although studies are lacking for this particular tumor location.

4 What is the prognosis for this patient? The prognosis for SCC in the oral cavity is thought to worsen as the location becomes more caudal. However, a recent study reported that tumor location, clinical stage, and histologic subtype were not associated with survival time in oral non-tonsillar SCC. In this patient, the prognosis is guarded because the location makes obtaining tumor-free margins with surgery difficult.

References

Fulton AJ, Nemec A, Murphy BG *et al.* (2013) Risk factors associated with survival in dogs with nontonsillar oral squamous cell carcinoma: 31 cases (1990–2010). *J Am Vet Med Assoc* **243**:696–702.

Grier CK, Mayer MN (2007) Radiation therapy of canine nontonsillar squamous cell carcinoma. *Can Vet J* **48**:1189–1191.

CASE 89

1 What is the diagnosis? Oral malignant melanoma.

2 What further tests need to be performed before treatment can be recommended? An MDB and evaluation of the mandibular lymph nodes are advised.

3 What treatment has the greatest chance for long-term survival? If staging is negative, surgical excision (rostral mandibulectomy) offers the best chance for long-term control or even cure.

4 What is the prognosis for this patient? Overall MST of patients undergoing curative intent surgery was 723 days in a recent report (818 days for patients presenting without metastasis). In a separate report, increasing size and patient age were negative prognostic factors. The MST was 630 days for patients whose tumors were <2 cm, 240 days if 2–4 cm, and 173 days for >4 cm. When only age was considered, MST of dogs <12 years old was 433 days, vs. 224 days for dogs ≥12 years of age. Based on the size of this lesion, age of patient, and ability to achieve complete surgical excision, a favorable prognosis is warranted.

References

Boston SE, Lu X, Culp WTN *et al.* (2014) Efficacy of systemic adjuvant therapies administered to dogs after excision of oral malignant melanomas: 151 cases (2001–2012). *J Am Vet Med Assoc* **245**:401–407.

Tuohy JL, Selmic LE, Worley DR *et al.* (2014) Outcome following curative-intent surgery for oral melanoma in dogs: 70 cases (1998–2011). *J Am Vet Med Assoc* **245**:1266–1273.

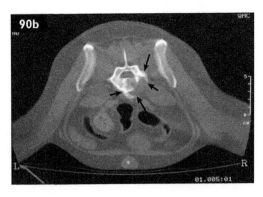

90b

CASE 90

1 Describe the CT image and list the differential diagnoses. There is a primarily lytic lesion that has destroyed a significant portion of the right ventral aspect of the vertebral body of L6 (**90b**). The soft tissue portion of the mass can be seen adjacent to the hypaxial muscles. There is new bone formation at the periphery of the lesion. A primary bone tumor or metastatic bone lesion are the primary considerations. Osteosarcoma, fibrosarcoma, chondrosarcoma, hemangiosarcoma, multiple myeloma and less frequently lymphoma, metastatic carcinoma, or liposarcoma are differentials for this lesion.

2 What is the most common primary vertebral body tumor diagnosed in the dog? Osteosarcoma is the most common primary vertebral body tumor diagnosed in dogs while lymphoma is the most common vertebral tumor diagnosed in cats. In one study, metastatic carcinomas were the most common secondary vertebral tumors and in a separate study, hemangiosarcoma was found most frequently.

3 What further testing is indicated? Complete staging of the patient is important to rule out the existence of a primary tumor in another location. Therefore, a complete MDB to include radiographs of the appendicular and axial skeleton and abdominal ultrasound to search for a primary tumor are advised. A biopsy (CT or ultrasound guided) should be performed for medical and surgical treatment planning. In this case, there was no further evidence of disease beyond the vertebral body. A CT-guided FNA was performed that was consistent with sarcoma. If possible, a needle core biopsy or surgical biopsy should be obtained to differentiate the tumor further.

4 What treatments are indicated? Given the patient's age, the owners did not wish to pursue surgery. What palliative options could be considered for this patient? RT +/– chemotherapy and/or bisphosphonate therapy can be used palliatively. For definitive therapy, surgery is recommended. Surgery is generally intralesional without curative intent. Gross resection of all visible tumor tissue is advised and decompression laminectomy is often necessary. Tumor-free margins are unlikely in this location, therefore postoperative radiation therapy is indicated. Aggressive multi-modality therapy (surgery, radiation, and chemotherapy) may improve the outcome; however, the overall median survival time of dogs with vertebral OSA remains poor. Patients presenting without serious neurologic deficits had better MST (330 days) than patients presenting with significant deficits (135 days). Postoperative neurologic status was a significant predictor of outcome.

Reference
Dernell WS, Ban Vechten BJ, Straw RC *et al.* (2000) Outcome following treatment of vertebral tumors in 20 dogs (1986–1995). *J Am Anim Hosp Assoc* **36**:245–251.

CASE 91

1 What is the diagnostic plan? In addition to the MDB, an abdominal ultrasound is indicated. Careful evaluation for peripheral lymph nodes should be a part of the physical examination, and FNA and cytology performed if lymphadenopathy is noted. An FNA of the mammary mass should be performed, followed by an incisional or excisional biopsy if possible. In this patient, FNA of the mammary mass revealed carcinoma.

2 What does the clinical presentation suggest? The clinical presentation is consistent with an inflammatory mammary carcinoma. In cats, this is very rare, but reported, and has a very aggressive clinical course. The rapid onset of a firm mass, erythema, and edema accompanied by significant pain are features of inflammatory mammary carcinoma. Histologically, dermal tumor embolization of superficial lymphatic vessels with severe secondary inflammation are considered to be hallmarks of this disease. The Ki67 labeling index is also often very high.

3 What is this patient's prognosis and how should treatment be approached? Because of the inflammatory nature of this carcinoma, a poor prognosis has to be given. Surgical intervention with a radical mastectomy is considered when there is no evidence of metastasis. Pet owners need to be aware of the potentially rapid clinical course of this cancer. Surgery alone can be palliative, but chemotherapy is recommended. There are no studies that have determined the optimal treatment for this uncommon clinical presentation of mammary carcinoma in cats. However, options for postoperative treatment include:

- Standard dosage chemotherapy (choices include doxorubicin, mitoxantrone, carboplatin).
- Metronomic (low dose) chemotherapy:
  - Cyclophosphamide and piroxicam or meloxicam.
  - Chlorambucil and piroxicam or meloxicam.
- The use of docetaxel (a semi-synthetic taxane similar to paclitaxel) has also been described. It appears to be safe for cats, but its benefit in inflammatory mammary carcinoma is not clear. The docetaxel can be given IV or orally in combination with cyclosporine (to improve oral bioavailability).

References

Castagnaro M, DeMaria R, Bozzetta E *et al.* (1998) Ki-67 index as indicator of the post-surgical prognosis in feline mammary carcinomas. *Res Vet Sci* **65**:223–226.

Hughes K, Dobson JM (2012) Prognostic histopathological and molecular markers in feline mammary neoplasia. *Vet J* **194**:19–26.

McEntee MC, Rassnick KM, Bailey DB *et al.* (2006) Phase I and pharmacokinetic evaluation of the combination of orally administered docetaxel and cyclosporine A in tumor-bearing cats. *J Vet Intern Med* **20**:1370–1375.

Perez-Alenza MD, Jimenez A, Nieto AL *et al.* (2004) First description of feline inflammatory mammary carcinoma: clinicopathological and immunohistochemical characteristics of three cases. *Breast Cancer Res* **6**:R300–R307.

Shiu KB, McCartan L, Kubicek L *et al.* (2011) Intravenous administration of Docetaxel to cats with cancer. *J Vet Intern Med* **25**:916–919.

Zappulli V, Rasotto R, Caliari D *et al.* (2015) Prognostic evaluation of feline mammary carcinomas: a review of the literature. *Vet Pathol* **52**:46–60.

CASE 92

1 Describe the lesions pictured. There is a large amount of crusty exudate around the vulva and rectum. In addition, there are visible coalescing, proliferative cutaneous lesions present.

2 Biopsies were taken in different areas of the perineum and all areas confirmed basal cell carcinoma (BCC). What treatment should be considered? BCCs usually present as solitary lesions and have a relatively benign biologic behavior. They are the most common skin tumors in the cat, but represent only approximately 5% of skin tumors in dogs. The disease in this case is behaving in a locally aggressive manner. Surgical excision is usually curative for most patients with BCC, but surgery is not possible in this case. Radiation therapy or chemotherapy (e.g. carboplatin) is a consideration, but reports of treatment for locally aggressive BCC in dogs are scarce.

Reference
Simeonov R, Simeonova G (2010) Comparative morphometric analysis of recurrent and nonrecurrent canine basal cell carcinomas: a preliminary report. *Vet Clin Pathol* 39: 96–98.

CASE 93

1 What is the probable cause of this lesion? Actinic keratitis is believed to result from UV light exposure.

2 What is the natural progression of disease? These UV light induced lesions are usually very slowly progressive, locally invasive, and rarely metastasize. In cats, a solar dermatitis progresses to actinic carcinoma in situ, which can progress to squamous cell carcinoma and may eventually become locally invasive. Pre-malignant lesions can be present for years before malignant transformation is seen. Although uncommon, spread to the mandibular and retropharyngeal lymph nodes can be seen with more invasive forms of SCC. This disease is most commonly seen in white-haired cats in areas where hair is thinner such as around the eyes, on the nasal planum, and on the ear pinnae.

3 How should this patient be managed? For pre-malignant lesions:
- Avoid further UV light exposure. Keeping cats indoors during daylight hours can reduce sun exposure. Sunscreens can be used, but products containing zinc oxide and octyl salicylate should be avoided. Fragrance-free, non-staining products with UVA and UVB barriers (SPF >15) are advised. There are products made especially for pets. Waterproof sunscreens made for babies are usually safe. Using "hats" or other means to protect sensitive areas can be useful. Figure **93b** shows innovative "ear covers" made by the owner of a cat with multiple pre-malignant lesions on the nasal planum and around the eyes, but that were worse on the ear tips.

Answers

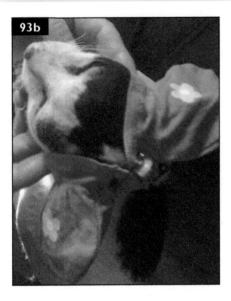

93b

- Topical anti-inflammatory agents (e.g. hydrocortisone) to alleviate inflammation.
- Systemic steroids if inflammation is severe.
- Antibiotics if secondary infection is suspected.
- Aldara® cream (imiquimod) may be used to treat a variety of keratoses. May be useful in preventing malignant transformation.

4 If the lesion progresses to SCC, what treatment is advised? For malignant lesions:

- Surgery is the treatment of choice, but in this cat, even with nasal planum resection, it may not be possible to obtain clean margins.
- Cryosurgery can be used to control smaller lesions.
- Radiation therapy: in cats, radiation appears to be far more effective for nasal planum SCC than it is in dogs.
- Strontium-90 plesiotherapy: overall response rate is reported as high as 98%, with 88% CR. Median progression-free survival was 1,710 days in one study, with an overall MST of 3,076 days.
- Photodynamic therapy.

References

Gill VL, Bergman PJ, Baer KE *et al.* (2008) Use of imiquimod 5% cream (Aldara) in cats with multicentric squamous cell carcinoma in situ: 12 cases (2002–2005). *Vet Comp Oncol* 6:55–64.

Goodfellow M, Hayes A, Murphy S *et al.* (2006) A retrospective study of (90) strontium plesiotherapy for feline squamous cell carcinoma of the nasal planum. *J Feline Med Surg* 8:169–176.

Hammond GM, Gordon IK, Theon AP *et al.* (2007) Evaluation of strontium Sr 90 for the treatment of superficial squamous cell carcinoma of the nasal planum in cats: 49 cases (1990–2006). *J Am Vet Med Assoc* 231:736–741.

Theon AP, Madewell BR, Shearn VI *et al.* (1995) Prognostic factors associated with radiotherapy of squamous cell carcinoma of the nasal plane in cats. *J Am Vet Med Assoc* 206:991–996.

CASE 94

1 What is the primary differential diagnosis for the findings on liver ultrasound? There are multiple hypoechoic lesions throughout the liver appearing to be cystic. Given the patient's breed, congenital hepatic cysts are likely. However, neoplasia cannot be entirely ruled out without a biopsy.

2 What is a possible cause of the azotemia and how should this be evaluated? The presence of hepatic cysts in a Persian cat is often associated with polycystic kidney disease (PKD). PKD is inherited in an autosomal dominant fashion in Persians and related breeds. Ultrasound of the kidneys should be performed in this patient given the breed, azotemia, and finding of multiple hepatic cysts.

3 What treatment should be considered? Unfortunately, there is no specific treatment for polycystic liver and kidney disease. The cysts are present at birth, but are typically undetectable until later in life when, after slow growth over years, hepatic or renal function is compromised. Larger or solitary liver cysts can be drained or surgically removed to palliate clinical symptoms. Treatment of PKD consists of medical management of renal failure.

References
Bosje JT, van den Ingh TS, van der Linde-Sipman JS (1998) Polycystic kidney and liver disease in cats. *Vet Q* 20:136–139.

Eaton KA, Biller DS, DiBartola SP *et al.* (1997) Autosomal dominant polycystic kidney disease in Persian and Persian-cross cats. *Vet Pathol* **34**:117–126.

Wills SJ, Barrett EL, Barr FJ *et al.* (2009) Evaluation of the repeatability of ultrasound scanning for detection of feline polycystic kidney disease. *J Feline Med Surg* **11**:993–996.

CASE 95

1 Describe the lesions noted in the ear. There are multiple cystic lesions, blue in color, occluding the ear canal.

2 What are the primary differential diagnoses for this cat's lesions? Ceruminous gland cysts or adenomas are most likely. Less common is ceruminous gland adenocarcinoma.

3 In addition to the MDB, what testing should be done to determine the course of treatment? Because this patient has failed medical management, a biopsy is advised. Regional lymph nodes should be evaluated if enlarged.

4 If these lesions are malignant, what treatment is recommended and what is this cat's prognosis? CT or MRI is used to determine whether the bulla is involved and whether disease extends beyond the bulla. Ear canal ablation with lateral bulla osteotomy is the surgical treatment recommended for ceruminous gland adenocarcinoma. Median survival times of patients treated with TECABO procedures (total ear canal ablation and bulla osteotomy) are 42 months, compared with only 10 months for patients undergoing more conservative lateral ear canal resection. Radiation therapy is reserved for patients whose disease extends beyond the ear canal and bulla. Reported median progression-free survival time with radiation therapy approaches 40 months.

Reference
Marino DJ, MacDonald JM, Matthiesen DT *et al.* (1994) Results of surgery in cats with ceruminous gland adenocarcinoma. *J Am Anim Hosp Assoc* **30**:54–58.

CASE 96

1 Describe the radiographs (96a, b) and give a clinical diagnosis. The heart shadow is enlarged and globoid in shape, suggestive of pericardial effusion.

2 What are the most common causes for the radiographic findings? The most common causes of pericardial effusion are neoplasia (e.g. hemangiosarcoma, mesothelioma, heart base tumor) and idiopathic pericardial effusion.

3 What further diagnostic tests are indicated? In addition to an MDB, abdominal ultrasound and echocardiography should be performed. A pericardiocentesis is recommended to help alleviate clinical symptoms. The lack of cancer cells seen on cytology, however, does not rule out a tumor because they do not exfoliate well into the pericardial fluid.

4 What is the likelihood of making a diagnosis based on the tests performed (listed in 3). What further non-invasive tests could be performed to help make a diagnosis? The sensitivity and specificity of echocardiography in finding a cardiac mass are 80% and 100%, respectively. The lack of visualization of a mass does not rule it out, however. Serum cardiac troponin I levels >0.1 ng/ml have been reported to be highly suggestive of hemangiosarcoma; however, cardiac troponin I is also elevated in dogs and cats with azotemic renal failure and non-cardiac systemic disease. Definitive diagnosis requires thoracotomy and biopsy. On echocardiography, a right atrial mass was found in this patient.

5 What therapy is advised? Pericardectomy is the treatment of choice for benign tumors or for idiopathic pericardial effusion. At the time of surgery, a biopsy can be obtained. For hemangiosarcoma, pericardectomy followed by doxorubicin chemotherapy is recommended. The MST for patients undergoing surgical resection of their right atrial HSA followed by doxorubicin chemotherapy was 175 days in one study. Patients not treated surgically but given doxorubicin were reported to have an MST of 139.5 days. Non-HSA heart base masses treated with pericardectomy have an MST of 730 days, vs. 42 days if no surgery is performed.

References
Ghaffari S, Pelio DC, Lange AJ *et al.* (2014) A retrospective evaluation of doxorubicin-based chemotherapy for dogs with right atrial masses and pericardial effusion. *J Small Anim Pract* 55:254–257.

MacDonald KA, Cagney O, Magne ML (2009) Echocardiographic and clinicopathologic characterization of pericardial effusion in dogs: 107 cases (1985–2006). *J Am Vet Med Assoc* 235:1456–1461.

Porciello F, Rishniw M, Herndon WE *et al.* (2008) Cardiac troponin I is elevated in dogs and cats with azotaemia renal failure and in dogs with non-cardiac systemic disease. *Aust Vet J* 86:390–394.

Shaw SP, Rozanski EA, Rush JE (2004) Cardiac troponins I and T in dogs with pericardial effusion. *J Vet Intern Med* 18:322–324.

Weisse C, Soares N, Beal MW *et al.* (2005) Survival times in dogs with right atrial hemangiosarcoma treated by means of surgical resection with or without adjuvant chemotherapy: 23 cases (1986–2000). *J Am Vet Med Assoc* 226:575–579.

Yamamoto S, Hoshi K, Hirakawa A *et al.* (2013) Epidemiological, clinical and pathological features of primary cardiac hemangiosarcoma in dogs: a review of 51 cases. *J Vet Med Sci* 75:1433–1441.

CASE 97

1 What does this picture suggest? The third eyelid is enlarged, pink, and appears to have a relatively smooth surface. Although it grossly appears to be an extreme prolapse of the tear gland of the third eyelid ("cherry eye"), the age of the patient makes this unlikely. Therefore, a tumor of the third eyelid is likely.

2 What is the recommended work-up for this patient?
- Evaluation of the regional lymph nodes.
- The third eyelid should be carefully examined by everting the lid and looking at the posterior surface as well as palpation using a lubricant to determine extent of attachment to the globe and underlying structures.
- Fluorescein stain.
- MDB to include thoracic radiographs.
- Orbital ultrasound, CT, and MRI are indicated if the tumor appears to be invasive beyond the third eyelid.
- For larger masses, a fine needle aspirate or incisional biopsy can aid in treatment planning. For smaller masses, excisional biopsy is recommended.

3 What are the differential diagnoses for this patient? Adenocarcinoma of the gland of the third eyelid is the most common conjunctival tumor in dogs, often appearing like the mass in the picture. Squamous cell carcinomas can occur but tend to have a more roughened, irregular surface than the mass shown here. Other considerations include mast cell tumor and lymphoma. Melanomas and hemangiosarcomas are also seen arising from the nictitans. In a recent retrospective study of 145 cases of third eyelid gland neoplasms of dogs (n = 127) and cats (n = 18), 85% of canine tumors were adenocarcinomas, 14.2% adenomas, and 0.8% squamous cell carcinomas. Non-malignant disorders include nodular granulomatosis and other inflammatory conditions. Cherry eye is highly unlikely given the patient's age.

4 What therapy is indicated? The treatment of choice for tumors confined to the third eyelid is surgical removal of the nictitans. This patient underwent successful surgical removal of the tumor and adenocarcinoma was diagnosed. Recurrence is common if the entire gland is not removed. Metastasis to the lymph nodes and orbit can also occur. If the mass extends beyond the nictitans, extent of disease should be confirmed with further imaging as described above. CT or MRI can help determine the type of surgery necessary to ensure adequate margins. For those whose disease is not surgical, radiation therapy can be considered.

Reference
Dees DD, Schobert CS, Dubielzig RR *et al.* (2015) Third eyelid gland neoplasms of dogs and cats: a retrospective histopathologic study of 145 cases. *Vet Ophthalmol* doi:10.1111/vop.12273.

CASE 98

1 What staging tests are indicated for this patient? In addition to the MDB, abdominal ultrasound is indicated. ASGAC has a high rate of metastasis to the sublumbar lymph nodes. In this case, the abdominal ultrasound was normal.

2 Surgical removal was accomplished to relieve obstructive symptoms; however, as expected given the large size of the tumor, margins showed tumor cells still present. What adjunctive therapy should be considered postoperatively and what is this patient's prognosis? Definitive therapy includes radiation to treat the localized disease and chemotherapy to control distant disease. The longest median survival times appear to be associated with multi-modality therapy using surgery, chemotherapy, and RT.

3 What side effect can be expected with postoperative therapy? Radiation therapy is associated with acute side effects (those that occur during or shortly after the completion of radiation) and late side effects (those that occur months to years after the completion of radiation). Acute side effects to the tissues in the treatment field can include hair loss, inflammation of mucous membranes and skin (including moist desquamation in more severe cases), and infection. Late side effects, although uncommon, can include fibrosis and anorectal stricture. In one study of 27 patients undergoing RT for AGASAC, 33% developed complications, including moist desquamation, tumor abscessation, and anorectal strictures. In another study of 15 dogs undergoing RT, 100% developed scooting/irritation, 80% tenesmus (in 20% it was persistent), 13% anorectal stricture, and 13% developed fecal incontinence.

References

Arthur JJ, Kleiter MM, Thrall DE *et al.* (2008) Characterization of normal tissue complications in 51 dogs undergoing definitive pelvic region irradiation. *Vet Radiol Ultrasound* 49:85–89.

Turek MM, Forrest LJ, Adams WM *et al.* (2003) Postoperative radiotherapy and mitoxantrone for anal sac adenocarcinoma in the dog: 15 cases (1991–2001). *Vet Comp Oncol* 1:94–104.

Williams LE, Gliatto JM, Dodge RK *et al.* (2003) Carcinoma of the apocrine glands of the anal sac in dogs: 113 cases (1985–1995). *J Am Vet Med Assoc* 223:825–831.

CASE 99

1 What staging tests should be performed? Despite the lower-grade nature of this tumor, thoracic radiographs and careful evaluation of the regional lymph nodes are recommended. Mitotic index, Ki67, and nuclear atypia have been reported to be strong indicators of biologic behavior in melanomas; a mitotic index of <4, Ki67 value of <19.5, and nuclear atypia score of <4 are associated with more benign behavior.

2 What further treatment is indicated? Curative-intent surgery has the greatest chance for a favorable outcome. In patients with stage I disease, MSTs are reported to be 874 days with surgery alone. Adjunct therapy is not advised.

3 How does the location of this lesion affect its biologic behavior? Melanomas arising from haired skin tend to have a more benign clinical course. When intraoral, their behavior is aggressive. When on the lip, however, a greater percentage of melanomas may behave in a lower-grade fashion. Because some lip melanomas can also be associated with a more aggressive clinical course, careful staging and assessment of histopathology are necessary.

References

Bergin IL, Smedley RC, Esplin DG *et al.* (2011) Prognostic evaluation of Ki67 threshold value in canine oral melanoma. *Vet Pathol* 48:41–53.

Boston SE, Lu X, Culp WTN *et al.* (2014) Efficacy of systemic adjuvant therapies administered to dogs after excision of oral malignant melanomas: 151 cases (2001–2012). *J Am Vet Med Assoc* 245:401–407.

Tuohy JL, Selmic LE, Worley DR *et al.* (2014) Outcome following curative-intent surgery for oral melanoma in dogs: 70 cases (1998–2011). *J Am Vet Med Assoc* 245:1266–1273.

CASE 100

1 What are the differential diagnoses for this patient? The clinical signs of pain in the jaw, inability to retropulse the eye normally into the socket, and the elevation in the third eyelid are suggestive of retrobulbar disease. The two primary considerations are abscess/infection and neoplasia.

2 What further diagnostics should be performed? Following an MDB, a CT scan should be performed. If a space-occupying lesion is identified on CT, it must be determined whether it is malignant or infectious. The CT can be used to evaluate tissue density in order to help with this distinction. If solid tissue is present, a biopsy should be performed at the time of the CT. If the lesion is consistent with an abscess or infection, it needs to be drained and cultured.

3 A CT image (100b) and cytology from a fine needle aspirate (100c) obtained at the time of the CT scan are shown. What is the diagnosis? The cytology is consistent with sarcoma. Histopathology will be necessary to determine the type and grade of sarcoma present.

4 Describe treatment options for this patient. Given the extent and location of disease, a clean surgical excision, even with enucleation, is not likely to result. Treatment options include surgical cytoreduction with radiation therapy to follow or RT alone. For patients with oral sarcomas treated with postoperative RT, MSTs were reported to be 540 days in one study. In another report, dogs treated for macroscopic canine oral soft tissue sarcoma that underwent curative-intent (full course) RT had an MST of 331 days, whereas dogs treated with palliative RT had an MST of 180 days. If the biopsy reveals a higher-grade sarcoma, chemotherapy could be considered, although data regarding the efficacy of chemotherapy are lacking for this type of tumor.

References

Forrest LJ, Chun R, Adams WM *et al.* (2000) Postoperative radiotherapy for canine soft tissue sarcoma. *J Vet Intern Med* **14**:578–582.

Poirier VJ, Bley CR, Roos M *et al.* (2006) Efficacy of radiation therapy for the treatment of macroscopic canine oral soft tissue sarcoma. *In Vivo* **20**:415–420.

CASE 101

1 What is the clinical syndrome shown in the picture of this patient? Pre-caval syndrome is present in this dog. Enlarged lymph nodes or a mass within the cranial thoracic cavity can obstruct lymphatic flow, resulting in diffuse swelling of the face, neck, and forelimbs.

2 Describe the ultrasound and cytology findings. The ultrasound picture of the spleen shows diffuse mottling of the splenic parenchyma. The cytology is characterized by a predominant population of lymphoblasts (all significantly larger than the segmented neutrophil present) with multiple prominent nucleoli exhibiting anisonucleosis. There are free nuclei and cytoplasmic fragments seen. These findings are supportive of lymphoma.

3 **What significant abnormality is noted in the blood work and how does this impact the patient's treatment and prognosis? What further testing is indicated before treatment is initiated?** An elevated white blood cell count is noted. A blood smear indicated a mature neutrophilia. There is significant hypercalcemia. The hypercalcaemia, in combination with the pre-caval syndrome, raises concern for T cell lymphoma. Given the possibility of a thoracic or mediastinal mass, thoracic radiography should be performed. Phenotyping (T vs. B cell) should be performed (immunohistochemistry, immunocytochemistry, PARR, or flow cytometry). T cell lymphoma has been shown to have a more aggressive clinical course in some patients. A urinalysis should be performed to determine whether the elevation in BUN indicates more than dehydration.

4 **How should this patient be managed?** The finding of pre-caval syndrome and extreme hypercalcemia constitutes a medical emergency. Hypercalcemia can cause renal failure, therefore treatment for lymphoma should not be delayed while waiting for biopsy or phenotyping results. Fluid diuresis with saline should be immediately instituted followed by initiation of chemotherapy. Radiation therapy can also be considered for rapid alleviation of symptoms caused by the pre-caval syndrome.

References

Avery AC, Olver C, Khanna C *et al.* (2013) Molecular diagnostics. In: Withrow SJ, Vail DM, Page RL, editors, *Small Animal Clinical Oncology*, 5th edition. St. Louis, Elsevier Saunders, pp. 131–142.

Friedrichs KR, Young KM (2013) Diagnostic cytopathology in clinical oncology. In: Withrow SJ, Vail DM, Page RL, editors, *Small Animal Clinical Oncology*, 5th edition. St. Louis, Elsevier Saunders, pp. 127–128.

Vail DM, Pinkerton ME, Young KM (2013) Canine lymphoma and lymphoid leukemias. In: Withrow SJ, Vail DM, Page RL, editors, *Small Animal Clinical Oncology*, 5th edition. St. Louis, Elsevier Saunders, pp. 608–637.

CASE 102

1 **What further diagnostic tests are indicated?** Prior to CT, an abdominal ultrasound should be performed to rule out another primary tumor site in the event that this lesion is not related to the OSA. If the ultrasound is negative, a CT scan should be performed to evaluate the full extent of disease in the lungs. A whole body technetium bone scan or PET/CT scan is strongly recommended to rule out skeletal metastatic disease prior to consideration of any surgical intervention.

2 **Are there any surgical options available for this patient?** The CT scan documented that there was only one lesion in the lungs. The mass in the lung could represent metastatic disease from the OSA or could possibly be a primary lung tumor.

Surgery was advised. Prognosis is dependent on the histopathology of the lesion. In this case, metastatic OSA was documented. Resection of pulmonary metastases in dogs with OSA can be considered; however, to give the best chance for longer-term survival, certain criteria have been suggested for patient selection:

- The primary tumor is in complete remission and metastasis has developed >300 days after the initial primary tumor was diagnosed.
- One or two nodules are visible on plain thoracic radiographs.
- Metastatic disease is only found in the lung (use a bone scan as described above to rule out bone metastasis).
- Ideally, a tumor doubling time of >30 days is seen with no new visible lesions within this time frame. Following the identification of a lung lesion, repeat radiographs in 30 days would help determine approximate tumor doubling time. Doubling times of <30 days have been associated with a poorer prognosis.

3 What is the prognosis for this patient if this is metastatic disease? Median disease-free intervals following metastatectomy for OSA were 176 days in a series of 36 patients (range, 20–1,495 days). This patient presented 5 months after metastatectomy for issues related to suspected arthritis. Further spread of cancer could not be documented radiographically, but a recommended CT scan or MRI was not pursued. The lungs remained clear on radiographs at that time. Owing to increasing difficulty in ambulating, the patient was euthanized.

References

Ehrhart NP, Ryan SD, Fan TM (2013) Tumors of the skeletal system. In: Withrow SJ, Vail DM, Page RL, editors, *Small Animal Clinical Oncology*, 5th edition. St. Louis, Elsevier Saunders, p. 486.

O'Brien MG, Straw RC, Withrow SJ *et al.* (1993) Resection of pulmonary metastases in canine osteosarcoma: 36 cases (1983–1992). *Vet Surg* **22**:105–109.

CASE 103

1 What recommendations should be made to this pet's owner? A CT scan could be performed to better determine the origin of the mass. An asymptomatic liver mass could be consistent with hepatoma or low-grade hepatocellular carcinoma. An asymptomatic stomach wall mass is unusual, but has the potential to carry a more guarded prognosis. Exploratory surgery is recommended because a diagnosis cannot be made on the basis of ultrasound appearance and an inconclusive aspirate.

2 Based on the dog's age and the appearance of this mass on ultrasound, cancer was suspected. What are other considerations? An abscess or granuloma secondary to previous foreign body and/or perforation of the stomach wall is possible, but seems unlikely owing to the lack of fever and a normal CBC. This patient was taken to surgery and a large mass removed that was arising from the stomach wall (**103b**). Histopathology confirmed that the mass was a granuloma, secondary to a previous migrating foreign body. This case illustrates the importance of not making conclusions without the benefit of a histopathologic diagnosis. It would have been very easy to assume cancer and

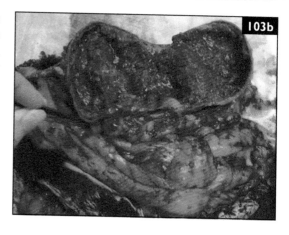

lead the owner into a decision not to pursue therapy based on a suspected poor prognosis. This patient is alive and well 4 years post-surgery.

CASE 104

1 The blue arrows outline the mass. What does the red arrow point to? The red arrow is pointing to the os penis.

2 What treatment is recommended? Despite the concern that the mass was firmly fixed to underlying tissues on palpation, it appeared separated from the body wall by a layer of fat or fascia on CT. However, it does appear closely associated with the prepuce and penis. Surgical excision with a penile amputation and perineal urethrostomy was performed. The margins were narrow (<2 mm) but clean. There were 2 mitotic figures per 10 hpf. Postoperative radiation therapy or metronomic chemotherapy could be considered because the margins were narrow. However, based on the low-grade nature of the tumor, close monitoring was advised.

3 What is the prognosis for this patient? Patients with histologically low-grade soft tissue sarcomas with a mitotic index of <9 had recurrence rates of approximately 7% even when tumors were narrowly excised. Metastatic rates for patients in this category ranged from 7 to 13% depending on the study referenced. Median survival time for dogs with low-grade STS (mitotic index <9) treated with surgery alone was 826–1138 days in one study.

References

Dennis MM, McSporran KD, Bacon NJ et al. (2011) Prognostic factors for cutaneous and subcutaneous soft tissue sarcomas in dogs. Vet Pathol **48**:73–84.

Kuntz CA, Dernell WS, Powers BE et al. (1997) Prognostic factors for surgical treatment of soft-tissue sarcomas in dogs: 75 cases (1986–1996). J Am Vet Med Assoc **211**:1147–1151.

CASE 105

1 Describe the cytology and give a presumptive diagnosis. There is a large cluster of epithelial cells exhibiting mild anisocytosis and anisokaryosis. The cytoplasm is angular in nature as seen in normal squamous epithelial cells; however, based on the size of the cells, the nuclei should be far more pyknotic. This is termed asynchronous nuclear to cytoplasmic differentiation and is a feature of squamous cell carcinoma.

2 What is the recommended staging for this patient and the likelihood of metastasis? The regional lymph nodes should be carefully evaluated. The incidence of metastatic disease is very low, but prior to any aggressive therapy, an MDB is recommended.

3 What therapeutic options are available? Given the location and the degree of invasion along the lower eyelid, surgical excision presents the challenge of obtaining clean margins while preserving function of the eyelid. A surgical procedure for the lower eyelid has been described where the lower eyelid is removed and replaced with lip tissue as a rotational graft. Non-surgical options for treatment are similar to those for nasal planum SCC in cats and can include external beam radiation therapy, strontium 90 plesiotherapy, cryotherapy, or photodynamic therapy. COX-2 inhibitors may be beneficial.

References

Bardagi M, Fondevila D, Ferrer L (2012) Immunohistochemical detection of COX-2 in feline and canine actinic keratoses and cutaneous squamous cell carcinoma. *J Comp Pathol* 146:11–17.

Cunha CSS, Carvalho LAV, Canary PC *et al.* (2010) Radiation therapy for feline cutaneous squamous cell carcinoma using a hypofractionated protocol. *J Feline Med Surg* 12:306–313.

Murphy S (2013) Cutaneous squamous cell carcinoma in the cat. Current understanding and treatment approaches. *J Feline Med Surg* 15:401–407.

CASE 106

1 Describe the CT findings. There is a soft tissue density, primarily in the right nasal cavity, causing destruction of the normal turbinate pattern. There also appears to be a small amount of abnormal tissue density on the left side.

2 What clinical signs are most commonly associated with nasal neoplasia? Cardinal signs of nasal neoplasia include epistaxis (beginning unilaterally and then progressing to bilateral), facial deformity (nasofrontal or palate abnormality), and epiphora. As the disease progresses, dyspnea from upper airway obstruction and exophthalmos can also be seen.

3 How should this patient be evaluated prior to biopsy? In addition to the MDB, aspiration and cytology of any enlarged regional nodes and a coagulation profile should be performed.

4 What procedures can be used for biopsy? Many nasal biopsy procedures have been described with varying degrees of success. Obtaining tissue through the nasal passage using a cup forceps or through a rhinoscopy using biopsy forceps is common. Blind biopsy techniques, advanced imaging-guided biopsy, and nasal hydropulsion are other techniques that have been evaluated. Second biopsies are often required to make a definitive diagnosis. Regardless of the type of procedure used, care needs to be taken not to approach the cribriform plate. In patients where there is significant facial deformity, a fine needle aspirate can sometimes be used to make a presumptive diagnosis. If a diagnosis cannot be obtained through transnostril techniques, a ventral rhinotomy can be utilized to obtain a tissue diagnosis. Patients with large tumor volumes have immediate symptom relief from this procedure.

5 What is the recommended treatment for this patient and the expected prognosis? Radiation therapy is considered the treatment of choice for nasal tumors. In general, the median survival times reported range from 14 to 19 months. The longest MSTs of 47 months were reported in a small number of dogs treated with curative intent RT followed by nasal cavity exenteration when residual tumor was noted at the time of recheck CT. Without treatment, MSTs are approximately 3 months.

References

Adams WM, Biorling DE, McAnulty JE et al. (2005) Outcome of accelerated radiotherapy alone or accelerated radiotherapy followed by exenteration of the nasal cavity in dogs with intranasal neoplasia: 53 cases (1990–2002). J Am Vet Med Assoc 227:936–941.

Ashbaugh EA, McKiernan BC, Miller CJ et al. (2011) Nasal hydropulsion: a novel tumor biopsy technique. J Am Anim Hosp Assoc 47:312–316.

Elliot KM, Mayer MN (2009) Radiation therapy for tumors of the nasal cavity and paranasal sinuses in dogs. Can Vet J 50:309–312.

Harris BJ, Lourenco BN, Dobson JM et al. (2014) Diagnostic accuracy of three biopsy techniques in 117 dogs with intra-nasal neoplasia. J Small Anim Pract 55:219–224.

Turek MM, Lana SE (2013) Canine nasosinal tumors. In: Withrow SJ, Vail DM, Page RL, editors, Small Animal Clinical Oncology, 5th edition. St. Louis, Elsevier Saunders, pp. 435–451.

CASE 107

1 Describe the cytologic findings. There is a predominant population of lymphocytes that are larger than neutrophils, with prominent and often large and irregular nucleoli. The cytology is suggestive of a high grade lymphoma.

2 Based on the presumptive diagnosis, what further diagnostics are indicated? In addition to the MDB described above, an abdominal ultrasound for staging should be performed. A tissue biopsy is needed for histologic confirmation and phenotyping.

3 **What treatment is advised?** The unusual finding of lymphoma as a primary tumor in the hock or carpus has been described and it is believed to behave in an aggressive manner. A recent study evaluated cats with cutaneous lymphoma of the tarsus. Tarsal lesions were most commonly described as subcutaneous or "mass-like". Patients were treated with either steroids alone (group 1), chemotherapy alone (group 2), a combination of radiation therapy and chemotherapy (group 3), or surgery with or without chemotherapy (group 4). The MST for all cats in the study was 190 days (range, 17–1,011). Group 1 had only two cats (surviving 22 days and 190 days), the MST for group 2 was 136 days, MST for group 3 was 216 days, and MST for group 4 was 410 days. There was no statistically significant difference between the treatment groups when compared individually; however, when the combined data from groups 1 and 2 was compared with the combined data from groups 3 and 4, the latter two groups had significantly improved survival times. An optimal treatment for tarsal lymphomas is not yet known. Chemotherapy should be considered for patients whose disease is found beyond the primary site. For localized disease, surgery (i.e. amputation) or RT +/- chemotherapy is recommended. In patients presented with disease confirmed to be localized to the hock area, amputation could provide excellent control.

Reference
Burr HD, Keating JH, Clifford CA *et al.* (2014) Cutaneous lymphoma of the tarsus in cats: 23 cases (2000–2012). *J Am Vet Med Assoc* **244**:1429–1434.

CASE 108

1 **List the differential diagnoses for this clinical presentation.** *Neoplastic*: most common are Sertoli cell tumor, interstitial cell tumor (Leydig cell tumor), and seminomas. *Non-neoplastic*: orchitis, testicular torsion, and epididymitis.
2 **Which of the common testicular tumors in dogs produce estrogen and what are the clinical manifestations of excess estrogen production?** Sertoli cell tumors produce estrogen in >50% of cases diagnosed. Feminization syndrome (bilateral symmetric alopecia and hyperpigmentation, gynecomastia, atrophy of the penis, pendulous prepuce) or pancytopenia can be seen as a result of the excess estrogen production.
3 **Based on the photograph alone, is this mass more likely to be malignant or benign?** Because the mass is present within a normally descended testicle, it is more likely to be benign. Sertoli cell tumors and seminomas are more likely to develop in patients with undescended testicles. Both interstitial cell tumors and seminomas tend to be incidental findings.
4 **What diagnostic tests are indicated for this patient and why?** An MDB and abdominal and testicular ultrasound should be performed. Hematologic

abnormalities that can be seen with hyperestrogenism are evaluated with the CBC. Although the metastatic rate of all three common testicular tumors tends to be low (<15%), thoracic radiographs and abdominal ultrasound are still indicated to rule out the presence of other malignancies or comorbidities, because the majority of patients with testicular tumors tend to be older. Testicular ultrasound is helpful in differentiating non-neoplastic processes from neoplastic ones, but is usually not able to differentiate among tumor types.

5 What are the treatment options? Surgery (castration/scrotal ablation) is the treatment of choice and is generally associated with an excellent outcome. This patient was diagnosed with a benign seminoma. Following surgery, no further treatment was indicated. In patients with metastatic tumors, treatment depends on the location of metastatic disease. For example, if regional lymph nodes are involved, radiation therapy can be considered. Chemotherapy is considered to be appropriate for more aggressive testicular tumors, but an optimal chemotherapeutic agent or protocol has not been established. Platinum-based protocols are used in humans with higher stages of disease, and cure rates are high.

References

Grieco V, Riccardi E, Greppi GF et al. (2008) Canine testicular tumours: a study on 232 dogs. *J Comp Pathol* **138**:86–89.

Johnston GR, Feeney DA, Johnston SD et al. (1991) Ultrasonographic features of testicular neoplasia in dogs: 16 cases (1980–1988). *J Am Vet Med Assoc* **198(10)**:1779–1784.

Liao AT, Chu PY, Yeh LS et al. (2009) A 12-year retrospective study of canine testicular tumors. *J Vet Med Sci* **71**:919–923.

CASE 109

1 Should an incisional biopsy or an excisional biopsy be performed and why? Given the location of the mass and the fact that it appears fixed to underlying tissues, it is unlikely that this is easily operable. Therefore, an incisional biopsy should be taken without attempting to do more aggressive surgery until a histologic diagnosis can be made.

2 How should this patient be further assessed? A CT scan is advised to determine the type of deep attachment present and to evaluate for bone invasion.

3 A new FNA was performed and again yielded fat, but scattered mesenchymal cells were also noted. What are the differential diagnoses? Lipoma, fibrolipoma, fibrosarcoma, or other soft tissue sarcoma is suspected. If bony changes are noted, tumors of the skull or orbital rim such as osteosarcoma, chondrosarcoma, or multilobular tumor of bone are possible.

4 How can this dog be treated? The incisional biopsy confirmed a fibrolipoma. The client declined a CT scan, so the patient was taken to surgery to have the

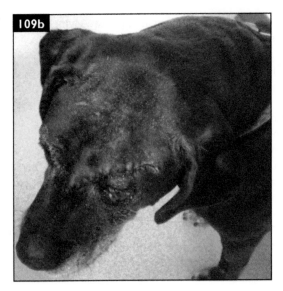

tumor debulked. Because of the long stable history and benign diagnosis, even if the tumor cannot be removed with clean surgical margins, vision could potentially be restored and quality of life improved for an extended period of time before regrowth is noted.

Follow up/discussion
Postoperatively, the patient was able to see normally from the affected eye. The tumor had not yet regrown at the last follow-up 8 months postoperatively (**109b**).

Reference
Liggett AD, Frazier KS, Styer EL (2002) Angiolipomatous tumors in dogs and a cat. *Vet Pathol* 39:286–289.

CASE 110

1 Describe the radiographic changes. There is significant osteolysis appearing to be localized within a section of the mandible and affecting the tooth roots and mandible. There are multiple punctate lesions present throughout the area of lysis. This pattern of lysis is often seen in multiple myeloma or in patients with localized plasma cell neoplasia.

2 A fine needle aspirate of the mass was taken. It yielded large pleomorphic round cells with occasional plasmacytoid differentiation. Based on the radiographic appearance and cytology, what further diagnostic tests are indicated before a treatment decision is made? Although not pathognomonic, the radiographic appearance and cytology raise strong suspicion for a solitary osseous plasmacytoma (SOP) or metastasis from systemic plasma cell neoplasia (i.e. multiple myeloma). The following diagnostic tests should be performed to rule out systemic disease:

- The physical examination should include a retinal examination to rule out hemorrhage.
- Careful staging is necessary to rule out systemic spread of disease. In addition to the MDB, bone survey radiographs looking for further lytic lesions or osteopenia are indicated.

- Bone marrow aspiration, serum and urine electrophoresis, and abdominal ultrasound should be performed, especially if serum globulin levels are increased.
- If there is no further evidence of disease beyond the mandible, a biopsy is indicated to obtain a definitive diagnosis.

3 The owner has declined mandibulectomy as a treatment option. What other therapy can be offered? Surgical removal through mandibulectomy offers the greatest chance of long-term control. Because this was declined, radiation therapy can be very effective in the treatment of SOP and can result in long-term control. Most patients with SOP eventually develop distant metastasis, but this can take months to years. Studies in humans have not shown any benefit to initiating chemotherapy prior to the onset of systemic spread.

Reference
Sternberg R, Wypij J, Barger AM (2009) Extramedullary and solitary osseous plasmacytomas in dogs and cats. *Vet Med* **104**:477–479.

CASE 111

1 What diagnostic tests should be performed? In addition to the MDB, a regional radiograph under anesthesia can determine bone changes and potentially rule out a tooth root abscess. A fine needle aspirate can give a presumptive diagnosis, but a tissue biopsy is preferred to obtain a definitive diagnosis. Careful evaluation of the regional lymph nodes with cytology or histopathology is indicated. Although regional radiographs are helpful in the preliminary evaluation, a CT scan is necessary to determine extent of involvement of the tumor, including nasal cavity or periorbitaol involvement, which is not uncommon in maxillary tumors.

2 List the most common tumors of the oral cavity in the dog. Melanoma, squamous cell carcinoma, and fibrosarcoma top the list of most common oral cavity tumors in dogs. Malignant tumors including, but not limited to, osteosarcoma, multilobular tumor of bone, chondrosarcoma, hemangiosarcoma, and lymphoma can also occur.

3 Based on the photograph, what parameters are visible that indicate that surgery is a consideration? Tumors that cross the midline on the palate are rarely surgical unless a palliative debulking procedure is considered. This tumor appears well away from the midline, indicating that this patient may be a good candidate for maxillectomy. Given the location of the tumor and the propensity for tumors in this region to be more invasive than can be observed on physical examination, CT is recommended for surgical planning.

4 This dog was diagnosed with an intermediate-grade fibrosarcoma. What treatment is indicated and what is the likelihood that this cancer will spread?

Treatment will ultimately depend on the CT results. If the tumor is localized, a maxillectomy should be performed. If margins are free of tumor with at least 1 cm of microscopically tumor-free margins, then surgery can be curative. When margins are narrow or have tumor cells still present, radiation therapy would be indicated. Chemotherapy is often used for higher-grade sarcomas, although several studies have failed to show a survival advantage for patients treated with chemotherapy postoperatively. No difference in survival time was noted between dogs with soft tissue sarcomas treated postoperatively with doxorubicin vs. those that underwent surgery alone. A survival advantage was also not appreciated for dogs treated with postoperative chemotherapy for oral fibrosarcomas. Oral fibrosarcomas tend to be locally invasive. Metastasis to the lungs or regional lymph nodes is seen in <30% of patients.

Reference

Gardner H, Fidel J, Haldorson G *et al.* (2013) Canine oral fibrosarcomas: a retrospective analysis of 65 cases (1998–2010). *Vet Comp Oncol* **13**:40–47.

CASE 112

1 What is the presumptive diagnosis? Lymphocytosis and thrombocytopenia are noted on the CBC. The peripheral blood smear shows a predominance of mature lymphocytes. The low platelet count was confirmed cytologically. Chronic lymphocytic leukemia should be considered.

2 What staging tests are indicated? In addition to the MDB, careful evaluation of peripheral lymph nodes and abdominal ultrasound are advised.

3 How is the definitive diagnosis made? In past years, bone marrow cytology was necessary to the make the diagnosis. In recent years, the use of flow cytometry for immunophenotyping has been shown to be a very effective method for diagnosing leukemia. This patient's flow cytometry revealed a CD8+ lymphocytosis. There are three major subtypes of chronic lymphocytic leukemia in dogs, in order of occurrence:

1 T-CLL: the majority of cells are CD8$^+$ granular lymphocytes
2 B-CLL: CD21+ or CD79+
3 Atypical CLL (combination of immunophenotypes).

4 Describe treatment options and prognosis for this patient. The initiation of chemotherapy in patients with CLL is largely dependent on several factors. First, if the patient were experiencing clinical symptoms such as lethargy, inappetence, or weight loss, treatment would be indicated regardless of the lymphocyte counts. If significant anemia or thrombocytopenia is present, treatment should also be initiated. However, in the absence of clinical symptoms or hematologic abnormalities beyond the lymphocytosis, the point at which chemotherapy should be initiated is somewhat controversial. Given the often indolent nature

Answers

of CLL, some oncologists advocate starting treatment only when absolute lymphocyte counts exceed 60,000/µl. Chlorambucil is considered the treatment of choice for canine CLL. In this patient, owing to the low platelet counts, initiating chemotherapy with vincristine and prednisone, followed by chlorambucil once platelet counts normalize, was recommended. Chlorambucil is given orally, in combination with prednisone. Survival times of >3 years can be seen in patients with uncomplicated CLL. The development of a blast crisis is associated with a poorer prognosis. In one study, dogs with CLL of the CD8+ immunophenotype had prolonged median survival times (1,098 days) when lymphocytes counts were <30,000/µl and 131 days if lymphocyte counts were >30,000/µl, although treatment information was limited. In a separate study, MST for atypical CLL was reported to be 22 days, for B-CLL 480 days, and for T-CLL 930 days.

References

Comazzi S, Gelain ME, Martini V *et al.* (2011) Immunophenotype predicts survival time in dogs with chronic lymphocytic leukemia. *J Vet Intern Med* **25**:100–106.
Williams MJ, Avery AC, Lana SE *et al.* (2008) Canine lymphoproliferative disease characterized by lymphocytosis: immunophenotypic markers of prognosis. *J Vet Intern Med* **22**:596–601.

CASE 113

1 Describe the radiograph shown and the procedure that was performed. The tumor bone was removed and replaced with a bone allograft (arrows in **113c** show proximal and distal ends of the allograft). A bone plate spans the repair and as a result the joint is immobilized. The surgery was performed at Colorado State University. This limb sparing procedure was well tolerated. In the patient's photograph, the stance is reflective of the carpal arthrodesis.

2 What was the probable diagnosis? Limb sparing procedures are generally used for osteosarcoma, but could be used for other types of primary bone tumor.

3 When is this procedure indicated? Limb sparing procedures can be used in

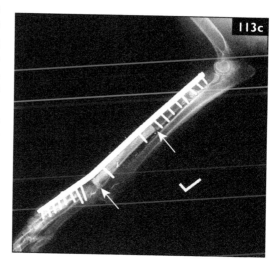

225

patients that have pre-existing orthopedic or neurologic problems that make them poor candidates for amputation, or in patients whose owners refuse to consider amputation. Distal radius and ulna sites are most amenable to limb sparing owing to preservation of good function following arthrodesis. Arthrodesis in other joints results in less favorable function. Allograft limb sparing (shown here) results in good to excellent function in at least 80% of patients. Complications include infection (40–50% infection rate reported), local recurrence of cancer, and implant failure. Other procedures include metal endoprosthesis limb sparing, ulna transposition limb sparing, pasteurized tumoral autograft, and longitudinal bone transport osteogenesis. There is no difference in survival times when these various procedures are combined with chemotherapy, but complications and morbidities differ.

4 How does the prognosis for this patient differ from that of patients undergoing amputation? The prognosis for patients undergoing limb sparing surgery and chemotherapy (cis-platin, carboplatin, doxorubicin, or combinations of cis-platin or carboplatin and doxorubicin) is similar to that of patients that undergo amputation and chemotherapy. Median survival times range from 230 to 366 days depending on the study cited. In a large series from Colorado State University, the 1-year recurrence-free survival rate was 76%. An interesting survival advantage was seen in patients whose allografts became infected. In fact, dogs that became infected were likely to live 250 days longer than those who did not experience infection in their allografts. Upregulation of antitumor immunity is a potential explanation for this occurrence.

References

Ehrhart NP, Ryan SD, Fan TM (2013) Tumors of the skeletal system. In: Withrow SJ, Vail DM, Page RL, editors, *Small Animal Clinical Oncology*, 5th edition. St. Louis, Elsevier Saunders, pp. 463–503.

Lascelles BD, Dernell WS, Correa MT *et al.* (2005) Improved survival associated with postoperative wound infection in dogs treated with limb-salvage surgery for osteosarcoma. *Ann Surg Oncol* **12**:1073–1083.

Liptak JM, Dernell WS, Ehrhart N *et al.* (2006) Cortical allograft and endoprosthesis for limb-sparing surgery in dogs with distal radial osteosarcoma: a prospective clinical comparison of two different limb-sparing techniques. *Vet Surg* **35**:518–533.

CASE 114

1 Describe the abnormality within the eye. There is a pigmented mass in the anterior uvea. It has slightly irregular "feathered" edges and is obstructing vision.

2 What recommendations can be made to the pet owner? Given the pigmented nature of the mass, this lesion is either a benign melanocytoma or a melanoma. The majority of intraocular melanomas in dogs are benign and most arise from the iris or ciliary body. Because of the low risk of spread (usually <4%), many oncologists and ophthalmologists will advise monitoring rather than immediately enucleating the eye. If, however, there are secondary complications such as glaucoma or severe uveitis, enucleation should be considered. Intraocular procedures (performed by a skilled ophthalmologist) are available that may potentially restore vision if a patient's melanoma is obstructing the ability to see. Even though this patient's vision is being affected by the tumor, her overall vision was poor to begin with because of the cataracts. A recommendation was made to monitor this patient for signs of increased intraocular pressure and development of severe inflammation, and only to enucleate if those occurred.

3 **What criteria are used to determine malignant behavior?** If a biopsy is performed, the mitotic index of the tumor cells appears to be the most important feature in determining biologic behavior of intraocular melanomas. The mitotic index is based on the number of mitotic figures observed in 10 hpf.
- An index of <2 is considered benign.
- An index of ≥4 with nuclear pleomorphism is considered malignant.

References

Grahn BH, Sandmeyer LS (2010) Diagnostic ophthalmology. *Can Vet J* **51**:105–106.
Wilcock BP, Peiffer RL (1986) Morphology and behavior of primary ocular melanomas in 91 dogs. *Vet Pathol* **23**:418–424.

CASE 115

1 **What are the differential diagnoses for this patient?** In this location, a tumor of the parotid salivary gland, an abscess, sialadenitis, lymphoma, or other metastatic neoplasia (submandibular lymph node involvement) are considerations.

2 **Cytology from a fine needle aspirate revealed the pictured cells (115b); what is your presumptive diagnosis?** A fine needle aspirate of the mass should be done first to attempt to differentiate benign from malignant disease. The cells pictured here are suggestive of carcinoma. The most likely diagnosis is salivary gland adenocarcinoma.

3 **What further diagnostics are indicated?** An MDB and fine needle aspirate of the regional lymph nodes should be performed next. If there is no further evidence of metastatic disease, a CT scan will help determine whether surgery is an option. At the time of the CT, a wedge or needle core biopsy is recommended to confirm the diagnosis. However, histologic grade has not been proven prognostic in cases of salivary gland adenocarcinoma.

4 **What treatment is recommended?** The treatment of choice for salivary gland adenocarcinomas is surgery. If the CT reveals a well-encapsulated mass, surgical excision should be considered. However, given the large size of the tumor in this

case, if there are indistinct borders on the CT, radiation therapy usually results in good local control. If radiation is successful at decreasing the tumor size, post-RT surgical excision may be possible.

5 What is this patient's prognosis? The prognosis for salivary gland adenocarcinoma is generally good. The metastatic rate to regional lymph nodes and lungs tends to be very low in dogs (<20% metastasizing to lymph nodes and <10% metastasizing to lungs). The MST for dogs diagnosed with salivary gland adenocarcinoma was 550 days in one study. Patients in this study were treated with a variety of modalities; however, surgery or surgery and RT was associated with a better outcome than surgery and chemotherapy. Another study reported an MST of only 74 days when surgical excision was used as the sole treatment modality. In the author's experience, good local control is achieved with surgery alone for smaller, encapsulated tumors where clean surgical margins are attained or with a combination of RT and surgery for larger tumors.

References

Hammer A, Getzy D, Ogilvie G *et al.* (2001) Salivary gland neoplasia in the dog and cat: survival times and prognostic factors. *J Am Anim Hosp Assoc* **37**:478–482.

Spangler WL, Culbertson MR (1991) Salivary gland disease in dogs and cats: 245 cases (1985–1988). *J Am Vet Med Assoc* **198**:465–469.

CASE 116

1 What are the differential diagnoses for this lesion? Benign processes can include ceruminous gland adenoma, sebaceous gland adenoma, polyps (although unlikely in this case based on appearance), and histiocytoma. The most common malignant tumors include ceruminous gland adenocarcinoma (most frequently diagnosed), undifferentiated carcinoma, squamous cell carcinoma, and less commonly round cell tumors, sarcomas, and melanoma.

2 In addition to the MDB, what diagnostic tests should precede treatment? Following the MDB and evaluation of mandibular lymph nodes, regional radiographs under anesthesia to evaluate the bulla for possible lysis are helpful if CT is not available, but a CT scan is the best way to evaluate for local extension of disease. A biopsy should be performed at the time of anesthesia for either of these procedures (radiography or CT).

3 What is the prognosis for this patient and how does the type of surgery performed affect the prognosis? The prognosis depends on the histologic diagnosis and extent of disease found on advanced imaging. In this case, a ceruminous gland adenocarcinoma was diagnosed. The CT scan showed that the tumor was invading throughout the vertical and horizontal canals and there was evidence of early lysis of the bulla. Studies have shown that patients treated with total ear canal ablation and lateral bulla osteotomy (TECABO) tend to have the best outcome. Patients that undergo lateral ear canal resection alone tend to experience recurrence of disease within 4 months of the original surgery, whereas patients undergoing TECABO do not tend to show recurrence, even when followed for an average of 3 years. Statistics for the use of radiation therapy for ceruminous gland adenocarcinoma are limited, but postoperative radiation was associated with a median progression-free survival time of 39.5 months in one report.

4 In addition to the presence of lymph node or lung metastasis, what are the negative prognostic indicators for this type of tumor? In dogs, extension of tumor into tissues surrounding the ear canal is associated with a more guarded prognosis. In addition to surgery, if disease is not confined to the ear canals and clean surgical margins are not achieved, postoperative radiation is recommended. Ideally, if the CT reveals disease extension outside of the ear canals, then RT could be used in the preoperative setting.

References
Moisan PG, Watson GL (1996) Ceruminous gland tumors in dogs and cats: a review of 124 cases. *J Am Anim Hosp Assoc* **32**:448–452.
Theon AP, Barthez PY, Madewell BR *et al.* (1994) Radiation therapy of ceruminous gland carcinomas in dogs and cats. *J Am Vet Med Assoc* **205**:566–569.

CASE 117

1 Describe the radiograph. Multiple, well-defined, "cannonball" lesions are present throughout all of the lung fields.

2 What are the differential diagnoses? The appearance of the lung lesions is most consistent with metastatic neoplasia from an extrapulmonary or intrapulmonary source. This pattern is often seen in cancers such as osteosarcoma, chondrosarcoma, or thyroid carcinoma, but can be seen with any neoplastic process. In additional to malignant disease, pulmonary lymphomatoid granulomatosis or fungal disease cannot be ruled out on the basis of radiographs alone.

3 What diagnostic tests should be performed? A thorough physical examination to include careful palpation of the neck for thyroid masses and an MDB should be performed. If no abnormalities are found on examination or on the MDB, survey radiographs of the appendicular and axial skeleton and abdominal ultrasound should be considered. A full body CT scan can be used to attempt to find a primary source for the lung disease. Ultrasound- or CT-guided fine needle aspiration of an accessible mass, surgical biopsy (although aggressive in the light of widespread metastasis), or biopsy during thoracoscopy can give a pretreatment diagnosis.

Answers

4 What is meant by "metastatic cancer of unknown primary" and how should it be treated? Metastatic cancer of unknown primary refers to a biopsy-proven malignancy without the identification of its primary tumor. In humans, metastatic carcinoma of unknown primary is the seventh most frequently occurring cancer and the fourth most common cause of cancer-related death. When possible, cytology or histopathology should be performed to determine the most appropriate course of therapy. Immunohistochemistry can often help in identifying a primary source. In the case of thyroid neoplasia, the use of thyroid transcription factor-1 IHC can be a useful diagnostic tool. With metastatic thyroid neoplasia, the prognosis can be more favorable, with patients having long survival times even in the face of lung metastasis. In order to determine prognosis and recommend an appropriate treatment course, knowledge of the type of cancer is critical. The most common metastatic cancers of unknown primary (with metastasis in the lungs) were fibrosarcoma, undifferentiated carcinoma, and undifferentiated · sarcoma in a recent retrospective study. Palliative therapy with broad-spectrum chemotherapy, tyrosine kinase inhibitors, and metronomic chemotherapy could be considered, but information is lacking on their efficacy. In general, for patients presenting with metastatic cancer with an unknown primary, survival times cited are approximately 30 days. A significant exception is metastatic thyroid cancer, because metastasis can be slow growing in nature and favorable survival times have been reported even in the face of the metastasis. In one study, patients that underwent radiation therapy for invasive thyroid tumors had an MST of 24 months and the presence of lung metastasis did not have a negative effect on survival.

References

Brearley MJ, Hayes AM, Murphy S (1999) Hypofractionated radiation therapy for invasive thyroid carcinoma in dogs: a retrospective analysis of survival. *J Small Anim Pract* 40:206–210.

Crews LJ, Feeney DA, Jessen CR *et al.* (2008) Radiographic findings in dogs with pulmonary blastomycosis: 125 cases (1989–2006). *J Am Vet Med Assoc* 232:215–221.

Rossi F, Aresu L, Vignoli M *et al.* (2013) Metastatic cancer of unknown primary in 21 dogs. *Vet Comp Oncol* 13:11–19.

CASE 118

1 Prior to the CT scan, what diagnostic tests should be performed? An MDB, coagulation profile (in the hope that a biopsy can be performed at the time of the CT scan), and a fine needle aspirate and cytology of the submandibular lymph node should be performed.

2 Describe the CT scan. There is a large, infiltrative mass obliterating the nasal cavity. The mass appears calcified throughout; it has destroyed the nasal septum and hard palate, and has broken into the frontal sinuses and periorbital tissues.

The right eye is being pushed laterally and dorsally by the mass. On further evaluation of the CT scan, there was lysis of the cribriform plate.

3 What is the clinical stage of disease? The WHO system for staging nasal tumors has not correlated well with clinical outcome. There are several staging systems that have been proposed, and the Adams or modified Adams staging system appears to be most helpful in predicting outcome (see below). This patient would be considered to have stage 4 disease based on the Adams staging system, owing to cribriform plate involvement.

4 A biopsy confirmed an undifferentiated carcinoma and cytology of the submandibular lymph node confirmed metastatic carcinoma. What are the negative prognostic indicators in this case? Negative prognostic indicators for dogs with nasal tumors have varied by the study cited, but include older age (>10 years), epistaxis, facial deformity, duration of clinical signs prior to diagnosis, advanced stage, cribriform plate involvement, failure to achieve resolution of clinical signs with treatment, and histologic type (worse are anaplastic carcinoma, undifferentiated carcinoma, and SCC). In this patient, the disease is locally extensive and invasive, there is metastasis to the submandibular lymph node, cribriform plate involvement (stage 4), and undifferentiated carcinoma cell type; all of these indicate a very poor prognosis. Dogs treated with radiation therapy that had evidence of cribriform plate extension had median survival times of <7 months.

Adams Staging System for Canine Nasosinal Neoplasia	
Stage 1	Involvement of one nasal passage, paranasal sinus, or frontal sinus with no bone involvement beyond the turbinates
Stage 2	Any bone involvement beyond turbinates, but no evidence of orbit/subcutaneous/submucosal masses
Stage 3	Orbit involved, or subcutaneous or submucosal mass
Stage 4	Extension into nasopharynx or osteolysis of cribriform plate.

MST for stages 1 and 2 with RT: 745 days; MST for stages 3 and 4: 315 days; MST for stage 4: approximately 200 days.

References
Adams WM, Kleiter MM, Thrall DE *et al.* (2009) Prognostic significance of tumor histology and computed tomographic staging for radiation treatment response of canine nasal tumors. *Vet Radiol Ultrasound* **50**:330–335.

Adams WM, Miller PE, Vail DM *et al.* (1998) An accelerated technique for irradiation of malignant canine nasal and paranasal sinus tumors. *Vet Radiol Ultrasound* **39**:475–481.

Kondo Y, Matsunaga S, Mochizuki M *et al.* (2008) Prognosis of canine patients with nasal tumors according to modified clinical stages based on computed tomography: a retrospective study. *J Vet Med Sci* **70**:207–212.

CASE 119

1 How should this patient be evaluated? In addition to a thorough physical examination and MDB, a digital vaginal examination followed by vaginoscopic examination should be performed. A contrast vaginourethrogram is often helpful in delineating extent of disease. Radiographs or ultrasound of the local area are usually not rewarding.

2 What information from the signalment helps in making a presumptive diagnosis? Because this is an older, intact female, the most likely diagnosis is a vaginal/perivulvar tumor. Tumors can occur within the vaginal lumen or arise from smooth muscle outside the vaginal lumen. Benign tumors are often pedunculated but can be non-pedunculated. The most common benign tumor of the vagina/vulvar area is a leiomyoma. Other benign tumors such as fibromas are also seen. Less commonly, malignant leiomyosarcomas can occur.

3 What further diagnostic tests are indicated? The majority of vaginal/vulvar tumors are benign, therefore pretreatment biopsies are not frequently performed. However, an MDB and abdominal ultrasound are still recommended before considering treatment to rule out comorbidities that may impact a treatment decision and to rule out metastasis from a potentially malignant vaginal tumor. In cases where the tumor has had a rapid clinical course and is non-pedunculated, malignancy should be ruled out through histopathology.

4 What is the recommended treatment and the prognosis for this patient? Surgical excision and ovariohysterectomy are advised. If tumors are pedunculated and intramural, they are often easily removed by transecting the pedicle. If non-pedunculated or extraluminal, partial or total vaginectomy with urethroplasty has been described and associated with an excellent outcome. Wide surgical excision is generally not needed as long as OHE is performed. If OHE is not performed, recurrence is more likely.

References

Herron MA (1983) Tumors of the canine genital system. *J Am Anim Hosp Assoc* **19**:981–994.

Nelissen P, White RAS (2012) Subtotal vaginectomy for management of extensive vagina disease in 11 dogs. *Vet Surg* **41**:495–500.

Thacher C, Bradley RL (1983) Vulvar and vaginal tumors in the dog: a retrospective study. *J Am Vet Med Assoc* **183**:690–692.

CASE 120

1 What could have been done differently at the time of the first surgery? Because this tumor was graded II with the Patnaik system (grade I, II, or III) histologically, further information was necessary to determine biologic behavior. Approximately 75% of canine mast cell tumors are graded II by this system and within that group a wide variation in biologic behavior is seen. Evaluation of the mitotic index as well as a mast cell tumor prognostic panel to include immunohistochemistry for c-KIT, AgNOR, and Ki67, and PCR to detect mutations in exon 8 or 11 would have added valuable information. With the narrow margins reported on the initial histopathology, further treatment could have been immediately recommended. A wider surgical excision, if possible, should have been performed. If further surgery was not considered possible, radiation therapy to the local site would have been another option. The biologic behavior of MCTs in the inguinal and perineal regions was previously believed to be more aggressive than that of similarly graded MCTs in other anatomic locations on the body. However, two large studies were performed that reported the biologic behavior to be similar to other anatomic locations. Many oncologists are still concerned about the behavior of MCTs in this location, but are more apt to rely on information gained from the prognostic panels, or at least the mitotic index, rather than relying on location alone. Evaluation of these parameters would have helped determine whether systemic therapy was necessary at that time and better defined the risk of not addressing the narrow margins.

2 What diagnostic tests are indicated in this patient? Full staging to include an MDB, abdominal ultrasound, and fine needle aspirate of the mass along the incision line as well as the mass palpated deep to that area should be performed. Given the history of confirmed MCT at the site and the erythema surrounding the tumor, pretreatment with diphenhydramine is advised before aspiration.

3 What is a potential tumor-related cause of the erythema noted? The local erythema is likely due to the tumor effects (release of vasoactive amines) on manipulation of the tumor; this phenomenon is referred to as "Darier's sign".

4 Describe treatment options for this patient. Based on the size of the mass, a complete surgical excision with wide margins would be difficult and would likely include a perineal urethrostomy. For this reason, knowledge of the current grade, staging results, mitotic index, proliferation analysis, and KIT status would be beneficial for treatment planning. A combination of treatment to include surgery, radiation therapy, and possibly systemic therapy will likely be necessary to treat this patient effectively. If a *c-KIT* mutation is present or the KIT staining pattern is 2 or 3, preoperative treatment with tyrosine kinase inhibitors may have a higher likelihood of helping to cytoreduce the tumor preoperatively. In the absence of *c-KIT* mutations, chemotherapy can be used.

References

Kiupel M, Webster JD, Kaneene JB *et al.* (2004) The use of KIT and tryptase expression patterns as prognostic tools for canine cutaneous mast cell tumors. *Vet Pathol* **41**:371–377.

Takeuchi Y, Fujino Y, Watanabe M *et al.* (2013) Validation of the prognostic value of histopathological grading or *c-kit* mutation in canine cutaneous mast cell tumours: a retrospective cohort study. *Vet J* **196**:492–498.

Webster JD (2015) Small molecule kinase inhibitors in veterinary oncology. *Vet J* **205**:122–123.

CASE 121

1 What is the presumptive clinical diagnosis? The clinical description and signalment of this dog suggest a benign perianal adenoma.

2 Describe the cytologic appearance. Cytologic evaluation of the aspirate reveals cohesive clusters of cells that are round to polygonal in shape. There is minimal anisocytosis or anisokaryosis. Perianal adenomas will typically have epithelial cells that are hepatoid in appearance. However, the differentiation between benign and malignant tumors can be a difficult distinction to make with cytology alone and therefore histopathology is recommended. An important reason to perform a fine needle aspirate is to rule out other, less common, malignancies that could occur in this region including lymphoma, mast cell tumor, SCC, TVT, to name a few.

3 If this dog had been neutered, how would that change the presumptive clinical diagnosis? Because perianal adenomas are considered to be sex hormone dependent, the presence of this mass on a neutered male would increase the suspicion for a malignant tumor (perianal adenocarcinoma).

4 What are the treatment recommendations and expected outcome? Surgical removal of perianal adenomas and castration are curative. However, if a tumor is large enough that conservative removal is difficult and risks disruption of the nerves of the anal sphincter, castration alone will result in gradual reduction in the size of the mass (this may take months), facilitating surgical removal when the tumor is smaller.

References

Turek MM, Withrow SJ (2013) Perianal tumors. In: Withrow SJ, Vail DM, Page RL, editors, *Small Animal Clinical Oncology*, 5th edition. St. Louis, Elsevier Saunders, pp. 423–431.
Vandis M, Knoll JS (2010) Canine circumanal gland adenoma: the cytologic clues. *Vet Med* 105:346–349.

CASE 122

1 Because the left submandibular lymph node is larger, is it safe to assume that the clinical symptoms 6 days after initiating chemotherapy are due to progressive lymphoma? No, this is not an assumption that can be made. All of the other lymph nodes have reduced significantly in size, indicating a partial remission. With the solitary lymph node having enlarged, the concern is that there is a resistant focus of cancer or, based on the fever and elevated white blood cell count, that the node has abscessed.

2 Should this patient be treated with chemotherapy today given the concern about progressive disease? Not without further diagnostics performed to rule out non-cancerous causes of the clinical symptoms.

3 A CBC was performed. What is the clinical assessment and what further diagnostics are indicated? The combination of fever and elevated white blood cell count can be seen with neoplasia, infection, or inflammation. A fine needle aspirate of the lymph node should be performed. On aspiration, pus was found with no evidence of lymphoma. The node was lanced, drained, and the patient placed on antibiotics (122). The fever resolved and within 5 days the patient was in complete remission. Lymph node abscessation due to rapid cancer cell death after chemotherapy can occur occasionally, especially in larger nodes that had already started to develop a necrotic center because of rapid growth of the cancer before treatment.

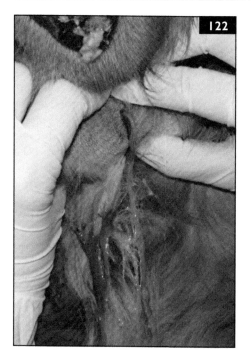

CASE 123

1 What diagnostic tests should be performed? Full staging, to include an MDB, abdominal ultrasound, and cytology from lymph node aspirates, is indicated. A tissue biopsy should be taken to determine grade and mitotic index. A mast cell tumor prognostic panel could also be requested.

2 What is known about mast cell tumors in the Shar Pei breed? The general impression among oncologists is that Shar Peis tend to have a greater percentage of biologically aggressive mast cell tumors, occurring commonly in younger patients. One study looked at cases of MCT in this breed and found that close to 50% of MCTs in the Shar Pei occurred in dogs <2 years of age; of these tumors, the majority were poorly differentiated. Biopsies are necessary to confirm mast cell neoplasia in the Shar-Pei because aspirates can be confusing in patients that have cutaneous mucinosis. Hyaluronic acid (HA) is a main component of mucin and CD44 is its major cell surface receptor. It appears that the binding of HA to its receptor CD44 may direct the terminal differentiation of mast cells in connective tissue, which could explain the Shar Pei's predilection for mast cell disease. The common finding of mast cells within mucin in the subcutaneous tissues of the

Shar Pei can make the differentiation between mucinosis and mast cell neoplasia more challenging with fine needle aspiration and cytology alone.

3 What treatment recommendations can be made? Based on the extremely invasive and aggressive nature of this lesion, surgery is not a consideration. If a *c-KIT* mutation exists or if the proliferation panel reveals a KIT pattern 2 or 3, tyrosine kinase inhibitors can be used. In the absence of these findings, chemotherapy should be considered. Radiation therapy, toceranib, and prednisone have shown efficacy for measurable mast cell tumors and could also be considered. Prednisone and an H1 blocker should be restarted. In addition, an H2 receptor antagonist blocker (e.g. cimetidine, famotidine, ranitidine) or proton pump inhibitor (e.g. omeprazole) to prevent gastric ulcers should also be used. With such a large, inflamed mass, degranulation as a result of treatment is a concern.

References

Carlsten KS, London CA, Haney S *et al.* (2012) Multicenter prospective trial of hypofractionated radiation treatment, toceranib, and prednisone for measurable canine mast cell tumors. *J Vet Intern Med* **26**:135-141.

Lopez A, Spracklin D, McConkey S *et al.* (1999) Cutaneous mucinosis and mastocytosis in a shar-pei. *Can Vet J* **40**:881–883.

Madewell BR, Akita GY, Vogel P (1992) Cutaneous mastocytosis and mucinosis with gross deformity in a Shar-pei dog. *Vet Dermatol* **3**:171–175.

Miller DM (1995) The occurrence of mast cell tumors in young Shar-Peis. *J Vet Diagn Invest* **7**:360–363.

Welle M, Grimm S, Suter M *et al.* (1999) Mast cell density and subtypes in the skin of Shar Pei dogs with cutaneous mucinosis. *Zentralbl Veterinarmed A* **46**:309–316.

CASE 124

1 Based on the evaluation thus far, what are the differential diagnoses? Based on the physical examination and aspirates, inflammation or seroma secondary to trauma, soft tissue sarcoma that is not exfoliating well, and lipoma (either infiltrative or intermuscular) are the most likely considerations.

2 A post-contrast CT scan of the hindlimbs is shown (124a). Describe the scan. The post-contrast image shows that the left limb is significantly larger than the right, due to a fat density infiltrating between the semitendinosus and semimembranosus muscles. Increased fat density between muscles of the left leg is seen (**124b**, arrow). These findings are most consistent with an intermuscular lipoma.

3 What treatments are advised and why? Intermuscular lipomas are benign but can cause significant compression of local structures as they grow and eventually lead to pain, lameness, and neurologic or vascular issues. Surgical resection is usually

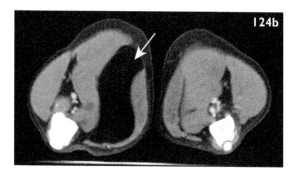

successful in curing intermuscular lipomas as they tend to be well circumscribed and can be removed even when large. Although surgical drains are typically discouraged when resecting malignant tumors, drains are necessary in this case to prevent seromas due to the large dead space that is created when the lipoma is removed.

References
Case JB, MacPhail CM, Withrow SJ (2012) Anatomic distribution and clinical findings of intermuscular lipomas in 17 dogs (2005–2010). *J Am Anim Hosp Assoc* 48:245–249.
Thomson MJ, Withrow SJ, Dernell WS *et al.* (1999) Intermuscular lipomas of the thigh region in dogs: 11 cases. *J Am Anim Hosp Assoc* 35:165–167.

CASE 125

1 Describe the character of the material obtained from FNA of the splenic mass. On cytology, malignant spindle cells with a proteinaceous background were observed. What is the likely diagnosis? The aspirate yielded a very thick, gelatinous mucoid material. Myxosarcoma is the most likely diagnosis.

2 What treatment is indicated? Surgical removal of the spleen and histopathologic evaluation of the tumor is advised. A diagnosis of myxosarcoma was confirmed.

3 What feature of the histopathology will help determine this patient's prognosis? The biologic behavior of non-lymphomatous non-angiomatous sarcomas most closely correlates with the mitotic index (MI). An MI of <9 was associated with an MST of approximately 9 months, whereas dogs whose MI was ≥9 had an MST of 1–2 months. There are no data regarding the efficacy of chemotherapy for this disease.

Reference
Spangler WL, Culbertson MR, Kass PH (1994) Primary mesenchymal (nonangiomatous/nonlymphomatous) neoplasms occurring in the canine spleen: anatomic classification, immunohistochemistry, and mitotic activity correlated with patient survival. *Vet Pathol* 31:37–47.

CASE 126

1 Describe the CT scan. There is a productive bone lesion at the caudal aspect of the mandible extending onto the vertical ramus. Although the lesion is primarily producing abnormal bone, there are areas of lysis within the mandible and vertical ramus of the mandible.

2 What are the differential diagnoses for this lesion? A primary bone tumor is likely, with multilobular tumor of bone, osteosarcoma, and chondrosarcoma the primary differentials.

3 A biopsy was performed, which confirmed multilobular tumor of bone. What important information from the histopathology is necessary in order to predict outcome? With complete surgical removal, what are the expectations for this patient? Histologic grade is an important predictor of outcome. In one study, the prognosis was highly dependent on the grade of the tumor, surgical margins, and tumor location, but it is generally excellent with complete excision. Patients with grade I tumors had MST of >897 days, grade II 520 days, and grade III 405 days. Mandibular sites and ability to achieve clean surgical margins were associated with a more favorable outcome.

References

Dernell WS, Straw RC, Cooper MF *et al*. (1998) Multilobular osteochondrosarcoma in 39 dogs: 1979–1993. *J Am Anim Hosp Assoc* **34**:11–18.

Hathcock JT, Newton JC (2000) Computed tomographic characteristics of multilobular tumor of bone involving the cranium in 7 dogs and zygomatic arch in 2 dogs. *Vet Radiol Ultrasound* **41**:214–217.

CASE 127

1 Describe the CT findings and possible diagnosis. There is a circumscribed mass of mixed echogenicity noted in the area of the left brachial plexus (**127b**, arrows). Peripheral nerve sheath tumors (PNSTs) have an affinity for the brachial plexus in dogs and therefore should be the primary consideration. Other tumors

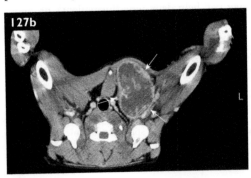

reported to occur in the region of the brachial plexus include other soft tissue sarcomas (STSs), lymphoma, hemangiosarcoma, and histiocytic sarcoma.

2 What diagnostic tests should be performed? A fine needle aspirate with CT or ultrasound guidance would provide a presumptive diagnosis, but a tissue biopsy would help determine tumor type and grade. A needle core biopsy was performed and confirmed PNST, low grade. Because PNSTs can extend into the spinal canal, an MRI is a better study to evaluate the full extent of disease.

3 What type of surgery would be recommended? With brachial plexus tumors, amputation is usually necessary to obtain a complete resection. The tumor appears to have well-defined margins on CT, but if this is a STS, there is a high probability that tumor-free margins would be difficult to achieve. For STS including PNST, radiation may be necessary postoperatively if clean margins are not attainable surgically. Metronomic chemotherapy has also been described as effective in delaying the onset of recurrence of incompletely excised STS, including brachial plexus tumors. Chemotherapy has not been shown to improve survival for patients with higher-grade tumors.

References
daCosta RC, Parent JM, Dobson H *et al.* (2008) Ultrasound-guided fine needle aspiration in the diagnosis of peripheral nerve sheath tumors in 4 dogs. *Can Vet J* 49:77–81.
Dennis MM, McSporran KD, Bacon NJ *et al.* (2011) Prognostic factors for cutaneous and subcutaneous soft tissue sarcomas in dogs. *Vet Pathol* 48:73–84.
Elmslie RE, Glawe P, Dow SW (2008) Metronomic therapy with cyclophosphamide and piroxicam effectively delays tumor recurrence in dogs with incompletely resected soft tissue sarcomas. *J Vet Intern Med* 22:1373–1379.
Kraft S, Ehrhart EJ, Gall D *et al.* (2007) Magnetic resonance imaging characteristics of peripheral nerve sheath tumors of the canine brachial plexus in 18 dogs. *Vet Radiol Ultrasound* 48:1–7.
Rose S, Long C, Knipe M *et al.* (2005) Ultrasonographic evaluation of brachial plexus tumors in five dogs. *Vet Radiol Ultrasound* 46:514–517.
Selting KA, Powers BE, Thompson LJ, *et al.* (2005) Outcome of dogs with high-grade soft tissue sarcomas treated with and without adjuvant doxorubicin chemotherapy: 39 cases (1996–2004). *J Am Vet Med Assoc* 227:1442–1448.

CASE 128
1 What diagnostic tests are necessary to determine whether further treatment is indicated? An MDB should first be performed. A CT scan is indicated to determine the extent of bony involvement and to determine whether surgery is possible. An incisional biopsy of the mass was performed and revealed osteosarcoma.

2 What is evident on the CT scan (128a)? There is an expansile lesion within the mandible which is lytic and productive, consistent with a bone tumor.

3 What treatment is advised? The lesion approached the vertical ramus of the mandible on CT, therefore a mandibulectomy will be required to obtain a clean surgical excision. Whether a caudal segmental mandibulectomy or hemimandibulectomy is required is dependent on the extent of disease noted on the CT. The role of chemotherapy postoperatively is far better defined for appendicular

Answers

OSA in dogs than for OSA of axial sites. Some studies have not shown that chemotherapy improves the outcome when surgical excision is incomplete. The role of chemotherapy as an adjunct to surgery when complete surgical excision is achieved has not been well defined.

4 With clean surgical excision, what are survival expectations? Mandibular OSA carries a good prognosis when a clean surgical excision is obtained. In comparison to appendicular OSA, metastatic rates tend to be lower (reported to be approximately 35% vs. >90% for appendicular sites).

5 What are favorable prognostic indicators for oral cavity osteosarcoma in dogs? Mandibular location, tumor-free margins after resection, and occurrence in smaller dogs are indicators of a more favorable prognosis. In a recent report of 50 dogs with mandibular OSA, tumor grade and mitotic index were significant in predicting outcome. Seventy-seven percent of dogs with grade I tumors were alive at 1 year while only 24% with grade II or III OSA were alive at 1 year. A mitotic index of >40 was also associated with a poorer outcome.

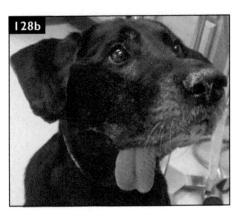

128b

Follow up/discussion
The patient is shown (128b) following a right hemi-mandibulectomy with his tongue hanging out on the side of the surgery, a common postoperative consequence of complete unilateral mandibulectomy. The opposite mandible will often drift medially, but in this patient it remained in a normal position.

References
Coyle VJ, Rassnick KM, Borst LB *et al.* (2015) Biological behaviour of canine mandibular osteosarcoma: a retrospective study of 50 cases (1999–2007). *Vet Comp Oncol* **13**:89–97.

Kosovsky JK, Matthiesen DT, Marretta SM *et al.* (1991) Results of partial mandibulectomy for the treatment of oral tumors in 142 dogs. *Vet Surg* **20**:397–401.

Selmic LE, Lafferty MH, Kamstock DA *et al.* (2014) Outcome and prognostic factors for osteosarcoma of the maxilla, mandible, or calvarium in dogs: 183 cases (1986–2012). *J Am Vet Med Assoc* **245**:930–938.

Schwarz PD, Withrow SJ, Curtis CR *et al.* (1991) Mandibular resection as a treatment for oral cancer in 81 dogs. *J Am Anim Hosp Assoc* **27**:601–610.

Straw RC, Powers BE, Klausner J *et al.* (1996) Canine mandibular osteosarcoma: 51 cases (1980–1992). *J Am Anim Hosp Assoc* **32**:257–262.

CASE 129

1 What are the differential diagnoses for this patient? The lesion appears well circumscribed on CT, with a fluid density surrounded by a thin wall. The appearance of the CT images and the fluid material obtained from the FNA support a cystic lesion. Thyroid neoplasia is also possible because aspirates will often be bloody and it may be difficult to obtain neoplastic cells. The differential diagnoses to consider are sebaceous cyst, carotid body tumor, salivary mucocele, thyroid adenoma or carcinoma, and a cystic thyroglossal duct remnant. An incisional or excisional biopsy is needed to make a definitive diagnosis. A thyroglossal duct cyst (TDC) was confirmed on incisional biopsy.

2 What is the cause and the biologic behavior of this lesion? This is a developmental abnormality. In the embryo, the thyroid gland originates in the mouth at the back of the tongue and then moves down the neck during embryonic development via the thyroglossal duct or tract. This tract usually degenerates by the 6th fetal week, but if this connection between the tongue and thyroid gland persists, a hollow tube remains, which can accumulate cystic material and can result in a TDC. Although the TDC is a benign lesion, carcinomas can arise from within these cysts. TDCs are usually not attached to other structures, making surgical excision the treatment of choice. Carcinomas arising from a TDC are reported but are very rare.

Reference

Giles JT, Rochat MC, Snider TA (2007) Surgical management of a thyroglossal duct cyst in a cat. *J Am Vet Med Assoc* **230**:686–689.

CASE 130

1 Describe the CT and cytology findings. *CT*: There is fluid or tissue density in the nasal cavity, worse on the right, with the right frontal sinus cavity affected. There is loss of turbinate detail, which is also worse on the right. A nasal tumor is suspected. *Cytology*: The predominant cell type is a lymphocyte. The medium to large lymphocytes present are suggestive of nasal lymphoma.

2 What is the diagnosis? Lymphoma is the most common nasal tumor diagnosed in cats, and the findings in this case are most suggestive of nasal lymphoma.

3 Is a tissue biopsy necessary? Cytology (squash-prep) was shown to have an excellent correlation with histopathology in >90% of cats with nasal tumors. However, it is more difficult to distinguish lymphoma from lymphoid inflammatory disease based on cytology alone. In another recent report, cytology was only diagnostic in 48% of cats with upper respiratory tract lymphoma. For this reason, a tissue biopsy with immunohistochemistry is advised. At this time, the prognostic significance of immunophenotype for this type of lymphoma has not been fully evaluated. The majority of cats with nasal lymphoma appear to have B cell lymphoma (~70%). T cell lymphoma (~30%) is diagnosed less frequently.

4 What treatment should be recommended and what are the survival expectations with treatment? Nasal lymphoma can be treated with radiation therapy alone, RT + chemotherapy, or chemotherapy alone. Nasal lymphoma is considered the variant of lymphoma that carries a good chance of long-term remission and potentially a cure. Response rates to treatment (chemotherapy and/or RT) are approximately 66–75%. MSTs of approximately 12–32 months have been reported. In one large study of 97 cats, the overall MST regardless of treatment modality was 536 days. There were three treatment groups evaluated: RT alone, RT + chemotherapy, and chemotherapy alone. Although there was no statistical difference among the groups, cats treated with RT alone or RT + chemotherapy that received total radiation dosages of >32 Gy had trends toward longer survival. In another study, 19 cats treated with RT + chemotherapy had an MST of 955 days. Despite the various reports that exist, a standard of care has not been established. This localized form of lymphoma does have the potential to become systemic. Systemic spread is seen in slightly below 20% of patients.

5 What are the most important prognostic factors for cats with nasal lymphoma? Negative prognostic indicators include the presence of anemia, cribriform plate involvement on CT, and anorexia. Positive prognostic factors are a complete clinical response and cats that received radiation dosages of >32 Gy (either with or without chemotherapy).

References

Haney SM, Beaver L, Turrel J et al. (2009) Survival analysis of 97 cats with nasal lymphoma: a multi-institutional retrospective study (1986–2006). *J Vet Intern Med* **23**:287–294.

Little L, Patel R, Goldschmidt M (2007) Nasal and nasopharyngeal lymphoma in cats: 50 cases (1989–2005). *Vet Pathol* **44**:885–892.

Moore A (2013) Extranodal lymphoma in the cat. Prognostic factors and treatment options. *J Feline Med Surg* **15**:379–390.

Santagostino SF, Mortellaro CM, Boracchi P et al. (2015) Feline upper respiratory tract lymphoma: site, cyto-histology, phenotype, FeLV expression, and prognosis. *Vet Pathol* **52**:250–259.

Sfiligoi G, Theon AP, Kent MS (2007) Response of nineteen cats with nasal lymphoma to radiation therapy and chemotherapy. *Vet Radiol Ultrasound* **48**:388–393.

CASE 131

1 What is being illustrated in this photograph? This patient has developed moist desquamation, which is an acute side effect of the radiation therapy to the skin. Hair loss in the treatment field is also evident, although the patient had been shaved for prior surgery. If moist desquamation develops, it is usually seen towards the end of the RT course. Regrowth of hair can take months, and in some patients hair loss is permanent. Hair color changes are common and hyper- or hypopigmentation of the skin can also be seen.

2 How should this patient be medically managed? Self-mutilation due to pruritus is the biggest challenge to overcome. Elizabethan collars or other means to keep patients from licking or rubbing at the sensitive skin are extremely important, as this can significantly delay healing. The area should be kept clean and dry. Gently rinsing with lukewarm water only and patting dry with a non-adherent dressing is helpful. Soap or other products should not be used. Bandaging the area should be avoided as this can cause further moisture build-up, which will delay healing. If the patient is scratching and rubbing the area and an E-collar is not helping, a loose T-shirt or sock can be used to cover the area. Anti-inflammatories (NSAIDs) and other pain medication will help alleviate discomfort. Antibiotics should be used if there is evidence of infection. The use of creams, oils, or powders can potentially interfere with the RT. However, once radiation has ended, the use of aloe vera, lanolin, and vitamin E can be considered. Other products such as A & D® Ointment, Aquaphor®, Biafine®, Radiacare®, or similar products designed to treat acute skin side effects from radiation in humans, can provide relief. Hydrocortisone cream can be helpful for some patients. Some patients get relief from gently using a hair dryer on the cool air setting (no heat) for several minutes. Blisters or scabs should not be disturbed because this will also delay healing. During and after healing, exposure to sun should be avoided.

Follow up/discussion
Figure **131b** is an example of hair color change following RT for a vaccine-associated sarcoma. Figure **131c** shows hair loss and hyperpigmentation following RT for nasal lymphoma.

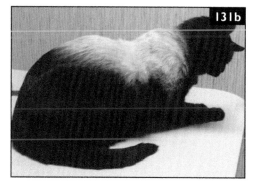 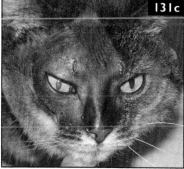

Answers

References

Carsten RE, Hellyer PW, Bachand AM *et al.* (2008) Correlations between acute radiation scores and pain scores in canine radiation patients with cancer of the forelimb. *Vet Anaesth Analg* 35(4):355–362.

Collen EB, Mayer NM (2006) Acute effects of radiation treatment: skin reactions. *Can Vet J* 47(9):931–932, 934–935.

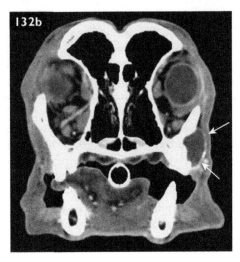

CASE 132

1 **Describe the CT findings.** There is a lesion on the right caudal maxilla that appears to be well defined and has a homogeneous center and a thin wall (**132b,** arrows). There is no bony invasion noted.

2 **A fine needle aspirate was performed and a proteinaceous fluid with evidence of mild hemorrhage was identified. In addition, there were occasional macrophages, neutrophils, and lymphocytes present. What is the clinical diagnosis?** The finding of a proteinaceous fluid combined with the CT appearance is suggestive of a cyst.

3 **What treatment is advised?** Draining the cyst will provide temporary relief, but surgical removal is required to prevent recurrence and to make a definitive diagnosis. Although suggestive of benign disease, malignancy needs to be ruled out. In this case, surgery was performed and histopathology revealed a squamous lined cyst with granulomatous inflammation and cholesterol clefts. These findings were considered diagnostic of a radicular cyst. Radicular cysts usually develop from a pre-existing periapical granuloma.

References

Beckman BW (2003) Radicular cyst of the premaxilla in a dog. *J Vet Dent* 20:213–217.

French SL, Anthony JM (1996) Surgical removal of a radicular odontogenic cyst in a four-year-old Dalmatian dog. *J Vet Dent* 13:149–151.

Lommer MJ (2007) Diagnostic imaging in veterinary dental practice. Periapical cyst. *J Am Vet Med Assoc* 230:997–999.

CASE 133

1 What is the clinical diagnosis? Rectal lymphoma.

2 What further staging tests should be performed? An MDB and abdominal ultrasound should be performed for staging. The majority of rectal lymphomas are B cell in origin, but a biopsy with IHC stains or ICC should be considered.

3 Assuming regional disease without evidence of distant disease, what is the prognosis for this patient? Lymphoma arising from the rectum/anal area at the initial presentation is uncommon. Treatment with chemotherapy is very effective, yielding mean survival times of 1,697 days in one study (MST not reached at time of publication). Patients with multicentric lymphoma can also present with rectal lesions or rectal prolapse and need to be differentiated from patients with primary rectal lymphoma on the basis of staging tests, because the prognosis is very different.

References

Fernandes NCCA, Guerra JM, Réssio RA *et al.* (2015) Liquid-based cytology and cell block immunocytochemistry in veterinary medicine: comparison with standard cytology for the evaluation of canine lymphoid samples. *Vet Comp Oncol*, doi:10.1111/vco.12137.

Sapierzynski R, Dolka I, Fabisiak M (2012) High agreement of routine cytopathology and immunocytochemistry in canine lymphomas. *Pol J Vet Sci* **15**:247–252.

Van Den Steen N, Berlato D, Polton G *et al.* (2012) Rectal lymphoma in 11 dogs: a retrospective study. *J Small Anim Pract* **53**:586–591.

CASE 134

1 Describe the ultrasonogram. In the apex of the bladder is a well-circumscribed lesion with a thick wall and hypoechoic center. Although not visible on this picture, the remainder of the bladder was normal.

2 What further tests would be indicated? An MDB should be performed, but as for other bladder tumor cases, a urinalysis should not be obtained by cystocentesis.

3 Is this patient a surgical candidate? The apical location of this tumor far away from the trigone makes this patient an excellent surgical candidate. At surgery, the mass was intimately attached to the bladder wall, but complete resection was possible (**134b**).

4 Does the gross appearance of the tumor give any indication about diagnosis? The smooth surface of the mass is not typical of TCC. Other considerations include sarcoma (fibrosarcoma, leiomyosarcoma, rhabdomyosarcoma) or benign leiomyoma. The diagnosis in this case was leiomyosarcoma.

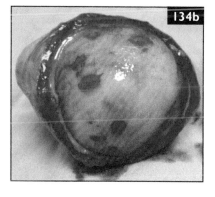

Reference
Knapp DW, McMillan SK (2013) Tumors of the urinary system. In: Withrow SJ, Vail DM, Page RL, editors, *Small Animal Clinical Oncology*, 5th edition. St. Louis, Elsevier Saunders, pp. 572–582.

CASE 135

1 How does the biologic behavior for this lesion differ from hemangiosarcoma that occurs in internally? Superficial purely cutaneous hemangiosarcoma carries a better prognosis than HSA of internal organs. However, the prognosis worsens for subcutaneous or intramuscular tumors. In one study, MST for patients with subcutaneous tumors treated with postoperative doxorubicin was 1,189 days, compared with 272 days for intramuscular sites. In another study, there was no difference in survival times between subcutaneous and intramuscular groups, both carrying a poor prognosis with an MST of 172 days.

2 This lesion is too large and broad based to achieve a complete surgical excision. What therapy should be considered? For this patient, treatment would most likely be palliative in nature. Chemotherapy (doxorubicin) has been studied in the setting of non-resectable subcutaneous HSA. The overall response rate was slightly less than 40% with a median response duration of only 53 days. Patients whose tumors decreased in size enough to have successful local resection had a median duration of response of 207 days. Radiation has also been described, with inconsistent results. In one study, palliative RT (<24 Gy total dose) was effective in reducing tumor burden and relieving pain in 75% of patients treated. Twenty percent of those patients evaluated achieved CR. MST was 95 days (range, 6–500 days).

3 What factors are believed to be negative prognostic indicators for subcutaneous HSA? Large tumor size (>4 cm associated with poorer outcome), presence of metastasis, clinical symptoms associated with the tumor, and anemia are all associated with poorer survival times. This patient's tumor was 10 cm at its largest dimension.

References
Bulakowski EJ, Philibert JC, Siegel S *et al.* (2008) Evaluation of outcome associated with subcutaneous and intramuscular hemangiosarcoma treated with adjuvant doxorubicin in dogs: 21 cases (2001–2006). *J Am Vet Med Assoc* **233**:122–128.
Hillers KR, Lana SE, Fuller CR *et al.* (2007) Effects of palliative radiation therapy on nonsplenic hemangiosarcoma in dogs. *J Am Anim Hosp Assoc* **43**:187–192.
Shiu KB, Flory AB, Anderson CL *et al.* (2011) Predictors of outcome in dogs with subcutaneous or intramuscular hemangiosarcoma. *J Am Vet Med Assoc* **238**:472–479.
Wiley JL, Rook KA, Clifford CA *et al.* (2010) Efficacy of doxorubicin-based chemotherapy for non-resectable canine subcutaneous haemangiosarcoma. *Vet Comp Oncol* **8**:221–233.

CASE 136

1 Describe the ultrasonogram. The spleen has multiple well-defined hypoechoic lesions throughout the parenchyma. In addition, a larger hypoechoic splenic mass is seen. The left medial iliac lymph node is enlarged. In addition to the pictured abnormalities, there were other markedly enlarged peritoneal lymph nodes.

2 An ultrasound-guided FNA of the spleen was performed and revealed a population of atypical histiocytic cells. What is a presumptive diagnosis? Lymphoma would be a primary consideration based on clinical and ultrasound findings, but the finding of the atypical histiocytic cells raises concerns for histiocytic sarcoma.

3 How should the diagnosis be confirmed? A definitive diagnosis requires histopathology with immunohistochemical staining. In this case, CD3, CD79a, and CD18 would be helpful. CD204 has also recently been shown to be a useful marker for canine histiocytic sarcoma. Given the widespread disease found on abdominal ultrasound, surgical intervention would be for diagnosis only. If surgery were declined, ICC for CD3 and CD79a could help rule out lymphoma.

4 How should this patient be treated? If histiocytic sarcoma is confirmed, chemotherapy with CCNU (+/− doxorubicin) would be recommended. However, the prognosis is considered poor. Median survival times were improved from 1 month without treatment to 3 months with treatment.

References
Cannon C, Borgatti A, Henson M *et al.* (2015) Evaluation of a combination chemotherapy protocol including lomustine and doxorubicin in canine histiocytic sarcoma. *J Small Anim Pract* **56**:425–429.

Kato Y, Murakami M, Hoshino Y *et al.* (2013)The class A macrophage scavenger receptor CD204 is a useful immunohistochemical marker of canine histiocytic sarcoma. *J Comp Pathol* **148**:188–196.

Moore PF (2014) A review of histiocytic disease of dogs and cats. *Vet Pathol* **51**:167–184.

Skorupski KA, Clifford CA, Paoloni MC *et al.* (2007) CCNU for the treatment of dogs with histiocytic sarcoma. *J Vet Intern Med* **21**:121–126.

CASE 137

1 What is the prognosis for this patient? The majority of melanocytic tumors arising from areas of haired skin are benign. The mitotic index is strongly linked to biologic behavior and, given that <1 mitotic figure was seen per 10 hpf, the prognosis for this dog is excellent.

2 What treatment options are available? Surgical excision is the treatment of choice; however, when multiple tumors are present, it is often difficult to control disease surgically. In these cases, removal of the largest lesions or lesions that are causing discomfort for the patient is recommended. Cryosurgery can be considered for smaller lesions (<1 cm) if surgical excision is not possible. The use of topical imiquimod (Aldara®) cream was successfully used in one report for cutaneous melanocytomas. Because of the slow growing nature of this type of tumor, monitoring for growth and only intervening surgically or medically if the tumors are progressing can be considered.

References

Coyner K, Loeffler D (2012) Topical imiquimod in the treatment of two cutaneous melanocytomas in a dog. *Vet Dermatol* **23**:145–149, e31.
Schultheiss PC (2006) Histologic features and clinical outcomes of melanomas of lip, haired skin, and nail bed locations of dogs. *J Vet Diagn Invest* **18**:422–425.

CASE 138

1 What is the cytologic diagnosis? There is a cluster of epithelial cells that exhibit anisocytosis and marked anisokaryosis and anisonucleoleosis, consistent with carcinoma.

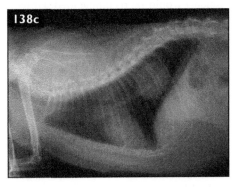

2 What diagnostic tests are indicated next? An MDB including thoracic radiographs is indicated. A thoracic radiograph is shown (**138c**).

3 What is the likely explanation for the clinical findings? Based on the presence of a solitary lesion in the lungs and a carcinoma of the digit, metastasis to the digit from the lung mass is suspected. There is a well-recognized syndrome of an unusual pattern of metastasis from pulmonary cancer in cats called the "lung–digit syndrome". Patients presenting for possible toe infections, especially those showing lysis of the bone on radiographs, should have thoracic radiographs performed to rule out primary pulmonary masses. Less commonly, other sites such as skin, eyes, skeletal muscle, bone, and internal organs are sites of metastasis. The weight bearing distal phalanges are most frequently affected. Involvement of multiple digits on multiple limbs is not uncommon.

4 What is the prognosis for this patient? Unfortunately, the prognosis for cats with the lung–digit syndrome is very poor. Median survival times are reported to be <2 months. Treatment is generally unrewarding.

References

Goldfinch N, Argyle DJ (2012) Feline lung–digit syndrome: unusual metastatic patterns of primary lung tumours in cats. *J Feline Med Surg* **14**:202–208.

Gottfried SD, Popovitch CA, Goldschmidt MH *et al.* (2000) Metastatic digital carcinoma in the cat: a retrospective study of 36 cats (1992–1998). *J Am Anim Hosp Assoc* **36**: 501–509.

CASE 139

1 What is being illustrated in this picture? This surgical specimen is being marked with colored ink in order to delineate the surgical margins more accurately. The different colors can help orient the pathologist to the rostral vs. caudal margins. Once colors have been used to mark specific areas, the remainder of the sample, including the deep margin, is marked with black ink. Inexpensive India ink can be used, or ink sets (**139b**) utilizing a color system can also be used. If all one color is used, sutures can be placed at the margins to orient the sample further. A full margin evaluation should be requested of the pathologist.

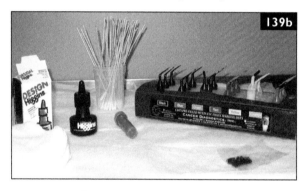

2 If this were a canine soft tissue sarcoma, what width of microscopic margins is required to be confident that a clean surgical margin has been achieved? In one study evaluating soft tissue sarcoma margins, if a 10 mm microscopic margin was achieved, the probability of cure approached 100%. It is more difficult to achieve a 10 mm deep margin. Removing the tumor at a depth one fascial plane below the tumor is usually adequate.

References

Banks T, Straw R, Thomson M *et al.* (2004) Soft tissue sarcomas in dogs: a study assessing surgical margins, tumour grade, and clinical outcome. *Aust Vet Pract* **34**:142–147.

Kamstock DA, Ehrhart EJ, Getzy DM *et al.* (2011) Recommended guidelines for submission, trimming, margin evaluation, and reporting of tumor biopsy specimens in veterinary surgical pathology. *Vet Pathol* **48**:19–31.

CASE 140

1 What is the anatomic location and character of the mass? What is the arrow pointing to in 140c? The mass measures 9.2 × 8.3 cm and appears homogeneous. The arrow is pointing to the trachea. The mass is causing moderate dorsal and marked rightward deviation of the trachea.

2 List the differential diagnoses for this mass. What tumor is most likely and why? Based on the echocardiogram, the tumor appears to be arising from the ascending aorta near the base of the heart. The most common tumors found at the heart base include aortic body tumor (chemodectoma), hemangiosarcoma, ectopic thyroid neoplasia, lymphoma, and connective tissue tumors. Given the location of the tumor, the long history of clinical symptoms, and lack of cavitation, a slow growing chemodectoma is likely. This patient was also previously diagnosed with laryngeal paralysis. Chronic hypoxia has been postulated to stimulate the development of chemoreceptor tumors in dogs and humans.

3 What further diagnostic tests should be performed? Electrocardiography (owing to possible electrical disturbances secondary to hypoxia or ischemia), coagulation profile, and ultrasound- or CT-guided aspirate. A fine needle aspirate should only be considered following careful evaluation of the patient's coagulation status. Cytology would help rule out lymphoma or soft tissue sarcomas, but will not necessarily differentiate chemodectoma from other neuroendocrine tumors such as an ectopic thyroid tumor because the cytologic appearance can be similar.

4 What treatment should be considered for this patient? Based on the locally invasive nature and location of this tumor, surgery is rarely possible. In patients with smaller and less invasive tumors, surgical excision should be accompanied by a pericardiectomy. Dogs with aortic body tumors have significantly improved outcomes if pericardiectomy is performed, even in patients without pericardial effusion. Radiation therapy can be considered. Although studies using RT for heart base masses are lacking, long-term control of inoperable chemodectoma has been reported.

References

Hardcastle MR, Meyer J, McSporran KD (2013) Pathology in practice. Carotid and aortic body carcinomas (chemodectomas) in a dog. *J Am Vet Med Assoc* **242**:175–177.

Obradovich JE, Withrow SJ, Powers BE *et al.* (1992) Carotid body tumors in the dog: eleven cases (1978–1988). *J Vet Intern Med* **6**:96–101.

Rancilio NJ, Higuchi T, Gagnon J *et al.* (2012) Use of three-dimensional conformal radiation therapy for treatment of a heart base chemodectoma in a dog. *J Am Vet Med Assoc* **241**:472–476.

CASE 141

1 An ultrasound-guided FNA of the intestinal mass was performed and the cytology is shown (141a). What is the cytologic diagnosis? The cytology is consistent with carcinoma. Based on the location, adenocarcinoma is suspected.

2 How does the presence of the enlarged lymph nodes affect survival expectations? Despite probable metastasis in the lymph nodes, surgery is still recommended because median survival times for patients whose tumors had metastasized beyond the primary site were approximately 1 year (358 days in one study) and the MST was close to 2.5 years (843 days) if no metastatic disease was found.

3 This patient was taken to surgery for resection and anastomosis of the primary tumor and removal of the lymph nodes. What significant prognostic factors can be obtained from the histopathology results? Margin evaluation is very important. Survival times were significantly longer in patients with documented clean surgical margins (1,320 days vs. 60 days if margins were incomplete).

4 What is the significance of this patient's breed? The Siamese breed has been shown to be the most common breed in multiple studies on intestinal neoplasia, including adenocarcinoma.

References
Green ML, Smith JD, Kass PH (2011) Surgical versus non-surgical treatment of feline small intestinal adenocarcinoma and the influence of metastasis on long-term survival in 18 cats (2000–2007). *Can Vet J* 52:1101–1105.
Rissetto K, Villamil JA, Selting KA *et al.* (2011) Recent trends in feline intestinal neoplasia: an epidemiologic study of 1,129 cases in the Veterinary Medical Database from 1964 to 2004. *J Am Anim Hosp Assoc* 47:28–36.

CASE 142

1 Describe the radiograph. Sternal lymphadenopathy is present. In cats, the sternal node is more caudal in location than in dogs.

2 Could this be considered a variation of normal? Normal sternal nodes cannot be seen radiographically, therefore this represents probable pathology.

3 What structures do the sternal nodes receive drainage from? The sternal node receives approximately 80% of the material drained from the peritoneal cavity. In addition, it drains the cranial and caudal mammary glands if malignancy is present. Also drained are the diaphragm, pleural spaces, cranial abdominal organs, and cranial ventral body wall.

4 What further diagnostics are indicated? An ultrasound of the abdomen should be performed.

Reference
Smith K, O'Brien R (2012) Radiographic characterization of enlarged sternal lymph nodes in 71 dogs and 13 cats. *J Am Anim Hosp Assoc* 48:176–181.

CASE 143

1 What abnormalities are noted on the thoracic radiograph? The sternal and mediastinal lymph nodes are enlarged.

2 Figure 143b shows a cross section of the small intestine and 143c is an image of the mid-abdomen. Describe these ultrasound images. The intestinal wall is extremely thickened (0.9 cm) and is devoid of the normal intestinal layering. Multiple enlarged mesenteric lymph nodes are seen.

3 Figure 143d shows the cytology obtained from an ultrasound-guided aspirate of the mesenteric lymph nodes. What is the diagnosis? The lymphocytes pictured are large (at least 1.5 times the size of the segmented neutrophil seen) and have enlarged and irregular nucleoli. The lymphoblasts make up at least 75% of the population of lymphocytes seen. This is suggestive of a high-grade lymphoma, but histopathology is required to establish a grade.

4 What further tests are indicated? ICC from the node aspirates can be performed to determine immunophenotype. Most reports suggest that the majority of intestinal lymphomas are of T cell origin. However, immunophenotype did not offer any insight into prognosis.

5 What is the treatment and prognosis for this patient? Chemotherapy for high-grade lymphoma is indicated. The prognosis for this form of lymphoma is generally poor. Although long-term survival has been reported, the median duration of response and overall survival time are generally in the 2–3-month range. Negative prognostic indicators have included diarrhea at initial presentation and failure to achieve a remission.

References
Frank JD, Reimer SB, Kass PH *et al.* (2007) Clinical outcomes of 30 cases (1997–2004) of canine gastrointestinal lymphoma. *J Am Anim Hosp Assoc* **43**:313–321.
Rassnick KM, Moore AS, Collister KE *et al.* (2009) Efficacy of combination chemotherapy for treatment of gastrointestinal lymphoma in dogs. *J Vet Intern Med* **23**:317–322.

CASE 144

1 What is the radiographic diagnosis? The right middle lung lobe is consolidated with air bronchograms, consistent with pneumonia. The presence of the megaesophagus and the right middle lung lobe location of the lung pattern make aspiration pneumonia the probable diagnosis.

2 Another radiograph (144c) was taken following a 2-week course of antibiotics. What is the revised radiographic diagnosis? The pneumonia has resolved, but now a mass is seen in the cranial mediastinum (**144d**, arrows). The megaesophagus is still present.

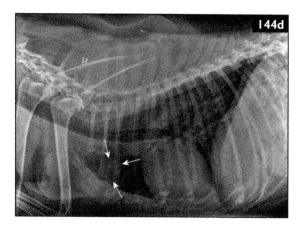

3 **What are the differential diagnoses?** Thymoma is the most common cranial mediastinal mass in the dog. Other considerations are:
- Lymphoma.
- Thymic branchial cyst.
- Ectopic thyroid tumor.
- Mediastinal/thymic carcinoma.
- Chemodectoma.
- Metastatic carcinoma.

4 **How is the megaesophagus related to the anterior mediastinal mass?** The presence of megaesophagus raises the concern for thymoma. Up to 40% of dogs with thymoma are affected by paraneoplastic syndromes, the most common of which are myasthenia gravis (MG) and megaesophagus.

5 **What further diagnostic tests should be performed?** Complete staging including abdominal ultrasound should be performed. Ultrasound of the mediastinal mass can be helpful in differentiating thymoma from lymphoma. Thymomas tend to be cystic in appearance and heterogeneous in echogenicity when compared with lymphoma. A fine needle aspirate or needle core biopsy with ultrasound guidance can be considered. A CT scan will determine the extent of disease for surgical planning. A CT-guided aspirate or needle core biopsy can also be considered. In addition, an acetylcholine receptor antibody serum titer should be run. This patient had a titer of 2.6 nmol/l (>0.6 is abnormal), indicating that he had an acquired MG.

6 **What are the potential treatment options?** The treatment of choice for thymoma is surgical excision. However, in patients with megaesophagus, there is an increased surgical complication rate due to postoperative aspiration pneumonia. In addition, paraneoplastic syndromes do not always resolve after surgery.

Answers

However, in several studies, patients did well with surgical excision of thymomas, including invasive thymomas and thymomas with paraneoplastic syndromes. In one report, MSTs with and without surgical treatment were 635 days and 76 days, respectively. In contrast to previous reports, the presence of MG or megaesophagus at the time of diagnosis was not associated with survival time. Patients with a higher percentage of lymphocytes in their masses appeared to survive longer than those that did not. Radiation therapy has been evaluated in dogs with thymoma and could be considered as primary or adjunctive therapy. Complete responses are uncommon but partial remissions or stabilization of disease resulted in an MST of 248 days in one report. Chemotherapy agents used to treat lymphoma can be used palliatively, but complete responses are also rare. Chemotherapy tends to result in reduction of the lymphoid component of the tumor, so can provide some relief.

References
Atwater SW, Powers BE, Park RD *et al.* (1994) Thymoma in dogs: 23 cases (1980–1991). *J Am Vet Med Assoc* 205:1007–1013.
Patterson MME, Marolf AJ (2014) Sonographic characteristics of thymoma compared with mediastinal lymphoma. *J Am Anim Hosp Assoc* 50:409–413.
Robat CS, Cesario L, Gaeta R *et al.* (2013) Clinical features, treatment options, and outcome in dogs with thymoma: 116 cases (1999–2010). *J Am Vet Med Assoc* 243:1448–1454.
Smith AN, Wright JC, Brawner WR *et al.* (2001) Radiation therapy in the treatment of canine and feline thymomas: a retrospective study (1985–1999). *J Am Anim Hosp Assoc* 37:489–496.

CASE 145

1 What does this mass likely represent? This lesion is most consistent with a pilonidal cyst (also referred to as dermoid cyst). A pilonidal cyst is a congenital midline closure defect. In embryonal development, a pilonidal cyst can result when there is incomplete separation of the skin from the neural tube. This creates an epithelialized fistula that connects the skin to the vertebral canal. In dogs, pilonidal cysts tend to be most common in Rhodesian Ridgebacks, and in cats the Burmese breed is over-represented. The cysts can clinically appear as a draining tract or recurring abscess. They can also present with an asymptomatic subcutaneous mass, as in this patient. Some patients appear to be painful in the area of the cyst, while others show no symptoms at all.

2 What are the possible complications that can occur if the external portion of the mass were to rupture? If there is a connection between the cyst and the spinal cord, then spinal fluid can leak from the tract. Retrograde infection of the central nervous system can result. This patient made a complete recovery.

Reference
Rochat MC, Campbell GA, Panciera RJ (1996) Dermoid cysts in cats: two cases and a review of the literature. *J Vet Diagn Invest* **8**:505–507.

CASE 146

1 What does the cytology reveal? The lymph node contains a mixed population of lymphocytes, predominantly small, with occasional intermediate to larger lymphocytes. An increased number of plasma cells and neutrophils are seen. There is a large cluster of cells exhibiting anisocytosis, anisokaryosis, and anisonucleoleosis that appear epithelial in origin. This is a reactive node with metastatic carcinoma.

2 What is the probable cause of the lymphadenopathy and what should be done to evaluate this patient further? A primary carcinoma in the oral cavity is suspected. A more caudal location is likely because nothing was seen in the rostral oral cavity on physical examination. The patient should be anesthetized so that a more thorough evaluation of the oral cavity and pharynx can be performed. In this patient, a mass was noted on the caudal soft palate.

CASE 147

1 What further staging tests should be performed? An MDB and abdominal ultrasound are indicated. Multiple mast cell tumors are sometimes found to be metastases from a visceral site in cats with more aggressive disease. In patients with multiple tumors and/or systemic symptoms, bone marrow involvement is possible. Therefore, a buffy coat analysis or bone marrow analysis should be performed as part of the staging.

2 What is the prognostic value of histopathology? In cats, the Patnaik grading system does not correlate well with the biologic behavior of MCTs. Two histologic forms are recognized in cats: the mastocytic form (further subdivided into well-differentiated, poorly differentiated, or pleomorphic forms) and the atypical form (previously known as the histiocytic form). The well-differentiated mastocytic form is the most common. The atypical form tends to occur in younger cats (especially Siamese) and spontaneous regression can be seen. While histologic grade does not provide reliable information, identification of poorly differentiated types can be predictive of more aggressive biologic behavior.

3 Do cats possess mutations in *c-KIT* as seen in dogs? Is evaluation of cytoplasmic KIT labeling beneficial in cats? *c-KIT* mutations occurred in >50% of cats with MCTs tested, but there was no association with survival time identified. In patients with multiple tumors, the mutation status of different tumors in the same cat can vary, making it more difficult to predict behavior on the basis of mutation status.

4 What are negative prognostic indicators for mast cell tumors in cats? Multiple tumors, poorly differentiated cell types, positive cytoplasmic KIT labeling, mitotic index >5, multiple nodules (>5), and visceral involvement are associated with a poorer prognosis. The value of proliferation markers in determining prognosis for cats with mast cell tumors is still under investigation, but increased Ki67 is believed to be predictive of a more guarded prognosis.

5 What treatment should be considered for this patient? In cats, a 50% response rate is seen with various chemotherapy agents (CCNU, vinblastine, chlorambucil have been used). Median duration of response is slightly better than 5 months when CCNU is used. Tyrosine kinase inhibitors have been reported to be beneficial in a limited number of cats, but this has not yet been widely studied. The aberrant KIT expression found in a significant portion of feline MCTs presents a potential therapeutic target. Response of feline MCT has been observed when the tyrosine kinase inhibitor imatinib mesylate (Gleevec®) was used in one report.

References

Isotani M, Tamura K, Yagihara H *et al.* (2006) Identification of a *c-kit* exon 8 internal tandem duplication in a feline mast cell tumor case and its favorable response to the tyrosine kinase inhibitor imatinib mesylate. *Vet Immunol Immunopathol* **114**:168–172.

Mallett CL, Northrup NC, Saba CF*et al.* (2012) Immunohistochemical characterization of feline mast cell tumors. *Vet Pathol* **50**:106–109.

Rassnick KM, Williams LE, Kristal O *et al.* (2008) Lomustine for treatment of mast cell tumors in cats: 38 cases (1999–2005). *J Am Vet Med Assoc* **232**:1200–1205.

Sabattini S, Bettini G (2010) Prognostic value of histologic and immunohistochemical features in feline cutaneous mast cell tumors. *Vet Pathol* **47**:643–653.

CASE 148

1 What does this picture demonstrate? The combination of miosis, enophthalmos, and third eyelid prolapse is consistent with Horner's syndrome. Horner's syndrome results from lesions interfering with the sympathetic nerve supply to the head and orbit.

2 What are the differential diagnoses for this abnormality? Trauma to the neck and chest, anterior mediastinal masses, and middle ear disease (infection, polyps) are the most common causes of Horner's syndrome in the cat. An idiopathic Horner's syndrome is also recognized.

3 What diagnostic tests are indicated? One of the most important tests to confirm the presence of Horner's syndrome is conducted during the initial physical examination. The miotic pupil will not dilate significantly in the dark, while the normal larger pupil will dilate. An MDB, to include neck radiographs, careful otic examination, and radiography of the skull, is indicated. In this patient, thoracic radiographs revealed a cranial mediastinal mass.

Reference
Penderis J (2015) Diagnosis of Horner's syndrome in dogs and cats. *In Pract* 37:107–119.

CASE 149

1 What are the possible causes for collapse? Causes of collapse can include hypoglycemia (insulinoma, sepsis, hepatoma), cardiac arrhythmias, and CNS disease.

2 How should this patient's work-up proceed? Although the heart rhythm was normal and no murmurs were heard, echocardiography and electrocardiography should be considered to rule out any evidence of arrhythmias, pericardial effusion, or cardiac masses. A Holter monitor may be necessary to identify an intermittent arrhythmia. If cardiac function is determined to be normal, MRI of the brain would be recommended to rule out a brain tumor as a cause of the collapse. Insulinomas can be difficult to confirm because they may not be evident on ultrasound of the pancreas and insulin levels may only increase episodically. It is often necessary to test glucose and insulin levels at the time of collapse to confirm insulinoma.

3 Based on the MRI findings (149a), what treatments can be considered? This patient has a contrast-enhancing lesion in the cerebellum, which explains the ataxia. The broad based attachment, smooth margins, and uniform contrast enhancement are consistent with the diagnosis of meningioma. Radiation therapy is recommended because this is a difficult location to approach surgically. In general, meningiomas in cats tend to be more easily excised and surgery can be used as the sole treatment. However, in dogs, tumors tend to be more difficult to remove owing to their locally invasive nature, and postoperative RT is usually necessary. Stereotactic radiotherapy could be considered, but this has not yet been fully evaluated in dogs. Chemotherapy with hydroxyurea or CCNU has been reported.

4 What is the prognosis for this patient? In one study, surgery alone was associated with a MST of 7 months in comparison with an MST of 16.5 months in patients treated with postoperative RT. In this patient, RT is advised. Reported median survivals for dogs with brain tumors treated with radiation vary. In general, dogs with meningiomas treated with RT have MSTs of approximately 1–2 years. When 3-dimensional conformal RT was used in one study, the MST was 577 days. However, when patients dying of causes other than meningioma were excluded, the MST was approximately 900 days. Chemotherapy has been used palliatively. CCNU as a primary treatment for meningioma failed to improve survival significantly over symptomatic therapy (e.g. corticosteroids with or without anticonvulsant drugs) alone.

Answers

References

Axlund TW, McGlasson MS, Smith AN (2002) Surgery alone or in combination with radiation therapy for treatment of intracranial meningiomas in dogs: 31 cases (1989–2002). *J Am Vet Med Assoc* **221**:1597–1600.

Bley CR, Sumova A, Roos M *et al.* (2008) Irradiation of brain tumors in dogs with neurologic disease. *J Vet Intern Med* **19**:849–854.

Keyerleber MA, McEntee MC, Farrely J *et al.* (2014) Three-dimensional conformal radiation therapy alone or in combination with surgery for treatment of canine intracranial meningiomas. *Vet Comp Oncol* **12**:67–77.

Motta L, Mandara MT, Skerritt GC (2012) Canine and feline intracranial meningiomas: an updated review. *Vet J* **192**:153–165.

Rossmeisl JH, Jones JC, Zimmerman KL *et al.* (2013) Survival time following hospital discharge in dogs with palliatively treated brain tumors. *J Am Vet Med Assoc* **242**:193–198.

Sturges BK, Dickinson PJ, Bollen AW *et al.* (2008) Magnetic resonance imaging and histological classification of intracranial meningiomas in 112 dogs. *J Vet Intern Med* **22**:586–595.

Van Meervenne S, Verhoeven PS, Devos J *et al.* (2014) Comparison between symptomatic treatment and lomustine supplementation in 71 dogs with intracranial, space-occupying lesions. *Vet Comp Oncol* **12**:67–77.

Wisner ER, Dickinson PJ, Higgins RJ (2011) Magnetic resonance imaging features of canine intracranial neoplasia. *Vet Radiol Ultrasound* **52**:S52–S61.

CASE 150

1 What is the probable diagnosis? Based on the clinical appearance, radiographs, and cytology, the most likely diagnosis is an infiltrative lipoma. Care must be taken to rule out an underlying sarcoma or other type of tumor.

2 What further work-up is indicated? In addition to an MDB, ultrasound of the leg can sometimes be helpful in confirming that the character of the mass is consistent with fat and determining whether the mass is an infiltrative lipoma or an intermuscular lipoma. CT is advised to determine the extent of disease and to plan surgery.

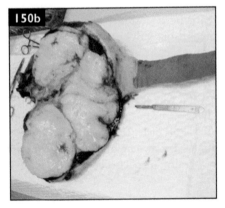

3 What is the best treatment for this patient? Infiltrative lipomas invade between muscle cells rather than between whole muscles, as in intermuscular lipomas. While intermuscular lipomas are usually treatable by removing the lipoma using blunt dissection between the muscles, infiltrative lipomas require more aggressive surgical excision. In this patient, CT was performed and amputation advised. Even with aggressive surgical resection, it was not a clean resection (**150b**). Infiltrative lipomas have been reported to be responsive to radiation therapy, therefore RT was recommended for this patient postoperatively.

References
McEntee MC, Page RL, Mauldin GN *et al.* (2000) Results of irradiation of infiltrative lipoma in 13 dogs. *Vet Radiol Ultrasound* **41**:554–556.
McEntee MC, Thrall DE (2001) Computed tomographic imaging of infiltrative lipoma in 22 dogs. *Vet Radiol Ultrasound* **42**:221–225.

CASE 151

1 Describe the CT images. There is a well-circumscribed mass that appears to be within the cranial mediastinum in **151a**; however, as the mass is followed caudally (**151b**) it can be seen originating in the pulmonary parenchyma of the right cranial lung lobe. The mass appeared to have a multilocular pattern. The mass measured 5.2 cm at its largest dimension.

2 What is the cytologic diagnosis? There is a clump of epithelial cells and scattered single epithelial cells. There is mild anisocytosis. In addition, there are pulmonary macrophages present. Carcinoma is suspected, but cannot be confirmed cytologically.

3 What are the differential diagnoses for this patient's mass? A primary lung tumor is likely. A mediastinal tumor that had invaded into the right cranial lung lobe is possible, but less likely. The multilocular appearance noted on CT is also commonly seen with thymomas.

4 This patient was taken to surgery and a right cranial lung lobe mass was found to be infiltrating into the mediastinum. The tumor was removed and the histologic diagnosis was well-differentiated papillary carcinoma with clean margins. What are the negative prognostic indicators for dogs with primary lung tumors? Factors associated with a poorer prognosis include the following:

- Large size (>5 cm associated with an MST of 8 months vs. 20 months for tumors <5 cm).
- Squamous cell histologic type (MST for SCC 8 months, vs. 19 months for adenocarcinoma).
- Lymph node positive (positive had MST 2–6 month vs. negative 12+ months).
- Histologically high grade (MST 6 months, vs. 16 months for low grade).
- Presence of clinical signs (MST 8 months, vs. 18 months for no symptoms).

Therefore, this patient's tumor type and grade, and node negative status, are all favorable. The size of the tumor at its largest dimension is right on the borderline prognostically and clinical signs were minor. A favorable prognosis is likely.

References

Barrett LE, Pollard RE, Zwingenberger A *et al.* (2014) Radiographic characterization of primary lung tumors in 74 dogs. *Vet Radiol Ultrasound* **55**:480–487.

Marolf AJ, Gibbons DS, Podell BK *et al.* (2011) Computed tomographic appearance of primary lung tumors in dogs. *Vet Radiol Ultrasound* **52**:168–172.

McNiel EA, Ogilvie GK, Powers BE *et al.* (1997) Evaluation of prognostic factors for dogs with primary lung tumors: 67 cases (1985–1992). *J Am Vet Med Assoc* **211**:1422–1427.

Ogilvie GK, Weigel RM, Haschek WM *et al.* (1989) Prognostic factors for tumor remission and survival in dogs after surgery for primary lung tumor: 76 cases (1975–1985). *J Am Vet Med Assoc* **195**:109–112.

Polton GA, Brearley MJ, Powell SM *et al.* (2008) Impact of primary tumour stage on survival in dogs with solitary lung tumours. *J Small Anim Pract* **49**:66–71.

CASE 152

1 Describe the CT scan and list the differential diagnoses for this lesion. There is a homogeneous mass obliterating the right nasal passage and frontal sinus and breaking through the osseous nasal septum into the left nasal passage. Dorsally, the mass has broken through the frontal sinus and destroyed the frontal bone. Laterally, the mass has destroyed the bone of the nasal cavity and is putting pressure on the right eye, causing distortion of the globe. Ventrally, the tumor appears to be invading into the nasopharynx. Owing to the degree of bone destruction and local invasiveness of this lesion, benign diseases (rhinitis, etc.) would be considered less likely. More than 90% of nasal tumors in cats are malignant. Among malignant tumors, approximately 45% are epithelial in origin (of these, 50% are adenocarcinoma, 50% SCC), approximately 30% lymphoma, and 25% sarcomas (FSA, CSA, OSA, etc.). These percentages vary depending on the sources cited.

2 What is the cytologic diagnosis? There is a cluster of epithelial cells with mild anisocytosis and prominent nucleoli. A tumor of epithelial origin is likely.

3 What further diagnostic tests should be performed? A tissue biopsy is necessary to provide a definitive diagnosis and establish an appropriate treatment plan. Trans-nostril techniques to obtain a core of tissue are preferred. Prior to biopsy, a coagulation profile should be performed. The diagnosis for this patient was adenocarcinoma.

4 What treatment options can be offered? Curative intent radiation therapy would be the treatment of choice for this patient. MSTs for patients with nasal adenocarcinoma treated with RT range from 12 to 19 months depending on the report.

References

Mellanby RJ, Herrtage ME, Dobson JM (2002) Long-term outcome of eight cats with non-lymphoproliferative nasal tumours treated by megavoltage radiotherapy. *J Feline Med Surg* **4**:77–81.

Mukaratirwa S, van der Linde-Sipman JS, Gruys E (2001) Feline nasal and paranasal sinus tumours: clinicopathological study, histomorphological description and diagnostic immunohistochemistry of 123 cases. *J Feline Med Surg* 3:235–245.

Sfiligoi G, Theon AP, Kent MS (2007) Response of nineteen cats with nasal lymphoma to radiation therapy and chemotherapy. *Vet Radiol Ultrasound* 48:388–393.

CASE 153

1 What is the interpretation of the IHC results? It rules out the possibility of T or B cell lymphoma and histiocytic sarcoma. The CD45+ result confirms round cell tumor origin, but this is poorly differentiated. A non-T or non-B lymphoma is possible, but cannot be confirmed with IHC tests.

2 The tumor goes to the midline. Is surgery an option? Surgical debulking is a consideration, but the mass is nearing the midline and a tongue amputation caudal to the tumor is not routinely performed because of functional compromise. Radiation therapy to the tongue, although infrequently described, could be considered. Total glossectomy (removal of ≥75% of the tongue) has also been described and was considered well tolerated.

3 What further diagnostics should be performed? Full staging to include an MDB and abdominal ultrasound should be performed.

References
Dvorak LD, Beaver DP, Ellison GW *et al.* (2004) Major glossectomy in dogs: a case series and proposed classification system. *J Am Anim Hosp Assoc* 40:331–337.

Syrcle JA, Bonczynski JJ, Monette S *et al.* (2008) Retrospective evaluation of lingual tumors in 42 dogs: 1999–2005. *J Am Anim Hosp Assoc* 44:308–319.

CASE 154

1 What are the differential diagnoses for this patient? Diagnostic considerations include:
- Ureteral obstruction/hydronephrosis.
- Pyelonephritis.
- Polycystic kidneys (although this is typically a bilateral finding).
- Compensatory hypertrophy.
- Neoplasia.

2 What diagnostic tests should be done? In addition to an MDB, an ultrasound of the abdomen should be performed. An ultrasound is needed to show the internal architecture of the kidney. Hydronephrosis is usually easily differentiated from pyelonephritis, polycystic disease, and neoplasia. Further diagnostics, such as urine culture, fine needle aspirate, or biopsy of the kidney, are dependent on the ultrasound findings. In this patient, hydronephrosis was found on ultrasound. A ureteral obstruction was diagnosed.

Answers

References

Cuypers MD, Grooters AM, Williams J *et al.* (1997) Renomegaly in dogs and cats. Part I: differential diagnoses. *Compend Contin Educ Vet* **19**:1019–1032.

Grooters AM, Cuypers MD, Partington BP *et al.* (1997) Renomegaly in dogs and cats. Part II: diagnostic approach. *Compend Contin Educ Vet* **19**:1213–1229.

CASE 155

1 What stage of disease is represented in this patient? There are circulating large lymphocytes in the peripheral blood suggesting stage V disease. The clinical symptoms are indicative of substage b. Therefore, this patient has stage Vb lymphoma.

2 What further diagnostics should be recommended? Blood work (CBC, serum chemistry panel) should be performed. Flow cytometry on the peripheral blood will help confirm leukemia and provide information regarding immunophenotype.

3 What factors in this patient's case are associated with a poorer prognosis? WHO substage b (clinically ill) and presence of bone marrow involvement have been associated with a poorer prognosis.

WHO Clinical Staging System for Lymphoma in Domestic Animals	
Stage I	Involvement limited to a single node or lymphoid tissue in a single organ (excluding bone marrow)
Stage II	Involvement of multiple lymph nodes in a regional area
Stage III	Generalized lymph node involvement
Stage IV	Liver and/or spleen involvement (+/– stage III)
Stage V	Involvement of blood and bone marrow and/or other organ systems (+/– stage IV)
Stage a	Without systemic signs
Stage b	With systemic signs

References

Marconato L (2011) The staging and treatment of multicentric high-grade lymphoma in dogs: a review of recent developments and future prospects. *Vet J* **188**:34–38.

Vail DM, Pinkerton ME, Young KM (2013) Canine lymphoma and lymphoid leukemia. In: Withrow SJ, Vail DM, Page RL, editors, *Small Animal Clinical Oncology*, 5th edition. St. Louis, Elsevier Saunders, pp. 608–638.

CASE 156

1 What is the purpose of using a transdermal device to deliver this vaccine? This delivery system concentrates the majority of the vaccine in the skin rather than in the subcutaneous tissues, as would a standard vaccine. The skin is heavily populated with Langerhans cells, which are potent antigen-presenting cells that are considered highly efficient for the initiation of humoral and/or cellular immune responses.

2 What are the major side effects noted when using this type of device? Side effects are minimal; occasionally a transient local irritation to the skin occurs. The device makes a relatively loud noise when engaged and can startle patients. Therefore, use of gentle restraint and distraction techniques (such as rubbing or scratching the head, etc.) are helpful for ease of administration.

Reference

Goubier A, Fuhrmann L, Forest L *et al.* (2008) Superiority of needle-free transdermal plasmid delivery for the induction of antigen-specific IFNγ T cell responses in the dog. *Vaccine* 26:2186–2190.

CASE 157

1 What is the most likely diagnosis? There is a mineralized mass in the retropharyngeal area causing ventral deviation of the trachea. The cytology shows clusters of epithelial cells exhibiting mild to moderate anisocytosis and mild anisokaryosis. This is most likely representative of a thyroid tumor, although metastasis to the retropharyngeal node from another primary tumor cannot be ruled out.

2 In addition to the MDB, what diagnostic tests are advised? A CT scan should be performed to determine the extent of disease for possible surgical planning. A tissue biopsy is needed to make a definitive diagnosis. A thyroid panel is indicated. Less than 10% of thyroid tumors in dogs are functional. Up to 30% will be hypothyroid due to probable destruction of the normal thyroid tissue by the tumor. The remainder are euthyroid.

3 What dictates the treatment decision? Based on the fixed nature of the tumor, surgical excision would be difficult. The CT would provide information regarding invasiveness. Freely moveable tumors are generally considered surgical.

4 What treatment options can be considered? Radiation therapy can be considered for tumors surgically removed but with incomplete margins, or for inoperable tumors. Progression-free survival times of 80% at 1 year and 72% at 3 years were noted in one study. Several chemotherapeutic agents have shown activity against canine thyroid carcinoma including doxorubicin, cis-platin, mitoxantrone, and actinomycin-D, although responses have been transient and generally partial rather than complete. In a recent study evaluating postoperative chemotherapy, the addition of chemotherapy to surgical excision did not improve survival. Radioactive iodine (I 131) has also been used for the treatment of non-resectable thyroid tumors, even when non-functional (i.e. normal serum thyroxine concentrations). In one study of 39 dogs, the MST for dogs with non-metastatic disease was 839 days. However, three dogs died of radioiodine-associated myelosuppression within 3 months of treatment. The use of toceranib phosphate (Palladia®) was associated with objective

response rates of 25% in dogs with thyroid carcinoma. Known targets of toceranib are expressed in some thyroid carcinomas including VEGFR and PDGFRα/β, KIT, and RET, making the use of Palladia® an attractive choice. Further investigation will better define the role of toceranib in treating thyroid carcinoma.

References
Barber LG (2007) Thyroid tumors in dogs and cats. *Vet Clin N Am Small Anim Pract* **37**:755–773.
Nadeau ME, Kitchell BE (2011) Evaluation of the use of chemotherapy and other prognostic variables for surgically excised canine thyroid carcinoma with and without metastasis. *Can Vet J* **52**:994–998.
Taeymans O, Penninck DG, Peters RM (2013) Comparison between clinical, ultrasound, CT, MRI, and pathology findings in dogs presented for suspected thyroid carcinoma. *Vet Radiol Ultrasound* **54**:61–70.
Theon AP, Marks SL, Feldman ES *et al.* (2000) Prognostic factors and patterns of treatment failure in dogs with unresectable differentiated thyroid carcinomas treated with megavoltage irradiation. *J Am Vet Med Assoc* **216**:1775–1779.
Turrel JM, McEntee MC, Burke BP *et al.* (2006) Sodium iodide I 131 treatment of dogs with nonresectable thyroid tumors: 39 cases (1990–2003). *J Am Vet Med Assoc* **229**:542–548.
Urie BK, Russell DS, Kisseberth WC *et al.* (2012) Evaluation of expression and function of vascular endothelial growth factor receptor 2, platelet derived growth factor receptors-alpha and -beta, KIT, and RET in canine apocrine gland anal sac adenocarcinoma and thyroid carcinoma. *BMC Vet Research* **8**:67.
Worth AJ, Zuber RM, Hocking M (2005) Radioiodide (131I) therapy for the treatment of canine thyroid carcinoma. *Aust Vet J* **83**:208–214.

CASE 158

1 What is the name of the object shown in 158a and 158b? A chemotherapy dispensing pin ("chemo-pin") is being used. A Luer-lok® syringe is used to access the drug through the pin.

2 What major contamination risk is this object attempting to overcome? One of the major concerns for exposure to chemotherapy during the reconstitution and dispensing process is the aerosolization of drug. The risk increases when a needle is withdrawn from a pressurized drug vial. The chemo-pin is a vented needle with a hydrophobic filter designed to eliminate dangerous aerosols.

3 What are the devices shown in 158c and 158d and what are their advantages? The closed system transfer device system shown here is the Equashield™ system. The closed system drug transfer devices such as Equashield™ and PhaSeal® are considered superior in preventing the escape of hazardous drugs and aerosolization of chemotherapeutic agents into the environment. The harmful effects of workplace exposure to antineoplastic agents were well recognized as early as the 1970s. Risks of handling these agents by healthcare personnel include damage to DNA, infertility, and a possible increased risk of cancer. Necessary precautions of personal protective equipment (chemotherapy gloves, gowns, etc.), chemotherapy hood, and a closed system drug-transfer device will greatly reduce the risk of workplace exposure.

References

Clark BA, Sessink PJM (2013) Use of a closed system drug-transfer device eliminates surface contamination with antineoplastic agents. *J Oncol Pharm Pract* **19**:99–104.

Falck K, Grohn P, Sorsa M *et al.* (1979) Mutagenicity in urine of nurses handling cytostatic drugs. *Lancet* **1**:1250–1251.

Kicenuik K, Northrup N, Dawson A *et al.* (2014) Treatment time, ease of use and cost associated with the use of Equashield™, PhaSeal®, or no closed system transfer device for administration of cancer chemotherapy to a dog model. *Vet Comp Oncol*, doi:10.1111/vco.12148.

Website for closed system transfer devices: www.bd.com/pharmacy/phaseal and equashield.com.

CASE 159

1 What are the causes of hypercalcemia in dogs? Causes of hypercalcemia include (but are not limited to) hypercalcemia of malignancy (e.g. lymphoma, anal gland tumors, mammary gland tumors, thymoma, multiple myeloma, thyroid carcinoma), hypoadrenocorticism, chronic kidney disease and acute kidney injury, hypervitaminosis D or A, primary hyperparathroidism, iatrogenic (excess calcium or oral phosphate binders), and false elevation due to lipemia or laboratory error.

2 What is the interpretation of these results? Although the concentration of parathyroid hormone is not numerically elevated, this result is viewed as being inappropriately elevated in response to the hypercalcemia. With this degree of hypercalcemia, the PTH level should be closer to 0. The results of this profile are consistent with a diagnosis of primary hyperparathyroidism. The normal, or negative, PTHrP result would be expected with this diagnosis.

3 What further diagnostic tests should be performed? Ultrasound evaluation by a skilled ultrasonographer of the neck is often useful in identifying a parathyroid mass. Parathyroid adenomas can occur in more than one gland in approximately 10% of patients. There are four parathyroid glands.

4 How should this dog be treated? Surgical removal of the affected parathyroid glands is considered the most effective treatment for primary hyperparathyroidism. Other procedures have been described (ultrasound-guided radiofrequency heat ablation or ethanol ablation) but success appears to be very dependent on the skill of the person performing the procedure.

5 What are the complications of treatment? Up to three of the four glands can be removed without the development of permanent hypoparathyroidism. However, hypocalcemia can be a result of atrophy of the normal glands caused by the chronic inhibition of PTH secretion by chronic hypercalcemia. Postoperatively, ionized

Answers

calcium levels should be checked at least twice daily for up to a week. Intravenous calcium is required if clinical symptoms of hypocalcemia occur or if calcium levels are low. Calcitriol is advised for subacute and chronic treatment if calcium levels fail to normalize. The recurrence rate after surgery is <10% and the prognosis is usually excellent.

References
Felman EC, Hoar B, Pollard R et al. (2005) Pretreatment clinical and laboratory findings in dogs with primary hyperparathyroidism: 210 cases (1987–2004). *J Am Vet Med Assoc* **227**:756–761.
Pollard RE, Long CD, Nelson RW et al. (2001) Percutaneous ultrasonographically guided radiofrequency heat ablation for the treatment of primary hyperparathyroidism in dogs. *J Am Vet Med Assoc* **218**:1106–1110.
Raso L, Pollard RE, Feldman EC (2007) Retrospective evaluation of three treatment methods for primary hyperparathyroidism in dogs. *J Am Anim Hosp Assoc* **43**:70–77.
Sakals S, Peta GRH, Fernandez NJ et al. (2006) Determining the cause of hypercalcemia in a dog. *Can Vet J* **47**:819–821.

CASE 160

1 What further diagnostic tests should be considered prior to treatment? An MDB and abdominal ultrasound are indicated.

2 What treatment and supportive care should be recommended? Treatment options include:

- CCNU (lomustine) is currently the most widely used chemotherapeutic agent for CTCL or mycosis fungoides.
- Retinoids such as the synthetic vitamin A derivative isotretinoin (Accutane®) have been beneficial for some patients.
- Fatty acid supplementation (Hollywood Brand Safflower oil is reported to be good source of linoleic acid – 3 ml/kg twice weekly).
- Antibiotics are usually intermittently used to control superficial infection.
- Corticosteroids.
- Topical steroids (triamcinolone spray, betamethasone, or hydrocortisone) can be used in earlier stages of disease.
- Antibiotic shampoos can be used to help control superficial secondary pyodermas.
- Responses can sometimes be seen using l-asparaginase and other chemotherapy agents typically used for lymphoma.

3 What is the prognosis for this patient? The prognosis for epitheliotropic lymphoma is generally poor. Initial overall response rates to CCNU have been reported to be high (~80%), but the duration of response is short (~3 months). Accutane® used at 3–4 mg/kg/day is associated with a 40–50% response rate, also short lived. Overall median survival times vary from several months to 2 years, depending on the study referenced. A retrospective analysis of 30 cases reported an MST of 6 months after diagnosis and, in this report, treatment with CCNU or prednisolone did not affect the outcome. Mycosis fungoides limited to mucosal sites is typically associated with a better outcome (MST 1,070 days vs. 274 for cutaneous sites in one study).

References

Fontaine J, Bovens C, Bettenay S et al. (2009) Canine cutaneous epitheliotropic T-cell lymphoma: a review. *Vet Comp Oncol* 7:1–14.

Fontaine J, Heimann M, Day MJ (2010) Canine cutaneous epitheliotropic T-cell lymphoma: a review of 30 cases. *Vet Dermatol* 21:267–275.

Iwamoto KS, Bennett LR, Normal A et al. (1992) Linoleate produces remission in canine mycosis fungoides. *Cancer Lett* 64:17–22.

Risbon RE, DeLorimier LP, Skorupski K et al. (2006) Response of canine cutaneous epitheliotropic lymphoma to lomustine (CCNU): a retrospective study of 46 cases (1999–2004). *J Vet Intern Med* 20:1389–1397.

Williams LE, Rassnick KM, Power HT et al. (2006) CCNU in the treatment of canine epitheliotropic lymphoma. *J Vet Intern Med* 20:136–143.

CASE 161

1 Name the breeds of dog that are more susceptible to chemotherapy-related hair loss. Dogs with continually growing hair coats are at the greatest risk for chemotherapy-related hair loss similar to that seen in humans, although the pattern of hair loss tends to be patchy. Complete baldness is very rare. Breeds that appear to be more susceptible to hair loss include Old English Sheepdogs, Poodles, Bichon Frises, and terrier breeds such as Soft Coated Wheaten Terriers and Bedlington Terriers. In other breeds, such as the Golden Retriever pictured here, hair loss tends to be less noticeable. In **161a** there was thinning of the hair on the back of the neck, believed to be accelerated by the collar rubbing in this area. Breeds with feathering (**161b**) on the tail and legs will show thinning of these hairs in some cases.

2 What hair loss patterns are seen in cats undergoing chemotherapy? It is uncommon to see alopecia from chemotherapy in cats. Cats can lose longer guard hairs and whiskers when undergoing chemotherapy, but this is usually subtle and often has to be pointed out to cat owners. Regrowth of these hairs and whiskers occurs after chemotherapy is stopped.

3 What chemotherapy agents are more likely to cause hair loss? The risk of hair thinning or hair loss appears greater with doxorubicin (Adriamycin®) than with other chemotherapy agents commonly used in pets, although any agent can potentially cause alopecia.

Answers

CASE 162

1 What are the primary side effects of doxorubicin seen in dogs? Infusion rate dependent hypersensitivity, gastrointestinal toxicity (vomiting, diarrhea), myelosuppression, and cumulative dose-related cardiotoxicity are recognized side effects. Doxorubicin is a potent vesicant, necessitating careful IV administration. An indwelling IV catheter should be placed, and patients should be restrained manually for the infusion. Do not hook a patient up to an IV drip and put them into a cage unattended. The drug is diluted in saline and administered over approximately 20–30 minutes. Some sources say that it can be administered as an IV push over 10 minutes, but this increases the risk of a hypersensitivity reaction.

2 How do the side effects of doxorubicin seen in cats differ from those in dogs? In cats, while any of the above listed toxicities for dogs are possible, in one study, renal toxicity appeared to predominate and cardiac effects were not clinically significant. In a later study, increased renal toxicity was not observed when two dosage schemes were compared.

References

O'Keefe DA, Sisson DD, Gelberg HB *et al.* (1993) Systemic toxicity associated with doxorubicin administration in cats. *J Vet Intern Med* 7:309–317.

Reiman RA, Mauldin GE, Mauldin GN (2008) A comparison of toxicity of two dosing schemes of doxorubicin in the cat. *J Feline Med Surg* 10:324–331.

CASE 163

1 Describe the radiograph and give the differential diagnoses. There is a lytic and productive lesion of the proximal humerus. A periosteal reaction is seen (more prominent on the caudal aspect of the bone). The lesion is consistent with a primary bone tumor. Osteosarcoma is the most common primary bone tumor in dogs; however, it is not as commonly seen in dogs that weigh <15 kg. In fact, less than 5% of dogs that are diagnosed with osteosarcoma weigh <12 kg. Chondrosarcoma, fibrosarcoma, hemangiosarcoma, plasma cell tumors, and lymphoma are also seen as primary tumors in bone. The proportion of these non-OSA primary tumors of bone is 5–10%. Bone lesions from systemic mycosis can occur in dogs but are typically associated with living or travelling to an endemic area and a history of respiratory illness. Bacterial osteomyelitis is rare when there is no history of previous surgery or a draining tract from a wound in close proximity to where the bone lesion exists.

2 What further diagnostic tests are indicated? A bone biopsy is recommended to obtain a definitive diagnosis. The center of the tumor is the location where there is the greatest diagnostic yield.

3 A biopsy revealed osteosarcoma, low grade. What treatment recommendations should be made? Amputation of the forequarter is recommended. Chemotherapy (e.g. carboplatin or cis-platin as single agent therapy, or either drug combined with doxorubicin) is commonly used in larger dogs with osteosarcoma; however, one study suggested that chemotherapy may not be indicated for smaller dogs.

4 How is the prognosis for this patient different from that of the majority of dogs diagnosed with osteosarcoma? Smaller dogs (≤15 kg) tend to have a lower mitotic index and histologic grade of osteosarcoma than larger breed dogs. When amputation alone was evaluated in smaller dogs, median survival times of 257 days were seen. With amputation and chemotherapy, MSTs were 415 days; however, there was no statistical difference between the amputation alone and amputation and chemotherapy groups, suggesting that chemotherapy may not provide a survival advantage. Proximal humeral location and elevated pretreatment serum alkaline phosphatase levels are associated with a poorer prognosis in larger breed dogs, but were not considered negative prognostic indicators in smaller dogs.

Reference
Amsellem PM, Selmic LE, Wypij JM *et al.* (2014) Appendicular osteosarcoma in small-breed dogs: 51 cases (1986–2011). *J Am Vet Med Assoc* **245**:203–210.

CASE 164

1 Describe the type of chemotherapy protocol that this represents. This is a metronomic chemotherapy (MC) protocol. MC refers to the use of uninterrupted administration of drugs at doses that are significantly lower than the maximum tolerated dose (MTD) of chemotherapy traditionally used. Most MC protocols use chemotherapy agents at dosages as low as one-tenth of the dosage of standard MTD. MC is not believed to kill tumor cells directly, but instead targets cells that are critical for blood vessel formation (anti-angiogenic therapy). Blood vessel formation is critical for the growth and metastasis of tumors. Therefore, targeting the endothelial cells and circulating endothelial progenitor cells should theoretically kill tumors indirectly by starving them of their blood supply. With the use of MTD protocols, chemotherapy is given with periods of rest in between treatments, allowing for repair of normal cells (such as bone marrow or GI epithelium). However, during this repair time, repair and repopulation of other endothelial cells is seen, including those critical to the angiogenesis involved in tumor growth and metastasis. With MC, there is no rest period to allow for repair of these endothelial cells. In addition to anti-angiogenic properties, MC is believed to modulate the immune system of tumor-bearing patients by inhibiting regulatory T cells (Treg). Treg are increased in the peripheral blood of dogs with various types of cancer.

In humans, increased numbers of Treg may be associated with a less favorable outcome for certain tumor types. In dogs, the prognostic significance of elevated Treg is unknown. However, it is known that low-dose cyclophosphamide selectively decreases Treg and inhibits angiogenesis in dogs with soft tissue sarcomas.

2 In what cancers in dogs and cats has this type of chemotherapeutic regimen been evaluated? MC has been evaluated in soft tissue sarcomas, TCC of the bladder, and hemangiosarcoma in the post-surgical setting and appears to delay the progression of disease. In metastatic cancer of various histologic types, MC has been evaluated as a first-line therapy and although this was only a pilot study, a benefit was shown.

References

Burton JH, Mitchell L, Thamm DH *et al.* (2011) Low-dose cyclophosphamide selectively decreases regulatory T cells and inhibits angiogenesis in dogs with soft tissue sarcoma. *J Vet Intern Med* **25**:920–926.

Elmslie RE, Glawe P, Dow SW (2008) Metronomic therapy with cyclophosphamide and piroxicam effectively delays tumor recurrence in dogs with incompletely resected soft tissue sarcomas. *J Vet Intern Med* **22**:1373–1379.

Lana S, U'ren L, Plaza S *et al.* (2007) Continuous low-dose oral chemotherapy for adjuvant therapy of splenic hemangiosarcoma in dogs. *J Vet Intern Med* **21**:764–769.

Marchetti V, Giorgi M, Fioravanti A *et al.* (2012) First-line metronomic chemotherapy in a metastatic model of spontaneous canine tumours: a pilot study. *Invest New Drugs* **30**:1725–1730.

Schrempp DR, Childress MO, Stewart JC *et al.* (2013) Metronomic administration of chlorambucil for treatment of dogs with urinary bladder transitional cell carcinoma. *J Am Vet Med Assoc* **242**:1534–1538.

CASE 165

1 The history and clinical appearance of this patient are suggestive of what paraneoplastic syndrome? This patient most likely has cancer cachexia. Cancer cachexia is defined by the loss of lean body mass and metabolic alterations noted in cancer patients in the face of adequate nutritional intake. This differs from cancer "anorexia", which results from a poor appetite and the resultant poor nutritional intake. Cancer cachexia is believed to be a result of excessive cytokine stimulation leading to insulin resistance, lipolysis, and proteolysis of tissues.

2 How common is this syndrome in pets with cancer? The incidence of true cancer cachexia in dogs and cats is unknown, but it is most likely uncommon. It is far more common to see cancer anorexia. Cachexia is also seen in patients with chronic kidney disease, congestive heart failure, and other chronic diseases.

3 How does the presence of this syndrome affect this patient's prognosis? Unfortunately, the metabolic alternations noted with cachexia are believed to occur before the clinical signs of the cancer, and even with successful treatment of the cancer can be difficult to reverse. Progressive wasting can occur and ultimately leads to a decline in quality of life. In humans, up to 20% of cancer deaths are due to cachexia and therefore it is a significant negative prognostic indicator. Treatment of the cancer and aggressive nutritional support can help decrease cachexia.

4 What is sarcopenia? Sarcopenia is defined as a loss of lean body mass that occurs with aging. It is similar to cachexia but is seen during aging in the absence of disease. In humans, sarcopenia actually begins earlier in life (at approximately 30 years of age) and can result in significant loss of lean body mass over time. Therefore, patients that were already losing lean body mass will be further compromised if later affected with cachexia secondary to disease.

References

Freeman LM (2012) Cachexia and sarcopenia: emerging syndromes of importance in dogs and cats. *J Vet Intern Med* **26**:3–17.

Michel KE, Sorenmo K, Shofer FS (2004) Evaluation of body condition and weight loss in dogs presented to a veterinary oncology service. *J Vet Intern Med* **18**:692–695.

CASE 166

1 Describe the cytology and give a preliminary diagnosis. The primary population of cells is that of well-differentiated fusiform mesenchymal cells in a proteinaceous background. There is minimal variation in the size and shape of the cells. There is mild anisokaryosis. A mesenchymal neoplasm, potentially of smooth muscle origin, is likely. It is often difficult to distinguish leiomyoma from its malignant counterpart, leiomyosarcoma, on the basis of cytology alone. Histologic confirmation is necessary.

2 What are the differential diagnoses? Based on the caudal abdominal location and vaginal discharge, a tumor of the reproductive tract is a primary consideration. The most common uterine tumor in the dog is a leiomyoma. Other mesenchymal tumors that can be seen are leiomyosarcomas, fibroma, fibrosarcoma, and hemangiosarcoma.

3 What further tests are indicated in order to determine the best treatment plan? Given the large size of this mass, a CT scan is recommended to determine invasiveness into surrounding tissues and help in surgical planning. A needle core biopsy at the time of CT is advised. In this case, leiomyoma was confirmed.

4 What is the best course of treatment? If the mass appears well circumscribed and is not invading into critical structures, surgical removal and complete OHE can potentially be curative. In this patient, the tumor appeared to be closely associated with the ureter and colon on CT (**166b**). A post-contrast CT image showed the mass (**166c**, blue arrows; the red arrow points to the urinary bladder, which is being pushed to one side with contrast agent pooling at bottom; the green arrows indicate contrast within portions of the ureter). Exploratory surgery is necessary to

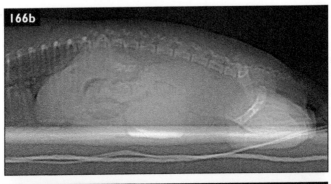

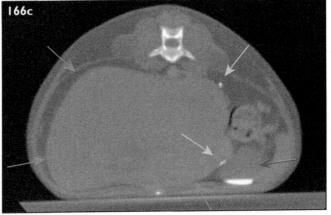

determine whether the mass is actually involving these structures or just pushing them aside.

Reference

Sapierzynski R, Malicka E, Bielecki W *et al.* (2007) Tumors of the urogenital system in dogs and cats. Retrospective review of 138 cases. *Pol J Vet Sci* **10**:97–103.

CASE 167

1 Describe the radiograph and ultrasound. The heart and trachea are being displaced dorsally by a space-occupying lesion, appearing to be of fat density. On ultrasound, the entire ventral third of the thorax was filled with tissue, also appearing to be fatty. The tissue is relatively homogeneous with bright echoes scattered throughout. The diaphragm was intact (ruling out a diaphragmatic hernia with falciform fat in the chest cavity).

2 What further diagnostics are indicated for this patient? An ultrasound-guided fine needle aspirate can help to rule out other potential tumors, but ultrasound findings are very consistent with fat. A CT scan is recommended for surgical planning.

3 What treatment is advised? Surgical removal is advised. Even though the tumor is likely to be benign, as it grows it will further compromise the cardiopulmonary system and may become necrotic as well.

4 What is the patient's prognosis? Intrathoracic lipomas are rare. They have been reported to occur in mediastinal, pleural, and pericardial sites. Excellent outcomes were seen in the majority of patients that underwent surgical excision. Tumors often were able to be "digitally removed" even when large. Adhesions and invasiveness were not typically encountered, but could allow for regrowth of the lipoma due to inability to obtain a clean surgical excision. Of those cases reported in the literature, most were removed and did not recur.

References

Ben-Amotz R, Ellison GW, Thompson MS *et al.* (2007) Pericardial lipoma in a geriatric dog with an incidentally discovered thoracic mass. *J Small Animal Pract* 48:596–599.

Lynch S, Halfacree Z, Desmas I *et al.* (2013) Pulmonary lipoma in a dog. *J Small Animal Pract* 54:555–558.

Mayhew PD, Brockman DJ (2002) Body cavity lipomas in six dogs. *J Small Animal Pract* 43:177–181.

CASE 168

1 What are the radiographic findings? There is lysis and destruction of P3. There is also significant soft tissue swelling of the digit.

2 What are the differential diagnoses for this patient? The most common causes for swelling of the digit and lysis of the underlying bone include infection, squamous cell carcinoma, malignant melanoma, malignant soft tissue tumors, benign soft tissue tumors, osteosarcoma, and hemangiopericytoma.

3 What additional tests should be performed? Fine needle aspirate of the toe mass and popliteal lymph node are indicated.

4 What is the treatment and prognosis for this patient? Digital amputation and lymph node removal are advised. Even if cytology confirms metastatic disease, amputation of the digit is still advised. Regardless of tumor type, overall survival times are not significantly negatively affected by age at diagnosis, gender, type or site of tumor, and stage of disease. Early surgical intervention is associated with the most favorable outcome. In this patient, a benign soft tissue tumor was diagnosed. A multilobulated proliferation of epithelial cells forming dense central clusters of keratin surrounded by fibrovascular interlobular stroma was consistent with a subungual keratoacanthoma. This is a benign tumor of nail bed epithelium often

Answers

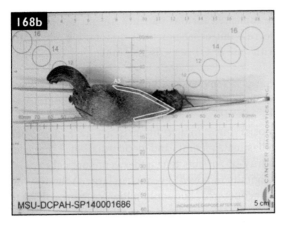

MSU-DCPAH-SP140001686

causing lysis of P3, as was seen in this case. These tumors are slow growing and are cured by amputation of the affected digit. The neoplastic cells widely replaced P3 and impinged on the ventral aspect of P2 and the P2–P3 interphalangeal joint, but did not invade P2 or enter the joint. The margins were free of neoplastic cells, and therefore excision should be curative. The amputated toe is shown (**168b**) in preparation for histopathologic evaluation of tumor tissue and margins. Bone margins were evaluated after decalcification.

Reference
Gardner HL, Cavanaugh RP (2014) What is your diagnosis? Keratoacanthoma. *J Am Vet Med Assoc* **244**:1031–1032.

CASE 169

1 Describe the cytology. There is a mixed population of lymphocytes, with small lymphocytes (less than the size of a segmented neutrophil) predominating. There are plasma cells, occasional large lymphocytes, and a single mitotic figure (red arrow). There is a large pigment-containing macrophage (blue arrow). The cytology is most consistent with a reactive lymph node.

2 What further diagnostic tests should be performed? Urinalysis, coagulation profile, and serum electrophoresis should be performed. Further testing would depend on the results of these tests. If clotting ability is normal, an ultrasound-guided aspirate of the spleen would be indicated. In the presence of a monoclonal gammopathy, additional testing would include evaluation of the urine for Bence Jones proteins, a bone marrow aspirate/biopsy, and testing for *Ehrlichia*. A polyclonal gammopathy would be more supportive of inflammatory causes.

3 What are the differential diagnoses for hyphema and hyperglobulinema? Multiple myeloma, lymphoma, ehrlichiosis, and chronic inflammatory disease are the primary considerations.

4 What is a possible mechanism of the hyphema? Hyperviscosity, due to the hyperglobulinemia, could be a cause of the hyphema in this patient. Vascular endothelial cells are compromised by blood sludging and infiltration of the excess proteins into the vascular wall. The excess globulins are associated with platelet and coagulation disorders, which can lead to hyphema. Alternatively, when hyperviscosity is not present, breakdown in the vascular integrity due to the direct effect of the cancer can occur. In this patient, a diagnosis of lymphoma was made from a splenic aspirate. Immunocytochemistry confirmed B cell lymphoma.

Reference
Komaromy AM, Ramsey DT, Brooks DE *et al.* (1999) Hyphema. Part I: pathophysiologic considerations. *Compend Contin Educ Vet* **21**:1064–1069.

CASE 170

1 Describe how the treatment plans would differ between these two patients. Chemotherapy is indicated post-amputation for dogs with osteosarcoma. However, the biologic behavior of OSA in cats is different. Metastasis is less common in cats and the use of postoperative chemotherapy is generally not recommended.

2 What are the primary toxicities associated with cis-platin use in dogs and in cats? *Dogs:* Cis-platin is highly nephrotoxic in dogs. Emesis during administration can be severe. Myelosuppression is typically mild. Care must be taken to evaluate renal function prior to using cisplatin. Cardiac function should also be evaluated to be certain aggressive saline diuresis would be tolerated. *Cats:* Cis-platin is CONTRAINDICATED IN CATS. In cats, fulminant pulmonary toxicity (dyspnea, hydrothorax, pulmonary edema, and death) precludes its use.

3 What is the administration protocol for cis-platin? In dogs, there are several administration protocols published. Saline diuresis is required before and after administration owing to the risk of renal toxicity. Prior to each treatment with cis-platin, a CBC, chemistry panel, and urinalysis should be performed. One protocol utilizes a fluid rate of 18.3 ml/kg/hour for 4 hours prior to administration of cis-platin. The drug is diluted in enough saline to maintain the same fluid rate over 20 minutes, and then continued for 2 hours post-treatment. An anti-emetic is administered prior to treatment. Maropitant, butorphenol, dexamethasone, and metoclopramide have all been used effectively. In the author's experience, maropitant has superior efficacy. Special precautions are required for handling cis-platin and patient wastes because up to 80% of the cis-platin is eliminated in the urine within the first 48 hours. Urine, feces, and vomitus should be handled as medical waste. Hospitalization for at least 24 hours following chemotherapy administration is often recommended to decrease the risk of exposure to pet owners. Owing to the ease of administration, decreased toxicity, and ability to use in cats, carboplatin is being used more frequently. However, there is still debate over which drug is more efficacious for osteosarcoma.

Answers

References

Dimopoulou M, Kirpensteijn J, Moens H *et al.* (2008) Histologic prognosticators in feline osteosarcoma: a comparison with phenotypically similar canine osteosarcoma. *Vet Surg* 37:466–471.

Gustafson DL, Page RL (2013) Cancer chemotherapy. In: Withrow SJ, Vail DM, Page RL, editors, *Small Animal Clinical Oncology*, 5th edition. St. Louis, Elsevier Saunders, p. 171.

Heldmann E, Anderson MA, Wagner-Mann C (2000) Feline osteosarcoma: 145 cases (1990–1995). *J Am Anim Hosp Assoc* 36:518–521.

Vail DM, Rodabaugh HS, Conder GA *et al.* Efficacy of injectable maropitant (Cerenia) in a randomized clinical trial for prevention and treatment of cisplatin-induced emesis in dogs presented as veterinary patients. *Vet Comp Oncol* 5:38–46.

CASE 171

1 What are the differential diagnoses for this patient? Causes for collapse and seizure include hypoxia (cardiac, pulmonary, anemia), neurologic (brain tumor, ischemic event, epilepsy), and hypoglycemia (insulin-secreting tumor, hepatoma).

2 In addition to the MDB, an abdominal ultrasound was performed. The ultrasound image of the region of the pancreas is shown (171). A 0.30 × 0.38 cm hypoechoic nodule is seen within the right limb of the pancreas. What further diagnostic tests are indicated? Blood drawn at the time of collapse is helpful in detecting hypoglycemia. Imaging with abdominal ultrasound and/or CT can aid in staging and localization of a pancreatic mass; however, the sensitivity of these tests is often low. Surgical exploratory is usually superior in identifying a pancreatic mass. Insulinomas are often very small and the inability to find a mass on ultrasound does not rule out the presence of an insulin-secreting tumor. An important aspect of ultrasound or CT is to look carefully for signs of metastatic disease. Over 50% of dogs have metastatic disease at presentation. Sites for possible metastasis include regional lymph nodes, liver, duodenum, omentum, and spleen.

3 The blood glucose at the time of collapse was 40 mg/dl. What further tests should be performed based on this finding? Insulin levels should be tested on blood at the time of the collapse. This is usually difficult because most patients experience intermittent episodes of collapse or seizures, and glucose and insulin levels are often normal at the time of examination. Fructosamine concentration can be evaluated to determine whether chronic hypoglycemia is present because these values can reflect blood glucose concentrations over the previous 1–2 weeks. If hypoglycemia is suspected but not detected, multiple samples for plasma glucose concentration should be collected (e.g. hourly) during a fasting period. When glucose levels start to fall below 60 mg/dl, insulin levels should be tested. Great care needs to be taken not to allow clinical symptoms to occur.

4 **How is the diagnosis of insulinoma made?** The presence of hypoglycemia in conjunction with inappropriately high levels of insulin supports the diagnosis of insulinoma. The finding of a pancreatic mass during abdominal ultrasound or CT is also supportive, but owing to the often small and solitary nature of insulinomas, imaging is not always helpful. A definitive diagnosis requires surgery and histopathologic evaluation.

5 **List the prognostic indicators for insulinoma in the dog.** The treatment used (medical rather than surgical), presence of metastatic disease, and persistent hypoglycemia after treatment have all been associated with poorer outcomes. Surgical management (partial pancreatectomy) appears to be superior to medical management of insulinoma (381 days vs. 74 days in one report; 785 days vs. 196 days in another report). Postoperative hypoglycemia has been reported as a negative prognostic indicator, although Tobin *et al.* did not observe a difference in survival times in patients treated surgically and those treated postoperatively with prednisone and diazoxide to control hypoglycemia. The presence of metastatic disease at the time of surgery is associated with a significantly shorter survival time. The addition of medical management postoperatively improved MSTs to 1,316 days in a recent study.

References

Goutal CM, Brugmann BL, Ryan KA (2012) Insulinoma in dogs: a review. *J Am Anim Hosp Assoc* **48**:151–163.

Polton GA, White RN, Brearley MJ *et al.* (2007) Improved survival in a retrospective cohort of 28 dogs with insulinoma. *J Small Anim Pract* **48**:151–156.

Robben JH, Pollak YWEA, Kirpensteijn J *et al.* (2005) Comparison of ultrasonography, computed tomography, and single-photon emission computed tomography for the detection and localization of canine insulinoma. *J Vet Intern Med* **19**:15–22.

Tobin RL, Nelson RW, Lucroy MD *et al.* (1999) Outcome of surgical versus medical treatment of dogs with beta cell neoplasia: 39 cases (1990–1997). *J Am Vet Med Assoc* **215**:226–230.

CASE 172

1 **What structure is the blue arrow pointing to?** The blue arrow is pointing to the frontal sinus cavity.

2 **What structure is the black arrow pointing to?** The black arrow is pointing to the olfactory lobe of the brain.

3 **What is the red arrow pointing to?** The red arrow is pointing to the nasopharynx.

4 **Describe the CT scan. What is the significance of the changes seen at the tip of the black arrow?** There is extensive bone lysis and proliferative new bone, and invasion of the tumor across the cribriform plate into the olfactory lobe of the

brain. Patients with tumors causing lysis and extension into the cribriform plate have been shown to have significantly shorter disease-free intervals and survival times following radiation therapy.

Reference

Adams WM, Kleiter MM, Thrall DE *et al.* (2009) Prognostic significance of tumor histology and computed tomographic staging for radiation treatment response of canine nasal tumors. *Vet Radiol Ultrasound* 50:330–335.

CASE 173

1 **Describe the lesion seen on MRI.** At the level of the L5 vertebra, there is an expansile mass that fills the left lateral aspect of the spinal canal and infiltrates or extends from the left lamina, pedicle, and lateral left aspect of the vertebral body. The spinal cord is displaced towards the right and is severely compressed.

2 **What are the differential diagnoses for this lesion?** The primary differential is vertebral neoplasia: chondrosarcoma, osteosarcoma, or plasma cell tumor. Less likely is neoplasia arising from the soft tissues within the spinal canal with secondary invasion into the vertebrae. Granulomatous inflammatory etiologies would be considered less likely.

3 **How should a definitive diagnosis be obtained?** Surgical biopsy and histopathology are recommended. Surgery was performed to relieve compression on the spinal cord and to obtain a definitive diagnosis. At surgery, the mass was arising from and involving the fifth lumbar vertebral body on the left side. On histopathology, cells exhibited moderate anisocytosis and anisokaryosis. The mitotic index was 5 per 10 hpf. Prominent trabeculae of osteoid were being formed throughout the mass. Within the medullary space of the bone, there were disorganized streams and bundles of spindle cells lining blood-filled vascular spaces and channels. Intramedullary sarcoma, most consistent with osteosarcoma, was reported. The histologic features of the tumor were consistent with a telangiectatic osteosarcoma, although hemangiosarcoma could not be completely excluded.

4 **What treatment options should be considered and what is this patient's prognosis?** The prognosis for dogs with primary vertebral tumors is considered very guarded. Median survival times of 135 days (range, 15–600 days) are reported regardless of treatment modality. Postoperative improvement of neurologic status, however, has a significant influence on outcome. In humans, radiation therapy plays an important role in the treatment of vertebral tumors. In dogs, it appears that RT may also play a role in treating vertebral tumors. Given the incomplete surgical margins in this patient, RT was pursued postoperatively.

Follow up/discussion

Post-operatively, this patient remained very painful as exhibited by her stance in this photograph (**173d**). Following RT, she is more comfortable, is ambulating normally and no longer hunched up in her back (**173e**).

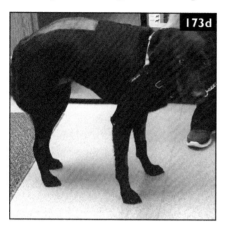

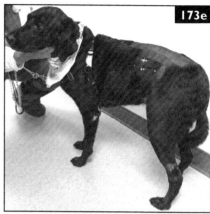

Reference

Dernell WS, Van Vecten BJ, Straw RC *et al.* (2000) Outcome following treatment of vertebral tumors in 20 dogs (1986–1995). *J Am Anim Hosp Assoc* **36**:245–251.

CASE 174

1 What is the cytologic diagnosis? There are large round cells with indistinct nucleoli, a moderate amount of lightly basophilic cytoplasm containing moderate numbers of coarse azurophilic granules. The cells are suggestive of a large granular lymphocyte (LGL) lymphoma.

2 What further diagnostic tests are indicated to make a definitive diagnosis and stage the patient? In addition to FeLV, FIV, abdominal ultrasound, and FNA of the mass, a CBC, serum chemistry panel, urinalysis, and thoracic radiographs are needed to complete the MDB. FNA of the liver and spleen will help confirm further organ involvement. Histopathology with immunohistochemistry, and cytology with immunocytochemistry or PCR for T cell receptor gene rearrangement to detect clonality will help to confirm the diagnosis. Feline LGLs are of cytotoxic T cell or natural killer cell origin. Feline LGL lymphoma is most commonly composed of T cells (CD3+) that express CD8αα and CD103.

3 What is the prognosis for this patient? LGL lymphoma is an uncommon but morphologically distinct variant of feline lymphoma. Unfortunately, LGL lymphoma in cats carries a grave prognosis. Median survival times post-diagnosis are less than months and response to chemotherapy is generally poor. Survival beyond 3 months is uncommon. Feline LGL lymphoma is believed to be of small intestinal origin and metastatic disease in the mesenteric lymph nodes, liver, spleen, and kidney is routinely seen. Involvement of the peripheral blood can also occur.

References
Krick EL, Little R, Patel R *et al.* (2008) Description of clinical and pathological findings, treatment and outcome of feline large granular lymphocyte lymphoma (1996–2004). *Vet Comp Oncol* **6:**102–110.
Roccabianca P, Vernau W, Caniatti M *et al.* (2006) Feline large granular lymphocyte (LGL) lymphoma with secondary leukemia: primary intestinal origin with predominance of a CD3/CD8(alpha)(alpha) phenotype. *Vet Pathol* **43:**15–28.

CASE 175

1 What is seen on the ultrasound image? The stomach wall is extremely thickened diffusely and measures up to 0.65 cm in width. Regional lymphadenopathy was also detected.

2 What are the primary differential diagnoses? Primary gastric cancer in dogs is uncommon. Approximately 70–80% of dogs with gastric cancer are diagnosed with adenocarcinoma. Lymphoma is the second most common cancer found in the stomach. There appears to be a genetic predisposition for gastric adenocarcinoma in some breeds, including Chow Chows. Other breeds affected are Rough Coated Collies, Belgian Shepherds, Staffordshire Bull Terriers, and Norwegian Lundehunds. Other far less common tumors that can occur in the stomach include leiomyoma, leiomyosarcoma, gastrointestinal stromal tumor, histiocytic sarcoma, mast cell tumor, plasmacytomas, and carcinoids.

3 How should a definitive diagnosis be obtained? An ultrasound-guided FNA can help rule out lymphoma, but is often not reliable because of the increased inflammation and necrosis often associated with gastric neoplasia. Endoscopy may be needed to obtain a histologic diagnosis. A surgical biopsy should be obtained for those patients whose tumors appear operable. Unfortunately, early symptoms of gastric neoplasia tend to be minimal and non-specific. For this reason, gastric cancer is often diagnosed very late in the course of the disease. Approximately 75% of dogs with gastric adenocarcinoma have metastasis at the time of diagnosis.

4 What is the prognosis for this patient? Given the local extent of disease and lymph node metastasis, the prognosis for this patient is poor. With no further treatment, survival for patients with inoperable gastric cancer rarely exceeds 3 months. In some patients, aggressive surgical resection (gastrojejunostomy or Bilroth I) can be palliative even if clean surgical margins are not obtained. In patients where palliative surgery is possible, survival times can be improved significantly (8 months in one study). Chemotherapy for gastric adenocarcinoma is not well documented in dogs. Protocols adapted from human medicine tend to be used (e.g. "FAC": 5-fluorouracil (5-FU), cyclophosphamide, doxorubicin; single agent carboplatin or cis-platin, 5-FU, doxorubicin). Although not yet studied, the use of TKIs may be considered palliatively.

References
Sullivan M, Lee R, Fisher EW *et al.* (1987) A study of 31 cases of gastric carcinoma in dogs. *Vet Rec* **120**:79–83.
Swann HM, Holt DE (2002) Canine gastric adenocarcinoma and leiomyosarcoma: a retrospective study of 21 cases (1986–1999) and literature review. *J Am Anim Hosp Assoc* **38**:157–164.

CASE 176

1 Describe the radiographs and ultrasound. The thoracic radiographs show a large mediastinal mass filling the cranial thoracic cavity, causing dorsal deviation of the trachea, and obscuring a significant portion of the heart shadow. On ultrasound, a soft tissue mass of mixed echogenicity is seen cranial to and above the heart shadow.

2 List the differential diagnoses for a mass in this location. Lymphoma, thymoma, ectopic thyroid tumor, branchial cysts, rare sarcoma, and metastatic cancer are the major differential diagnoses.

3 What diagnosis is most likely based on the testing performed thus far? The results of the cytology support the diagnosis of thymoma.

4 What further diagnostic tests can provide a definitive diagnosis and establish the extent of disease? Histopathology is the only way to establish a definitive diagnosis. It is important, however, to rule out lymphoma before surgery is considered, because lymphoma would be treated medically rather than surgically. The success rate in obtaining a diagnostic sample from transthoracic biopsy was only 50% in one report. Flow cytometry has been shown to be useful in differentiating lymphoma from thymoma in dogs, which can often be difficult because of the significant lymphoid component possible with thymomas. Canine thymic lymphocytes can be differentiated from peripheral lymphocytes by their simultaneous expression of CD4- and CD8-positive cells. In cases of thymoma, 10% of lymphocytes co-expressed CD4 and CD8, whereas in lymphomas, <2% contained CD4+CD8+ lymphocytes in one study. Flow cytometry may prove useful in the future, but currently has not been validated in cats. A CT scan or MRI can help determine the degree of invasiveness. In humans, MRI is considered superior to CT for this purpose.

5 What are the treatment options for this patient? Surgical excision is the treatment of choice for non-invasive thymomas. For more invasive tumors whose surgical risks are considered high, radiation therapy has been shown to be very effective in cats with thymoma.

6 List the positive and negative prognostic indicators for this disease. In a recent report that evaluated 32 cats undergoing excision of thymic epithelial tumors, there were no significant predictors of survival times. In contrast, the presence of paraneoplastic syndromes or incomplete histologic margins was associated with decreased survival times in dogs. In the same report of 32 cats undergoing surgery, the risk of perioperative death was 22%, but median survival time was 3.71 years and the 1- and 4-year survival rates were 70% and 47%, respectively. In another report, MST for cats treated surgically for invasive thymomas was 790 days and with non-invasive thymomas 1,825 days. In a retrospective study of seven cats treated with radiation therapy instead of surgery, the MST was 720 days.

7 What paraneoplastic syndromes can be seen in cats with this diagnosis? Approximately 40% of all dogs and cats diagnosed with thymoma have paraneoplastic syndromes. These include myasthenia gravis, megaesophagus, exfoliative dermatitis, erythema multiforme, hypercalcemia, T cell lymphocytosis, anemia, polymyositis, and other immune-mediated diseases.

References

Garneau MS, Price LL, Withrow SJ et al. (2015) Perioperative mortality and long-term survival in 80 dogs and 32 cats undergoing excision of thymic epithelial tumors. *Vet Surg* **44**:557–564.

Gores BR, Berg J, Carpenter JL et al. (1994) Surgical treatment of thymoma in cats: 12 cases (1987–1992). *J Am Vet Med Assoc* **204**:1782–1785.

Hague DW, Humphries HD, Mitchell MA et al. (2015) Risk factors and outcomes in cats with acquired myasthenia gravis (2001–2012). *J Vet Intern Med* **29**:1307–1312.

Lana S, Plaza S, Hampe K et al. (2006) Diagnosis of mediastinal masses in dogs by flow cytometry. *J Vet Intern Med* **20**:1161–1165.

Smith AN, Wright JC, Brawner Jr. WR et al. (2001) Radiation therapy in the treatment of canine and feline thymomas: a retrospective study (1985–1999). *J Am Anim Hosp Assoc* **37**:489–496.

Zitz JC, Birchard SJ, Couto GC et al. (2008) Results of excision of thymoma in cats and dogs: 20 cases (1984–2005). *J Am Vet Med Assoc* **232**:1186–1192.

CASE 177

1 What further diagnostic tests are indicated? The finding of gastric ulcers in association with possible metastatic disease in the liver and abdominal lymph nodes is suggestive of a gastrinoma. With gastrinoma, fasting serum gastrin levels are usually over 3 times the reference range (20–104 pg/ml for dogs). This patient's gastrin level was 1,730 pg/ml. Gastrin levels can also be increased with renal or hepatic disease and in patients being treated with antacid therapy, but are not usually elevated to this degree. Histopathology is necessary to make a definitive diagnosis.

2 There is evidence of metastatic disease on ultrasound. Would surgery be indicated? In the case of metastatic gastrinoma, surgery can still be therapeutic because debulking the tumor will decrease the gastrin secretion. In addition, resection of deep or perforating ulcers can significantly improve clinical signs. This patient underwent exploratory laparotomy. A 0.5 cm mass was found in the right lobe of the pancreas. Abdominal lymph nodes and liver nodules were biopsied and confirmed metastatic gastrinoma.

3 What is Zollinger–Ellison syndrome and how should it be medically managed? Zollinger–Ellison syndrome refers to a triad of a non-beta cell neuroendocrine tumor in the pancreas, hypergastrinemia, and GI ulceration. Therapy should be directed at supportive care with IV fluids if dehydration is present, H2 receptor antagonists (e.g. cimetidine, ranitidine, or famotidine), proton pump inhibitors (e.g. omeprazole), and sucralfate. Octreotide, a somatostatin analog, has been used in dogs, but efficacy is not well established. Somatostatin inhibits gastrin secretion.

4 What is the prognosis for this patient? Gastrinoma carries a very guarded to poor prognosis, primarily due to the fact that its small size precludes early diagnosis. Over 85% of patients have metastatic disease by the time the tumor is identified. The liver is the most common site of metastasis, but regional lymph nodes, omentum, spleen, mesentery, and other serosal surfaces can also be affected. With medical management, reported survival times range from days to >2 years. Some patients initially present with severe symptoms secondary to GI perforation and peritonitis, in which case the prognosis is extremely poor.

References
Hughes SM (2006) Canine gastrinoma: a case study and literature review of therapeutic options. *N Z Vet J* 54:242–247.
Lunn KF, Page RL (2013) Tumors of the endocrine system: gastrointestinal endocrine tumors. In: Withrow SJ, Vail DM, Page RL, editors, *Small Animal Clinical Oncology*, 5th edition. St. Louis, Elsevier Saunders, p. 521.

CASE 178

1 Describe the ultrasound and cytology findings. What is the presumptive diagnosis? The ultrasound shows a 2.04 cm mass at the caudal pole of the right kidney. The mass has a mixed echogenicity. On cytology, there is a large clump of epithelial cells that exhibit significant anisocytosis and anisokaryosis. Based on the cytology, carcinoma is most likely.

2 What is the treatment of choice for primary renal tumors? Primary renal tumors (excluding lymphoma) are very rare in cats. The majority of tumors diagnosed are renal carcinomas (tubular renal carcinoma, tubulopapillary carcinoma, TCC). Because primary renal carcinomas are rare, care should be taken to stage the patient to be certain that this does not represent metastatic disease. The majority of cats diagnosed with renal carcinoma in one report had evidence of metastasis at the time of presentation. If no further disease is identified, nephrectomy is the treatment of choice, but a decision to pursue surgery is dependent on renal function.

3 What is recommended for this patient? This cat has had a history of early chronic kidney disease. However, renal values at the time of diagnosis were similar to previous tests. Because renal function was considered stable, a nephrectomy was performed. A tubulopapillary carcinoma was diagnosed. No further treatment was elected because of concern regarding preservation of the function of the remaining kidney. This patient lived another year before succumbing to renal failure.

References

Henry CJ, Turnquist SE, Smith A *et al.* (1999) Primary renal tumours in cats: 19 cases (1992–1998). *J Feline Med Surg* 1:165–170.

Klainbart S, Segev G, Loeb E *et al.* (2008) Resolution of renal adenocarcinoma-induced secondary inappropriate polycyhthaemia after nephrectomy in two cats. *J Feline Med Surg* 10:264–268.

CASE 179

1 What are the differential diagnoses for hematochezia in this patient? Colorectal polyp, colorectal tumor, trauma, foreign body, infection (parasitic, viral, bacterial), coagulopathy or thrombocytopenia, idiopathic (hemorrhagic gastroenteritis).

2 What is the likely cause for the blood being eliminated immediately after the rectal examination? The blood most likely had pooled in the rectum and this was emptied when the rectal examination was performed.

3 What diagnostic tests should be pursued next? An MDB is indicated. In addition to routine blood work (CBC, chemistry panel), a coagulation panel should be performed to rule out a coagulopathy. A peripheral blood smear should be obtained for careful evaluation of platelets. Abdominal ultrasound should be performed and, if available, transrectal ultrasound can be helpful in identifying colorectal tumors. A colonoscopy is indicated and biopsies taken if lesions are noted.

4 What are the most common malignancies found in the rectum? In one study of patients with primary rectal tumors, 50% were found to be malignant. Of those that were malignant, adenocarcinoma was the most common. Carcinomas, plasmacytomas, mucinous carcinoma, and papillary carcinoma were also identified. Polyps were the most common benign lesions found. Adenomas and leiomyomas were seen, but were less common. This patient was diagnosed through colonoscopy to have a rectal carcinoma in situ. With surgical removal, median survival time in one study was 1,006 days. Sublumbar metastasis tends to be rare.

5 A rectal pull-through surgery was advised for this patient. What complications can be associated with this type of surgery? While patients with rectal tumors that undergo rectal pull-through surgery tend to have good local tumor control and survival times, the complication rate is high. Post-surgical complications were reported in a retrospective analysis of 74 patients undergoing rectal pull-through surgeries for the removal of rectal masses. Complications included fecal incontinence (56.8%), which is transient in about half of the patients experiencing this complication. Other complications included diarrhea, tenemus, stricture formation, rectal bleeding, constipation, dehiscence, and infection.

References

Holt PE, Lucke VM (1985) Rectal neoplasia in the dog: a clinicopathological review of 31 cases. *Vet Rec* **116**:400–405.

Kupanoff PA, Popovitch CA, Goldschmidt MH (2006) Colorectal plasmacytomas: a retrospective study of nine dogs. *J Am Anim Hosp Assoc* **42**:37–43.

Nucci DJ, Liptak JM, Selmic LE *et al.* (2014) Complications and outcomes following rectal pull-through surgery in dogs with rectal masses: 74 cases (2000–2013). *J Am Vet Med* **245**:684–695.

CASE 180

1 What procedure is being illustrated here (180)? Phlebotomy is being performed. Following removal of blood, fluid therapy is used to restore vascular volume.

2 What are the differential diagnoses for this patient? The elevated hematocrit, hemoglobin, and RBC count indicate an increased RBC mass. An increased red cell mass is defined as polycythemia. Polycythemia can be either relative or absolute. Relative polycythemia is the result of hemoconcentration (dehydration) and is by far the most common form of polycythemia seen in cats. The normal serum protein level in this patient makes hemoconcentration less likely, however. Absolute polycythemia can be either secondary or primary. Secondary polycythemia can result from inappropriate increased production of erythropoietin, as can occur in rare cases of renal disease or renal neoplasia. It can also occur when there is reduced oxygenation to the tissues (e.g. lung pathology, cardiac shunts), which results in an appropriate increased production of erythropoietin. Primary absolute polycythemia (polycythemia vera) is a very rare myeloproliferative disorder. Causes of absolute polycythemia include decreased tissue oxygenation (cardiac disease), inappropriate erythropoietin production (renal neoplasia, cysts), and polycythemia vera.

3 What further diagnostic tests are indicated? Thoracic radiographs, ECG, and echocardiography to rule out cardiac disease, abdominal ultrasound to rule out renal pathology, and arterial O_2 are indicated. Erythropoietin levels are not always helpful in cats in differentiating absolute secondary polycythemia from primary polycythemia. Although it is very rare, lack of cardiac or renal disease and a normal arterial O_2 support a diagnosis of polycythemia vera. The diagnosis of polycythemia vera is based on the exclusion of causes of secondary polycythemia. Bone marrow aspirates will be consistent with erythroid hyperplasia, but there are no characteristic cytologic features of the red cells or precursors in the bone marrow that are specific to the diagnosis of myeloproliferative disease. Myeloid:erythroid ratios are normal.

4 How should this patient be managed? Periodic phlebotomy and/or hydroxyurea chemotherapy can be used to control the polycythemia. Formulas for the removal of blood volumes have been described.

References
Evans LM, Caylor KB (1995) Polycythemia vera in a cat and management with hydroxyurea. *J Am Anim Hosp Assoc* **31**(5):434–438.

Nitsche EK (2004) Erythrocytosis in dogs and cats: diagnosis and management. *Compend Contin Educ Vet* **26**(2):104–118.

Watson ADJ, Moore AS, Helfand SC (1994) Primary erythrocytosis in the cat: treatment with hydroxyurea. *J Small Anim Pract* **35**(6):320–325.

CASE 181

1 What is the diagnosis? The histopathology and immunohistochemical staining are consistent with histiocytic disease. Cutaneous histiocytosis is a histiocytic proliferative disorder that presents with single or multiple lesions, which tend to wax and wane and may even regress spontaneously. It is typically a disease of young dogs. Some cases will respond to corticosteroids, while others may require more aggressive immunosuppressive therapy. The lesions occur as multiple cutaneous and subcutaneous nodules up to ~4 cm in diameter. They may regress spontaneously and then occur in other sites. E-cadherin expression is unique to Langerhans' cells (epithelial dendritic antigen-presenting cells), therefore this case most closely resembles Langerhans' cell histiocytosis (LCH).

2 What further diagnostics should be performed? In addition to the MDB, abdominal ultrasound is indicated to rule out systemic histiocytosis.

3 What is the cause of this disease? LCH is an extremely rare disorder of uncertain etiology, characterized by abnormal proliferation of cells of the dendritic cell lineage and associated with a wide clinical spectrum and varied behavior. In humans, the condition can also have a marked clinical variation in its behavior and in some patients it can be characterized by rapid systemic spread. There is considerable debate as to whether this represents a malignancy or a disorder of immune regulation. Recent studies in people with LCH have shown that 60% have a mutation in an oncogene (the *BRAF* oncogene), which is evidence of a clonal neoplastic disorder.

4 How should this patient be managed? In children with LCH limited to the skin that have minimal clinical symptoms, monitoring is advised. Likewise in dogs, as the lesions may spontaneously regress, patients may be monitored. However, in this case it was felt that the lesions were "non-regressing" and therefore therapeutic intervention earlier on was pursued. In one study, a combination of tetracycline and niacinamide was effective for approximately 80% of patients with cutaneous histiocytosis. Other treatments described include azathioprine and cyclosporine A. Prednisone is effective in only about 10% of patients. This patient was treated with tetracycline and niacinamide for its immunomodulating effects.

References

Moore PF (2014) A review of histiocytic diseases of dogs and cats. *Vet Pathol* 51:167–184.
Palmeiro BS, Morris DO, Goldschmidt MH *et al.* (2007) Cutaneous reactive histiocytosis in dogs: a retrospective evaluation of 32 cases. *Vet Dermatol* 18:332–340.

CASE 182

1 Describe the radiograph and CT scan. The plain radiograph shows no evidence of bony changes associated with the zygomatic arch. The CT scan reveals temporal muscle atrophy (**182c**, blue arrow) and masseter muscle atrophy (**182c**, purple arrow). The left trigeminal canal is widened and there is a contrast-enhancing mass located within the calvarium just dorsal to the left trigeminal canal that extends ventrally, following the trigeminal nerve (**182c**, gold

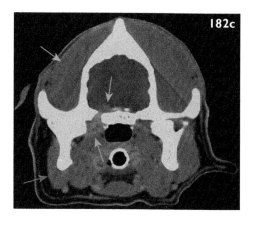

arrows). Additional CT slices showed extension of the mass along the path of the maxillary and mandibular branches of the trigeminal nerve.

2 What are the differential diagnoses for this lesion? Based on the CT findings, left trigeminal nerve neoplasia such as a nerve sheath tumor is considered most likely. Trigeminal neuritis is less likely but cannot be entirely ruled out. There is pressure resorption of the trigeminal canal, which is more common with neoplasia than with neuritis. A tissue biopsy would be necessary to make a definitive diagnosis. An MRI would be better able to help differentiate neoplasia from neuritis.

Reference

Bagley RS, Wheeler SJ, Klopp L *et al.* (1998) Clinical features of trigeminal nerve-sheath tumor in 10 dogs. *J Am Anim Hosp Assoc* 34:19–25.

CASE 183

1 Describe the radiograph (183c). There is severe lysis of the zygomatic arch extending into the maxilla. There is a small amount of new bone production and significant soft tissue swelling. A CT scan would be necessary to delineate the lesion further.

2 What are the differential diagnoses for this lesion? Considerations for this lesion include a primary bone tumor such as osteosarcoma, chondrosarcoma, or fibrosarcoma. Carcinomas, such as squamous cell carcinoma, and oral malignant melanoma can also cause bone lysis. A fine needle aspirate of the lesion was performed and cytology revealed sarcoma, most consistent with osteosarcoma. A biopsy and CT scan would be useful to make a definitive diagnosis and determine extent of disease.

3 What palliative options could be recommended? Palliative radiation would top the list of considerations for pain relief for all of the listed differential diagnoses. Bisphosphonates have been used in the palliative setting, but radiation appears superior in its analgesic effects. Provided renal function is acceptable, NSAIDs could be considered concurrently.

References

Fan TM, Charney SC, de Lorimier LP *et al.* (2009) Double-blind placebo-controlled trial of adjuvant pamidronate with palliative radiotherapy and intravenous doxorubicin for canine appendicular osteosarcoma bone pain. *J Vet Intern Med* **23**:152–160.

Fan TM, de Lorimier LP, O'Dell-Anderson K *et al.* (2007) Single-agent pamidronate for palliative therapy of canine appendicular osteosarcoma bone pain. *J Vet Intern Med* **21**:431–439.

Farcas N, Arzi B, Verstraete FJM (2014) Oral and maxillofacial osteosarcoma in dogs: a review. *Vet Comp Oncol* **12**(3):169–180.

McDonald C, Looper J, Greene S (2012) Response rate and duration associated with a 4 Gy 5 fraction palliative radiation protocol. *Vet Radiol Ultrasound* **53**:358–364.

CASE 184

1 What are the differential diagnoses for a monoclonal gammopathy? Multiple myeloma, lymphoma or other lymphoid malignancy, and chronic antigenic stimulation (atopy, tick-borne infection, heartworm) are all considerations for a monoclonal gammopathy.

2 What further diagnostic tests should be performed? A thorough physical examination to include blood pressure and retinal examination are indicated. CBC, chemistry panel, urinalysis (evaluation for Bence Jones proteinuria), skeletal radiographs, coagulation assessment, and bone marrow aspirate/biopsy should be performed.

3 What criteria need to be met to make a diagnosis of multiple myeloma? At least two of the following criteria must be met to diagnose multiple myeloma: bone marrow plasmacytosis (>20% plasma cells), osteolytic bone lesions, monoclonal gammopathy, and light chain (Bence Jones) proteinuria.

4 What treatment and prognosis can be provided for this pet? The treatment of choice for dogs with multiple myeloma is oral melphalan and prednisone. Median survival times are favorable, reported to be 540 days. The extreme hypercalcemia noted in this patient is considered a medical emergency. Aggressive saline diuresis should be initiated.

5 What are the negative prognostic indicators? The presence of extensive osteolytic bone lesions, Bence Jones proteinuria, and hypercalcemia are associated with a poorer prognosis.

Reference
Sternberg R, Wypij J, Barger AM (2009) An overview of multiple myeloma in dogs and cats. *Vet Med* 104:468–476.

CASE 185

1 What is the diagnosis? Lymphoma.

2 Describe the radiograph. What is the probable cause of the cough? The heart appears enlarged (**185d**). There is a lymph node in the cranial thorax (black

arrow) and the trachea is deviated to the right (red arrow), suggesting possible mediastinal lymphadenopathy. The parenchyma of the lungs appears normal.

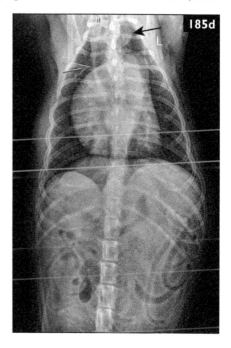

3 What further diagnostics should be performed? To complete the staging process, a urinalysis, abdominal ultrasound, and immunocytochemistry or node biopsy with immunohistochemistry are indicated. Given the cardiac enlargement and presence of a heart murmur, an echocardiogram is also indicated.

4 What is the stage of disease and how does it affect the prognosis? The subcutaneous metastasis is representative of stage V lymphoma. This dog is not exhibiting any clinical symptoms, therefore he would be considered to have stage Va disease.

While the assessment of spleen and liver with ultrasound is not necessary to assign a stage for this dog, it is important to provide a thorough evaluation and baseline of the extent of disease in this patient. The most reliable negative prognostic indicators for dogs with multicentric lymphoma include WHO substage (b worse), stage V disease with significant bone marrow involvement, high-grade histology, and T cell phenotype. Results of the immunophenotyping in this patient will help provide more prognostic information, but the presence of extensive subcutaneous involvement warrants a guarded prognosis.

5 Describe a treatment plan for this patient taking into consideration the blood work. Given the low platelet count, chemotherapy can safely be initiated with vincristine and prednisone. A multi-agent, sequential protocol is advised.

References

Jagielski D, Lechowski R, Hoffmann-Jagielska M *et al.* (2002) A retrospective study of the incidence and prognostic factors of multicentric lymphoma in dogs (1998–2000). *J Vet Med A Physiol Pathol Clin Med* **49**:419–424.

Marconato L, Stefanello D, Valenti P *et al.* (2011) Predictors of long-term survival in dogs with high-grade multicentric lymphoma. *J Am Vet Med Assoc* **238**:480–485.

Rao S, Lana S, Eickhoff J *et al.* (2011) Class II major histocompatibility complex expression and cell size independently predict survival in canine B-cell lymphoma. *J Vet Intern Med* **25**:1097–1105.

CASE 186

1 Based on the ultrasound appearance and cytology description, what is the diagnosis and stage of disease? The most likely diagnosis is gastric lymphoma. Although a biopsy or FNA and cytology of the lymph node would be needed for confirmation, the presence of regional lymph node enlargement would be consistent with stage II disease.

2 What is the most common type of lymphoma diagnosed in the stomach of cats? Primary gastric lymphoma is uncommon, with less than 20% of cats presenting with disease limited to the stomach. In contrast to other forms of GI lymphoma in cats, low-grade lymphoma is uncommon. Intermediate to high-grade lymphoma is more commonly diagnosed and B cell lymphomas appear to be more common.

3 What are the best indicators of prognosis for this form of lymphoma? In a recent study, castrated males did better than spayed females. The most reliable prognostic indicator is response to treatment. Cats achieving a complete remission had a median survival time of 431 days, in comparison to those achieving a partial remission having an MST of 138 days.

Staging of Feline Gastric Lymphoma	
Stage I	Single tumor (extranodal) or single anatomic area (nodal)
Stage II	Single tumor (extranodal) with regional lymph node involvement
Stage III	Extensive unresectable intra-abdominal disease or two or more nodal areas cranial and caudal to the diaphragm
Stage IV	I–III with liver and spleen involvement
Stage V	I–IV with initial involvement of the central nervous system and/or bone marrow

References

Gustafson TL, Villamil A, Taylor BE *et al.* (2014) A retrospective study of feline gastric lymphoma in 16 chemotherapy-treated cats. *J Am Anim Hosp Assoc* **50:**46–52.

Pohlman LM, Higginbotham ML, Welles EG *et al.* (2009) Immunophenotypic and histologic classification of 50 cases of feline gastrointestinal lymphoma. *Vet Pathol* **46:**259–268.

CASE 187

1 What is the mechanism of action of this drug? Palladia® is a small molecule inhibitor that blocks a variety of receptor tyrosine kinases (RTKs) on the cell surface. RTKs are receptors for extracellular growth factors that enable signaling to the cell interior, allowing for functions such as cell growth, survival, invasion, and angiogenesis. Dysregulation of these RTKs can lead to uncontrolled cell growth and survival, which is considered to be an underlying cause for many malignancies. The targeting of these RTKs by tyrosine kinase inhibitors such as Palladia® can inhibit tumor growth indirectly through disruption of angiogenesis or have direct anti-tumor activity. Examples of RTKs targeted by toceranib include vascular endothelial growth factor receptor (VEGFR), platelet-derived growth factor receptor (PDGFR), and KIT (stem cell factor receptor). Inhibiting VEGFR and PDGFR is believed to result in anti-angiogenic effects. Inhibition of KIT is associated with inhibition of development, survival, and proliferation of mast cells.

2 What are the indications for using Palladia®? Palladia® is labeled for use in Patnaik grade II or III, or recurrent cutaneous mast cell tumors in dogs with or without lymph node involvement. However, it has also been shown to have some activity against a variety of malignancies including anal sac gland adenocarcinoma, thyroid carcinoma, nasal carcinoma, metastatic osteosarcoma, and head and neck carcinoma. Owing to its anti-angiogenic properties, Palladia® is also used as part of metronomic chemotherapy protocols.

3 While this drug is not considered to be a chemotherapeutic agent, significant toxicities can be associated with its use. Describe the potential side effects and the management of these side effects. The most commonly reported side effects include decreased appetite, vomiting, diarrhea, lethargy, lameness, and weight loss. Less commonly, hepatotoxicity, nephrotoxicity, proteinuria, and systemic hypertension are reported. Careful evaluation of renal and liver function to include serum chemistry profile and urinalysis should be performed prior to its use. Blood pressure should be monitored before and during therapy. Dogs with mast cell tumors appear to be more susceptible to side effects because of potential complicating factors associated with the cancer itself (such as clinical or subclinical GI ulceration). Concurrent use of famotidine or omeprazole, and diphenhydramine is recommended for patients with MCT. Prednisone is indicated in some cases to decrease tumor inflammation and to decrease the release of vasoactive amines associated with tumor side effects. Other medications that can help alleviate inappetence, vomiting, or diarrhea include reglan, ondansetron, immodium, sucralfate, and metronidazole. Some authors suggest that it is best to avoid NSAIDs, especially on the same day as Palladia® is administered owing to the potential to increase gastrointestinal toxicity significantly. However, a recent report provides evidence for the safety of co-administration of toceranib and piroxicam. If melena or hematochezia is noted, Palladia® should be stopped and the patient given symptomatic therapy (e.g. sucralfate). The manufacturer recommends weekly veterinary assessment for the first 6 weeks of therapy and every 6 weeks thereafter. CBC, serum chemistry panel, urinalysis, blood pressure, body weight, and assessment of tumor for efficacy are advised for ongoing monitoring. Temporary discontinuation of the Palladia® may be necessary if anemia, azotemia, hypoalbuminemia, hyperphosphatemia, neutropenia, or significant side effects occur. Resumption of therapy at a lower dosage may be possible. The manufacturer provides parameters to monitor and also provides recommendations regarding dosage adjustments.

4 What safety precautions do pet owners need to be aware of when giving their pets Palladia®? Clients need to be advised of proper handling of this anti-cancer drug:

- Store out of the reach of children.
- Keep children away from feces, urine, or vomitus of treated dogs.
- Avoid contact with Palladia® if pregnant or nursing (can cause birth defects).
- Seek immediate medical advice if accidental ingestion occurs.
- Wear protective gloves when handling Palladia® and wash hands after use.
- Do not split or break tablets.
- Wear protective gloves when cleaning up stool, urine, or vomitus. Use disposable towels and place them in a sealable plastic bag for disposal.
- Wash any items soiled with stool, urine, or vomitus separately from other laundry.

References

Chon E, McCartan L, Kubicek LN *et al.* (2012) Safety evaluation of combination toceranib phosphate (Palladia®) and piroxicam in tumour-bearing dogs (excluding mast cell tumours): a phase I dose-finding study. *Vet Comp Oncol* 10(3):184–193.

London C, Mathie T, Stingle N *et al.* (2012) Preliminary evidence for biologic activity of toceranib phosphate (Palladia®) in solid tumors. *Vet Comp Oncol* 10(3):194–205.

CASE 188

1 What is the diagnosis? The cytology is consistent with a well-granulated mast cell tumor.

2 What factors seen in these photographs help predict the biologic behavior of this tumor? The well-granulated mast cells and long clinical history suggest a lower-grade tumor. Although histopathology is needed to grade MCTs accurately, cytologic grading can be helpful in predicting histologic grade with reasonable accuracy (94% in one study). In addition, the biologic behavior of MCTs in Pugs tends to be less aggressive than in many other breeds. One study evaluated outcome of purebred Pugs diagnosed with MCTs. It was found that over half of the Pugs had multiple tumors, and that 94% were low to intermediate grade (Patnaik system). Only high-grade (grade III) tumors behaved aggressively, with an MST of 182 days. The remainder of the MCTs exhibited relatively benign biologic behavior, even when multiple tumors were present. The median time to follow up was approximately 2 years and the MST had not been reached at publication.

3 What further diagnostic tests should be performed in order to develop a treatment plan? Complete staging is indicated. An MDB to include abdominal ultrasound should be performed. Histopathology to determine grade and mitotic index is necessary to plan treatment. In the patient pictured, the tumor is large and the ability to obtain a clean surgical excision is in question. With lower-grade tumors, more conservative margins can be considered, but this tumor is very broad based and excision may be difficult. Radiation therapy to cytoreduce the tumor may be effective with the intent to remove surgically any residual disease following radiation. Alternatively, surgical debulking followed by RT could be considered. In addition to local control of disease, for higher-grade tumors, assessment of a prognostic panel (PCR for *c-KIT* mutations, KIT staining patterns, Ki67, AgNOR, Ki67 × AgNOR) would be helpful to determine whether systemic treatment is indicated. Tyrosine kinase inhibitors may be helpful for cases possessing a *c-KIT* mutation or grade II or III KIT staining patterns, and chemotherapy for others.

Answers

References

McNiel EA, Prink AL, O'Brien TD (2006) Evaluation of risk and clinical outcome of mast cell tumours in Pug dogs. *Vet Comp Oncol* 4(1):2–8.

Scarpa F, Sabattini S, Bettini G (2014) Cytological grading of canine cutaneous mast cell tumors. *Vet Comp Oncol*, doi:10.1111/vco.12090.

Webster JD, Yuzbasiyan-Gurkan V, Miller RA *et al.* (2007) Cellular proliferation in canine cutaneous mast cell tumors: associations with *c-KIT* and its role in prognostication. *Vet Pathol* 44:298–308.

CASE 189

1 What further information should be obtained from the clinical history? It is important to know the patient's vaccination history. The American Association of Feline Practitioners recommends vaccinating cats subcutaneously as follows: rabies – below the right stifle; FeLV – below the left stifle; feline viral rhinotracheitis, calicivirus, and panleukopenia and others below the right elbow. The reason, sadly, for the more distal limb vaccination sites is to allow for complete excision by amputation of any vaccine-associated tumors. Although it is recommended to inject below the stifle, it is always possible that a vaccine has been administered in a more proximal location. More recently, subcutaneous injection in the tail has been described as a well-tolerated vaccination site.

2 What diagnostic tests are indicated? In addition to an MDB, thoracic radiography and abdominal ultrasound should be performed for staging purposes. Given the location and possible extension on the flank/abdominal body wall area, a CT scan is advised to determine the extent of disease. An incisional biopsy is advised to obtain a definitive diagnosis and can sometimes be helpful in distinguishing non-injection site sarcomas from injection site sarcomas. Vaccine-associated sarcomas are more accurately referred to as feline injection site sarcomas (FISSs), because sarcomas can occur secondary to any type of injection that induces inflammation and are not solely a result of vaccination. Inflammation is a common feature of these tumors, with lymphocytes and macrophages frequently noted at the periphery. They are frequently necrotic and have an increased mitotic index compared with non-injection site sarcomas. The cells are typically very pleomorphic. Fibrosarcoma is the most common histologic type of FISS, but other tumors such as malignant fibrous histiocytoma, undifferentiated sarcoma, osteosarcoma, rhabdomyosarcoma, liposarcoma, and chondrosarcoma have been identified.

3 What treatment options should be offered? The treatment recommendations would be dependent on the CT imaging and biopsy results. Surgical margins of 5 cm laterally and two fascial planes below the tumor have been described as the criteria for successful clean excision, but this can be difficult to achieve in most cats, especially on body wall sites. While recurrence rates were <15% and an

MST of 901 days was seen in a report describing these more radical surgeries, major complications were noted in 11% of patients. Recurrence rates tend to be high when criteria of 3 cm margins and one fascial plane below the tumor are used, even when margins appear free of tumor cells on histopathology. Wide surgical excision followed by radiation therapy is advised because recurrence rates of FISS treated with surgery alone range from 30 to 70%. The median DFI when tumor-free margins were obtained in one study was 16 months, compared to only 4 months when excision was incomplete. In patients treated with surgery and adjunct RT, median PFIs of approximately 3 years are reported. FISSs appear sensitive to chemotherapy and it is often used as an adjunct to surgery or to surgery and RT. Doxorubicin and liposome-encapsulated doxorubicin (Doxil) have been evaluated with mixed results. Epirubicin given prior to and after surgical excision provided superior rates of tumor-free survival and DFI when compared with historic controls. Immunotherapy (e.g. interleukin-2) is also currently being evaluated and appears promising. FISS cell lines are effectively inhibited by masitinib *in vitro*, suggesting a possible future role for masitinib in the treatment of FISS *in vivo*.

References

Cronin KL, Page RL, Spodnick G *et al.* (1998) Radiation therapy and surgery for fibrosarcoma in 33 cats. *Vet Radiol Ultrasound* **39**:51–56.

Hartmann K, Day MJ, Thiry E *et al.* (2015) Feline injection-site sarcoma: ACD guidelines on prevention and management. *J Fel Med Surg* **17**:606–613.

Kobayashi T, Hauck ML, Dodge R *et al.* (2002) Preoperative radiotherapy for vaccine associated sarcoma in 92 cats. *Vet Radiol Ultrasound* **43**:473–479.

Lawrence J, Saba C, Gogal R Jr *et al.* (2011) Masitinib demonstrates anti-proliferative and pro-apoptotic activity in primary and metastatic feline injection-site sarcoma cells. *Vet Comp Oncol* **10**(2):143–154.

Martano M, Morello E, Ughetto M *et al.* (2005) Surgery alone versus surgery and doxorubicin for the treatment of feline injection-site sarcomas: a report on 69 cases. *Vet J* **170**:84–90.

McEntee MC, Page RL (2001) Feline vaccine-associated sarcomas. *J Vet Intern Med* **15**:176–182.

Phelps HA, Kuntz CA, Milner RJ *et al.* (2011) Radical excision with five-centimeter margins for treatment of feline injection-site sarcomas: 91 cases (1998–2002). *J Am Vet Med Assoc* **239**:97–106.

Poirier VJ, Thamm DH, Kurzman ID *et al.* (2002) Liposome-encapsulated doxorubicin (Doxil) and doxorubicin in the treatment of vaccine-associated sarcoma in cats. *J Vet Intern Med* **16**:726–731.

Richards JR, Elston TH, Ford RB (2006) The 2006 American Association of Feline Practitioners Feline Vaccine Advisory Panel Report. *J Am Vet Med Assoc* **119**:1405–1441.

CASE 190

1 What is the presumptive diagnosis? Based on the blood smear, lymphoproliferative disease (lymphoid leukemia) is suspected.

2 What further diagnostics are needed to confirm the diagnosis? In addition to the MDB, FNA of the peripheral lymph nodes and abdominal ultrasound are indicated. Flow cytometry should be performed on the peripheral blood. Flow cytometry will help determine whether a clonal expansion of lymphocytes exists. Phenotype can be determined. The differentiation between chronic lymphocytic leukemia and acute lymphoblastic leukemia is important because the prognosis is very different. Assessing thyroid hormone status would also be indicated.

3 What are the possible reasons for the facial nerve paralysis? General causes of facial nerve paralysis include idiopathic, middle ear infections, neoplasia (nerve sheath tumors, tumors causing pressure on nerves, or brainstem lesions may affect the facial nerve), traumatic, metabolic, and inflammatory. Hypothyroidism has been proposed to be a cause of facial nerve paralysis. In this case, the leukemia is a primary consideration as a cause. Facial nerve paralysis has been described as a complication of leukemia in humans. Leukemia can affect the cranial nerves. A leukemic infiltrate around the cranial nerves can occur, or CNS spread of the disease can cause facial nerve paralysis. Resolution of the facial nerve paralysis can be seen in some cases that respond to treatment; however, it may be a permanent change.

4 How should this patient be treated? The prognosis and chemotherapy protocol are ultimately based on the results of the flow cytometry. CLL is treated with chlorambucil and prednisone and is associated with a favorable prognosis, whereas acute lymphoblastic leukemia would be treated with more aggressive chemotherapy and is associated with a poor prognosis. Because the patient was declining rapidly, vincristine and prednisone were initiated pending the results of the flow cytometry. Drugs that cross the blood–brain barrier such as CCNU can be considered if neurologic symptoms do not improve. Artificial tears are important to help prevent exposure keratitis. Ointments are generally preferred when there is no blink reflex and should be used every 4–6 hours.

References

Avery PR, Burton J, Bromberek JL *et al.* (2014) Flow cytometric characterization and clinical outcome of CD4+ T-cell lymphoma in dogs: 67 cases. *J Vet Intern Med* 28:538–546.

Bilavsky E, Scheuerman O, Marcus N *et al.* (2006) Facial paralysis as a presenting symptom of leukemia. *Pediatr Neurol* 34(6):502–504.

Christopher MM, Metz AL, Klausner J *et al.* (1986) Acute myelomonocytic leukemia with neurologic manifestations in the dog. *Vet Pathol* 23:140–147.

Comazzi S, Gelain V, Martini F *et al.* (2011) Immunophenotype predicts survival time in dogs with chronic lymphocytic leukemia. *J Vet Intern Med* 25:100–106.

Reggeti F, Bienzle D (2011) Flow cytometry in veterinary oncology. *Vet Pathol* 48(1):223–235.

CASE 191

1 What abnormality is noted in the oral cavity? There is bilateral severe tonsillar enlargement and inflammation.

2 Describe the cytology of the submandibular node. The sample consists of lymphoid tissue with increased numbers of plasma cells and reactive lymphocytes, moderate numbers of neutrophils, and clusters of very atypical epithelial cells. The epithelial cells are generally large cells with small to large amounts of moderately basophilic cytoplasm. Anisocytosis and anisokaryosis are marked. Nuclei are round with very prominent, multiple, and pleomorphic nucleoli. The cytology is consistent with a reactive lymph node with metastatic carcinoma and neutrophilic inflammation; the type of carcinoma is not clear.

3 What is the most likely diagnosis? Based on the bilateral tonsillar enlargement, tonsillar carcinoma is likely. The most common primary tonsillar cancer is squamous cell carcinoma. Cervical lymphadenopathy is a common presenting sign, even with very small primary cancers. Thoracic radiographs are positive for metastasis in 10–20% of cases at presentation. Over 90% of patients have some form of regional or distant metastasis at diagnosis.

4 What treatment options can be offered? The most aggressive treatment for tonsillar squamous cell carcinoma consists of surgical removal if localized and amenable to surgery or radiation therapy for control of local disease and chemotherapy for treatment of metastatic disease. Regional RT of the pharyngeal region and cervical lymph nodes is capable of controlling disease in >75% of cases, but overall survival times remain poor owing to metastatic disease. Therefore, treatment is generally palliative. Piroxicam has been used, with an overall response rate of <20%, in patients with bulky head and neck squamous cell carcinomas.

5 What is the prognosis for this patient? Regardless of treatment, the prognosis for tonsillar SCC remains poor with only 10% of patients alive 1 year after the diagnosis is made.

References
Mas A, Blackwood L, Cripps P *et al.* (2011) Canine tonsillar squamous cell carcinoma – a multi-centre retrospective review of 44 clinical cases. *J Small Anim Pract* 52:359–364.
Murphy S, Hayes A, Adams V *et al.* (2006) Role of carboplatin in multi-modality treatment of canine tonsillar squamous cell carcinoma – a case series of five dogs. *J Small Anim Pract* 47:216–220.

CASE 192

1 What further diagnostic/staging tests are indicated and why? Regional radiographs should be performed to evaluate for possible bone involvement. Thoracic radiographs and abdominal ultrasound are needed to rule out metastasis. In addition to the mitotic index, further evaluation of the biopsy specimen should include immunohistochemistry for Ki67, degree of nuclear atypia, and degree of pigmentation. A mitotic index of >4, increased nuclear atypia, and >50% of cells pigmented are all indicators of more aggressive disease. While most studies were done on oral malignant melanomas, these indicators can be helpful in other forms of malignant melanoma.

2 Describe a treatment plan for this patient. The prescapular lymph node should be removed. A negative aspirate does not rule out metastasis, in fact, in a study of OMM with metastasis to the regional lymph nodes, 30% of those nodes considered to be "normal" had histologic evidence of metastasis. Given the narrow margins, further local therapy is necessary. Removal of the two medial toes could achieve clean margins, but these are the weight-bearing toes. Radiation therapy should be considered. The melanoma vaccine can also be considered. Recent studies show favorable survival times in dogs with digital melanomas receiving the vaccine in conjunction with local and regional disease control.

3 What is this patient's prognosis? In this patient, histopathology of the prescapular node did not show any evidence of metastasis, and regional radiographs were normal. Interdigital melanomas that do not involve the nail bed or paw pads can have variable biologic behavior. Some behave as haired skin melanomas with a more favorable prognosis, while others behave in a more aggressive fashion. Predicting biologic behavior just by location of the tumor can be difficult, therefore histologic characteristics are important in making decisions regarding treatment. The overall MST of patients with loco-regional control of digital melanomas treated with the melanoma vaccine was 476 days, with 1-year survival rates of 63%. The MST for patients presenting without evidence of metastasis was 533 days. In this group (no metastasis), 48% were still alive at 2 and 3 years. MSTs are reported to be 365 days in patients treated with surgery alone.

References

Henry CJ, Brewer WG, Whitley EM *et al.* (2005) Canine digital tumors: a Veterinary Cooperative Oncology Group retrospective study of 64 dogs. *J Vet Intern Med* **19**:720–724.

Manley CA, Leibman NF, Wolchok IC *et al.* (2011) Xenogeneic murine tyrosinase DNA vaccine for malignant melanoma of the digit of dogs. *J Vet Intern Med* **25**:94–99.

Marino DJ, Matthiesen DT, Stefanacci JD *et al.* (1995) Evaluation of dogs with digit masses: 117 cases (1981–1991). *J Am Vet Med Assoc* **20**:726–728.

CASE 193

1 What is the interpretation of the protein electrophoresis? There is a marked monoclonal gammopathy in the gamma region.

2 What are the differential diagnoses for this patient? The monoclonal gammopathy is consistent with plasma cell myeloma or myeloma-related disorder. Rarely, ehrlichiosis or B cell lymphoma may produce a similar pattern. Ehrlichiosis is very uncommon in cats and usually is accompanied by fever and anemia. Lymphoma cannot be ruled out with the testing done thus far. Other causes of monoclonal gammopathies can include chronic pyoderma, FIP, amyloidosis, Waldenström's macroglobulinemia, and monoclonal gammopathy of unknown significance.

3 What further tests should be done to help make a definitive diagnosis? In addition to completion of an MDB (thoracic radiographs, urinalysis, FeLV/FIV testing), a fine needle aspirate of the enlarged and mottled spleen is advised. Skeletal survey radiographs looking for osteolytic lesions are indicated. A bone marrow aspirate or biopsy is also indicated. Retinal examination, coagulation profile, evaluation for Bence Jones proteinuria, blood pressure measurement, and echocardiography would complete the evaluation. The results of the splenic aspirate in this case revealed plasma cell neoplasia. The traditional criteria used to diagnose multiple myeloma include the presence of a monoclonal gammopathy, bone marrow plasmacytosis, lytic bone lesions, and Bence Jones proteinuria. Based on the common finding of extramedullary disease in cats, it has been proposed that the presence of atypical plasma cells and splenic, liver, and lymph node plasmacytosis be added to the list of diagnostic criteria for multiple myeloma in cats. When contrasting feline myeloma-related disorder with human myeloma, extramedullary involvement was determined to be more common (67% of cats affected; <5% of humans) and bone lesions less common (80% of humans affected; only 8% of cats). Other authors have reported bone lesions in cats to occur in ≤67% of patients. Other than the monoclonal gammopathy and atypical plasmacytosis in this patient's spleen, there was no further evidence of disease.

4 What treatment is indicated? Although it is not curative, patients with a significant volume of disease in the spleen may benefit from splenectomy. Chemotherapy using prednisolone and melphalan, chlorambucil, or cyclophosphamide has been described. Melphalan causes significant myelosuppression in cats and can result in a significant and prolonged thrombocytopenia. Melphalan was discontinued in >70% of cats with myeloma-related disorder in one study because of significant myelosuppression. The use of prednisolone and cyclophosphamide or chlorambucil yielded similar response rates with less toxicity.

References

Cannon CM, Knudson C, Borgatti A (2015) Clinical signs, treatment, and outcome in cats with myeloma-related disorder receiving systemic therapy. *J Am Anim Hosp Assoc* **51**:239–248.

Hanna F (2005) Multiple myelomas in cats. *J Fel Med and Surg* **7**:275–287.

Mellor PJ, Haugland S, Murphy S *et al.* (2006) Myeloma-related disorders in cats commonly present as extramedullary neoplasms in contrast to myeloma in human patients: 24 cases with clinical follow-up. *J Vet Intern Med* **20**:1376–1383.

Mellor PJ, Haugland S, Smith KC *et al.* (2008) Histopathologic, immunohistochemical, and cytologic analysis of feline myeloma-related disorders: further evidence for primary extramedullary development in the cat. *Vet Pathol* **45:**159–173.

Patel RT, Caceres A, French AF *et al.* (2005) Multiple myeloma in 16 cats: a retrospective study. *Vet Clin Pathol* **24:**341–352.

CASE 194

1 Is this patient a good candidate for further chemotherapy? Having been off all chemotherapy for 11 months, this patient is an excellent candidate for further chemotherapy, because resistance to previously used chemotherapeutic agents has not yet been demonstrated.

2 What chemotherapy recommendations should be made? The choice of a chemotherapy protocol should be made with careful consideration of the patient's general health at this time. Evaluation of renal and hepatic function is indicated to determine whether any abnormalities are present now that were not noted at the initial diagnosis. A multi-agent sequential chemotherapy protocol such as the University of Winsconsin protocol can be re-instituted, but cumulative lifetime dosage of doxorubicin has to be kept in mind. This patient received four doses of doxorubicin in the initial protocol (120 mg/m^2 total cumulative dosage) and could potentially safely receive two to four more doses for a total of 180–240 mg/m^2 total cumulative dosage. Treatment beyond this dose will significantly increase the risk of congestive heart failure. Reasonable substitutions for doxorubicin in the protocol include epirubicin, actinomycin-D, or mitoxantrone. In cases where doxorubicin appears to be the only effective agent, continued use with an iron chelator (dexrazoxane) can be considered. ECG and echocardiography are relatively insensitive predictors of doxorubicin cardiotoxicity. Routine echocardiography in conjunction with ECG prior to doxorubicin administration will detect pre-existing cardiac abnormalities, which limit doxorubicin administration in <10% of dogs, therefore the addition of echocardiography to pre-doxorubicin screening was considered a low-yield test in one study. This author recommends pre-doxorubicin screening with echocardiography and ECG in breeds with increased risk for dilated cardiomyopathy (e.g. Boxers, Dobermanns) or in patients with cardiac arrhythmias or radiographic abnormalities suggesting pre-existing heart disease.

Reference

Ratterree W, Gieger T, Pariaut R *et al.* (2012) Value of echocardiography and electrocardiography as screening tools prior to doxorubicin administration. *J Am Anim Hosp Assoc* **48:**89–96.

CASE 195

1 What is the presumptive diagnosis? The left kidney is hydronephrotic. The bladder wall is infiltrated with an irregular soft tissue mass that is affecting the trigone area and the ventral aspect of the bladder. The cytology shows a population of epithelial cells that are exhibiting significant anisocytosis, anisokaryosis, and anisonucleosis. Care must be taken in differentiating malignant epithelial cells from dysplastic cells that can be present in severe inflammation. The ultrasound and cytology findings are most consistent with transitional cell carcinoma.

2 What other staging/diagnostic tests are important in the assessment of this patient? An MDB should be performed to evaluate thoracic radiographs for possible metastasis. A urinalysis should be obtained by free-catch or urinary catheter only – because of the infiltrative disease along the bladder wall, cystocentesis should be avoided. Renal function should be assessed (BUN, creatinine, phosphorus, urine specific gravity). On ultrasound, careful attention should be paid to the contralateral kidney, ureters, prostate, and sublumbar nodes.

3 What measures can be taken to help prevent further damage to the kidney? In this case, the left kidney has become hydronephrotic because of an outflow obstruction caused by the tumor in the trigone. A ureteral stent should be considered for this patient.

CASE 196

1 What is the diagnosis for this patient? The CD21 lymphocytosis represents a clonal expansion of B cells, which is consistent with a primary leukemia or stage V lymphoma.

2 What is the significance of the size of the lymphocytes? Studies have shown that, with a CD21 lymphocytosis, the cell size is prognostic. Small lymphocytes are associated with a significantly better prognosis than large lymphocytes. A criterion of the size of lymphocytes in comparison to red blood cells has been used:
- Small lymphocytes: the nucleus of the cell is 1× the diameter of a canine RBC.
- Intermediate: 1.5–2× the diameter of an RBC.
- Large: 2–2.5× diameter of an RBC.

3 What does the lack of CD34+ cells mean? CD34 is a marker for undifferentiated progenitor cells. CD34+ lymphocytes indicate an acute lymphoblastic leukemia and are associated with a grave prognosis.

4 What treatment should be offered? With the borderline classification, a multi-agent CHOP-based protocol should be considered.

Reference
Williams MJ, Avery AC, Lana SE *et al*. Canine lymphoproliferative disease characterized by lymphocytosis: immunophenotypic markers of prognosis. *J Vet Intern Med* 22:596–601.

CASE 197

1 Describe the thoracic radiograph and the fluid obtained on thoracocentesis.
Pleural effusion with no obvious masses present. Post-thoracocentesis radiographs
did not reveal an etiology for the effusion. The fluid is milky white. The primary
considerations are a chylous effusion or a pseudo-chylous effusion.

**2 Based on the appearance of the fluid, what are the primary considerations? The
analysis of the fluid is shown. What is your diagnosis?** The analysis of the fluid
shown here was consistent with a true chylous effusion. It is thought that chylous
effusion results when there is abnormal flow or pressures in the thoracic duct
leading to leaking of chyle from the duct rather than from a ruptured duct. Trauma
is considered an unlikely cause. Causes of chylous effusion include any disease
that increases systemic venous pressure (right heart failure, mediastinal neoplasia,
cranial vena cava thrombi, or granulomas). The chylomicrons present give the fluid
the milky white appearance. In patients that are anorexic, a chylous effusion may
not have the characteristic white appearance because there are fewer chylomicrons
present. Triglyceride and cholesterol levels can be evaluated. In chylous effusion,
the triglyceride levels are increased and cholesterol levels decreased when compared
with serum levels.

3 What are the next diagnostic steps following the fluid analysis? Echocardiography
should be performed. In this case, the heart was normal and no obvious masses
were detected on ultrasound. After documenting that the heart function is normal,
a CT scan should be performed to evaluate for the possibility of neoplasia. A small
lymph node was noted in the mediastinum at the time of CT scan and an ultrasound-
guided aspirate confirmed lymphoma. Immunocytochemistry documented B cell
lymphoma. The patient responded very well to chemotherapy and the effusion
resolved. In some patients, the chylous effusion does not resolve immediately on
treatment, but can persist for several weeks or more.

Reference
Birchard SJ, Fossum TW (1987) Chylothorax in the dog and cat. *Vet Clin North Am Small
Anim Pract* **17**:271–283.

CASE 198

1 What additional tests should be performed prior to a CT scan? An abdominal
ultrasound is indicated to look for a primary tumor. In this case, a gastric mass
was seen. Based on this finding, a CT scan was performed of both the thoracic and
abdominal cavities.

**2 A CT image at the level of the stomach is shown (198c, orange arrow indicates
stomach wall, green arrows point to mass). In addition to the solitary thoracic mass,**

a mass in the gastric wall was confirmed. FNA of the lung mass was attempted but was non-diagnostic. What should be done to obtain a definitive diagnosis? Following the CT scan, it was not certain whether the gastric mass was related to the lung mass. The symptoms related to the stomach mass were significant and the prognosis for gastric neoplasia tends to be very guarded, so a decision was made to remove the gastric mass first to obtain a histologic diagnosis. However, this left the lung mass undiagnosed.

3 The symptoms attributable to the gastric mass predominated, therefore an exploratory laparotomy was performed in order to remove the gastric mass. There was a well-circumscribed mass in the gastric wall (198d). Histopathology revealed an undifferentiated round cell tumor. CD3 and CD79a were negative and CD18 was positive. What is the diagnosis? The IHC supports the diagnosis of histiocytic sarcoma. Based on this diagnosis, it was suspected that the lung mass was also HS.

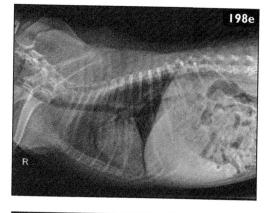

4 What is the suggested course of treatment and the prognosis for this patient? Based on the diagnosis of HS, CCNU chemotherapy was started and, 3 weeks post-treatment, radiographs of the thorax were taken that showed significant reduction in the size of the lung mass (198e, f). On the lateral thoracic radiograph, the mass is barely visible. On the VD view, the arrow points to remaining mass tissue. Despite the excellent response to CCNU, the prognosis for HS remains poor. MSTs with CCNU for HS are approximately 3 months.

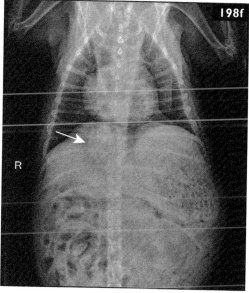

Answers

References

Caccon C, Borgatti A, Henson M *et al.* (2015) Evaluation of a combination chemotherapy protocol including lomustine and doxorubicin in canine histiocytic sarcoma. *J Small Anim Pract* **56**:425–429.

Moore PF (2014) A review of histiocytic disease of dogs and cats. *Vet Pathol* **5**:167–184.

Rassnick KM, Moore AS, Russell DS *et al.* (2010) Phase II, open-label trial of single-agent CCNU in dogs with previously untreated histiocytic sarcoma. *J Vet Intern Med* **24**:1528–1531.

Skorupski KA, Clifford CA, Paoloni MC *et al.* (2007) CCNU for the treatment of dogs with histiocytic sarcoma. *J Vet Intern Med* **21**:121–126.

CASE 199

1 What is the diagnosis? The spleen has a moth-eaten appearance consistent with infiltrative disease. In addition to peripheral blood, the majority of cells obtained from the splenic aspirate were poorly to moderately granulated mast cells. This represents splenic metastasis of the mast cell tumor.

2 What further diagnostic tests are indicated? Because this patient already had a confirmed high-grade mast cell tumor with a proliferation panel done, further histopathology of the spleen will not necessarily change the treatment plan. Ultrasound evaluation of the liver for metastatic mast cell disease is not sensitive for detecting metastatic MCT. For example, even if the ultrasound appearance of the liver is normal, aspiration is needed to rule out mast cell disease. Studies have shown that the sensitivity of ultrasound in detecting splenic mast cell disease is approximately 43%, but it is 0% for the liver. Buffy coat analysis or a bone marrow aspirate will help in determining bone marrow involvement. However, documentation of liver or bone marrow infiltration in this case is not likely to change the treatment recommendation. In some patients with extremely large spleens, splenectomy can help reduce the tumor burden, but chemotherapy is still required.

3 What treatment should be considered for this patient? Because the patient has failed chemotherapy with CCNU, vinblastine, and prednisone, the treatment choices are limited. Additional chemotherapy drugs/protocols can be considered. Chlorambucil and prednisolone have been described for the treatment of inoperable MCTs; protocols utilizing cyclophosphamide and single-agent hydroxyurea have also been described. A combination of vinblastine and toceranib phosphate has been evaluated for safety. The initial tumor in this patient was of KIT pattern 2, therefore the use of toceranib phosphate could be considered.

Answers

References

Book AP, Fidel J, Wills T *et al.* (2011) Correlation of ultrasound findings, liver and spleen cytology, and prognosis in the clinical staging of high metastatic risk canine mast cell tumors. *Vet Radiol Ultrasound* 52:548–554.

Camps-Palau MA, Leibman NF, Elmslie R *et al.* (2007) Treatment of canine mast cell tumours with vinblastine, cyclophosphamide and prednisone: 35 cases (1997–2004). *Vet Comp Oncol* 5:156–167.

Hayes A, Adams V, Smith K *et al.* (2007) Vinblastine and prednisolone chemotherapy for surgically excised grade III canine cutaneous mast cell tumours. *Vet Comp Oncol* 5:168–176.

Rassnick KM, Al-Sarraf R, Bailey DB *et al.* (2010) Phase II open-label study of single-agent hydroxyurea for treatment of mast cell tumours in dogs. *Vet Comp Oncol* 8:103–111.

Rassnick KM, Bailey DB, Russell DS *et al.* (2010) A phase II study to evaluate the toxicity and efficacy of alternating CCNU and high-dose vinblastine and prednisone (CVP) for the treatment of dogs with high-grade, metastatic or nonresectable mast cell tumours. *Vet Comp Oncol* 8:138–152.

Taylor F, Gear R, Hoather T *et al.* (2009) Chlorambucil and prednisone chemotherapy for dogs with inoperable mast cell tumours: 21 cases. *J Small Anim Pract* 50:284–289.

Thamm DH, Turek MM, Vail DM (2006) Outcome and prognostic factors following adjuvant prednisone/vinblastine chemotherapy for high-risk canine mast cell tumors: 61 cases. *J Vet Med Sci* 68:581–587.

CASE 200

1 Describe the findings on abdominal radiographs, blood work, and ultrasound. Lateral abdominal radiograph: there is a circumscribed mass in the mid abdomen. There is a mild anemia, moderate thrombocytopenia, and moderate neutropenia present. Bleeding from the intestinal mass is a likely cause of the anemia and thrombocytopenia. The abdominal ultrasound revealed a 3.32 × 3.55 cm mass associated with the duodenum.

2 What further tests should be performed? If deemed accessible based on ultrasound, a fine needle aspirate could be considered. In this case, FNA was performed and yielded a population of mesenchymal cells. Prior to consideration of surgery, coagulation parameters should be assessed.

3 A surgical exploratory was performed. A lobulated, firm mass was found associated with the anti-mesenteric border of the proximal duodenum opposite the pancreatic duct. The mass was well encapsulated. A marginal resection was performed owing to the proximity of the mass to the pancreatic duct. Histopathology was consistent with a soft tissue spindle cell sarcoma. There was a normal thin rim of connective tissue microscopically, but clean margins could not be confirmed. **What are the diagnostic considerations?** Based on the biopsy results and the location of the mass, a soft tissue sarcoma of smooth muscle origin is likely. Differential diagnoses include leiomyoma, leiomyosarcoma, and gastrointestinal stromal tumor (GIST).

4 **How would results of immunohistochemistry be helpful in this patient?** Immunohistochemistry staining for KIT is helpful in diagnosing GIST. Immunolabeling for KIT protein was positive, consistent with GIST. Approximately 90% of neoplastic cells showed strong positive cytoplasmic labeling for KIT protein. Based on this finding, treatment with tyrosine kinase inhibitors should be considered, especially with incomplete surgical margins.

5 **What is the prognosis for this patient?** GISTs are associated with an excellent prognosis in comparison with leiomyosarcoma or undifferentiated carcinoma. Median survival time with surgery was 37.4 months in one study. GISTs are a unique group of mesenchymal tumors that arise from the interstitial cells of Cajal, which regulate gastrointestinal motility. They were previously commonly misdiagnosed as leiomyosarcomas, a problem overcome by the use of immunohistochemical staining.

References

Gregory-Bryson E, Bartlett E, Kiupel M *et al.* (2010) Canine and human gastrointestinal stromal tumors display similar mutations in *c-KIT* exon 11. *BMC Cancer* **10**:559–568.

Hayes S, Yuzbasiyan-Gurkan V, Gregory-Bryson E *et al.* (2013) Classification of canine nonangiogenic, nonlymphogenic, gastrointestinal sarcomas based on microscopic, immunohistochemical, and molecular characteristics. *Vet Pathol* **50**:779–788.

Hobbs J, Sutherland-Smith J, Penninck D *et al.* (2015) Ultrasonographic features of canine gastrointestinal stromal tumors compared to other gastrointestinal spindle cell tumors. *Vet Radiol Ultrasound* **56**:432–438.

Morini M, Bettini G, Preziosi R *et al.* (2004) C-kit gene product (CD117) immunoreactivity in canine and feline paraffin sections. *J Histochem Cytochem* **52**:705–708.

Russell KN, Mehler SJ, Skorupski KA *et al.* (2007) Clinical and immunohistochemical differentiation of gastrointestinal stromal tumors from leiomyosarcomas in dogs: 42 cases (1990–2003). *J Am Vet Med Assoc* **230**:1329–1333.

CASE 201

1 **Interpret the radiograph and cytology.** On the radiograph, soft tissue swelling is noted, but there is no evidence of bone involvement. On cytology, individual to stellate nucleated cells exhibiting moderate to marked anisocytosis and anisokaryosis are seen. There is a finely stippled chromatin pattern, with multiple medium to large nucleoli present. There are multinucleated cells with marked intracellular anisokaryosis. Some of the cells have very large and irregularly shaped nucleoli (blue arrow). There are several mitotic figures (arrows). The cytology is consistent with sarcoma.

2 **What are the differential diagnoses for this patient?** Considerations based on tumor location and cytologic appearance include histiocytic sarcoma (HS), synovial cell sarcoma, or an undifferentiated neoplasm.

3 **What further diagnostics should be performed?** In addition to the MDB, an abdominal ultrasound and tissue biopsy are recommended. The treatment of choice based on the location and local invasiveness of the patient's tumor would be amputation.

4 **What is this patient's prognosis?** The prognosis can vary significantly depending on histologic tumor type and stage (localized vs. disseminated). Periarticular HS (PAHS), if localized at the time of initial diagnosis, carries a far better prognosis than other forms of HS that are disseminated. One study evaluated synovial cell sarcoma and PAHS treated with amputation alone. In the synovial cell sarcoma group, MST was 30.7 months, vs. 5.3 months for the HS group. Another more recent study looked at the difference in MST for dogs with PAHS in comparison with HS at other sites when treated with aggressive local therapy (amputation or radiation) and chemotherapy (CCNU). PAHS had an MST of 980 days (32.6 months) when disease was initially localized, and HS of other sites had an MST of 128 days (4.2 months). PAHS patients that had metastasis at diagnosis had an MST of 253 days (8.4 months). In this study, Rottweilers and Golden Retrievers were the most common breeds diagnosed with PAHS.

References

Klahn SL, Kitchell BE, Dervisis NG (2011) Evaluation and comparison of outcomes in dogs with periarticular and nonperiarticular histiocytic sarcoma. *J Am Vet Med Assoc* **239**:90–96.

Vail DM, Powers BE, Getzy DM *et al.* (1994) Evaluation of prognostic factors for dogs with synovial sarcoma: 36 cases (1986–1991). *J Am Vet Med Assoc* **205**:1300–1307.

CASE 202

1 **Describe the ultrasound findings.** The kidney is enlarged and abnormal in shape. There is hypoechoic subcapsular thickening present. The cortex of the kidney appears hyperechoic and is being distorted by the mass.

2 **Based on the ultrasound alone, what are the differential diagnoses for this patient?** The finding of hypoechoic subcapsular thickening is highly suggestive of renal lymphoma. In fact, approximately 80% of patients with this ultrasound finding are ultimately confirmed to have renal lymphoma. Other tumors (undifferentiated cancers, renal carcinoma) are possible but less likely given the bilateral renal changes. Non-malignant diseases that can present with this ultrasound appearance include chronic active nephritis and FIP-associated necrotizing vasculitis.

3 **Cytology obtained from an FNA of this renal mass is shown (202b). What is your diagnosis?** Aspiration with ultrasound guidance of the subcapsular material is consistent with lymphoma.

4 What impact does the azotemia have on predicting outcome for this patient? The azotemia in this case is mild and the specific gravity is normal. With rehydration and treatment of the lymphoma, there is an excellent chance that the azotemia will resolve. Even in patients with more severe azotemia, renal function can return to normal following treatment. In some patients whose kidneys have been severely compromised, renal function may not improve.

5 How do the neurologic symptoms relate to this cancer? In one study, up to 50% of patients with renal lymphoma suffered extension of disease into the CNS. For this reason, some oncologists advocate the inclusion of chemotherapy agents that are capable of crossing the blood–brain barrier (e.g. CCNU, cytosine arabinoside, prednisone) in chemotherapy protocols. The CNS spread of lymphoma can occur within the brain, the spine, or both. Cats with spinal lymphoma often have renal involvement, so it is not clear where the lymphoma actually originated when CNS involvement is seen. Full clinical staging of the lymphoma is important, as the majority of renal patients have multi-organ involvement.

6 How has this disease changed over time? In the past, 75% of cats diagnosed with renal lymphoma were young and FeLV positive. More recently, the median age of diagnosis is at least 9 years and it is most commonly not associated with FeLV.

7 What is this patient's prognosis? In one report, MST for cats treated with chemotherapy was 7 months. A response rate of approximately 60% has been noted.

References
Mooney SC, Hayes AA, Matus R *et al.* (1987) Renal lymphoma in cats: 28 cases (1977–1984). *J Am Vet Med Assoc* **191**:1473–1477.

Moore A (2013) Extranodal lymphoma in the cat. Prognostic factors and treatment options. *J Feline Med Surg* **15**:379–390.

Taylor SS, Goodfellow MR, Browne WJ *et al.* (2009) Feline extranodal lymphoma: response to chemotherapy and survival in 110 cats. *J Small Anim Pract* **50**:584–592.

Valdes-Martinez A, Cianciolo R, Mai W (2007) Association between renal hypoechoic subcapsular thickening and lymphosarcoma in cats. *Vet Radiol Ultrasound* **48**:357–360.

CASE 203

1 What is the association between the clinical symptoms and the mediastinal mass? The clinical symptoms described in this patient are most likely due to myasthenia gravis (MG), a paraneoplastic syndrome that can occur in patients with thymoma. MG is the most common paraneoplastic syndrome seen with thymoma and is an immune-mediated process caused by the formation of antibodies against the acetylcholine receptors at the neuromuscular junction.

2 What further diagnostic tests should be performed? Demonstration of the acetylcholine receptor antibodies through immunoprecipitation radioimmunoassay

(University of California, San Diego) is necessary to confirm the diagnosis of MG. Distinguishing between lymphoma and thymoma can often be difficult clinically. Thoracic ultrasound can be helpful in differentiating lymphoma from thymoma, but does not provide a definitive diagnosis. Mediastinal lymphoma tends to be more solid and thymoma more cystic on ultrasound. Ultrasound-guided fine needle aspiration or needle core biopsy can be performed for a preoperative diagnosis. Flow cytometry on mediastinal aspirates is a useful tool for preoperative diagnosis. All cases of thymoma in one study consisted of ≥10% lymphocytes co-expressing CD4 and CD8, a phenotype that is characteristic of thymocytes. In comparison, the majority of lymphomas contained <2% CD4+CD8+ lymphocytes. Thoracic CT can be helpful for surgical planning, especially when tumors are very large and appear invasive.

3 What preoperative management should be instituted? Pyridostigmine bromide (Mestinon®) should be instituted preoperatively. For patients with evidence of megaesophagus, a high calorie semi-solid diet fed in an upright position should be utilized. Pro-motility drugs and H2 receptor blockers will help decrease the risk of aspiration pneumonia.

References
Lana S, Plaza S, Hampe K *et al.* (2006) Diagnosis of mediastinal masses in dogs by flow cytometry. *J Vet Intern Med* **20**:1161–1165.

Patterson MME, Marolf AJ (2014) Sonographic characteristics of thymoma compared with mediastinal lymphoma. *J Am Anim Hosp Assoc* **50**:409–413.

Shelton GD, Schule A, Kass PH (1997) Risk factors for acquired myasthenia gravis in dogs: 1,154 cases (1991–1995). *J Am Vet Med Assoc* **211**:1428.

Warzee CC (2012) Hemolymphatic system. In: Kudnig ST, Séguin B, editors, *Veterinary Surgical Oncology*, 1st edition. Chichester, Wiley-Blackwell, pp. 449–454.

Index

Note: References are to case numbers, not page numbers.

Index

Index

Index

Also available in the Self-Assessment Color Review series

Brown & Rosenthal: *Small Mammals*
Elsheikha & Patterson: *Veterinary Parasitology*
Forbes & Altman: *Avian Medicine*
Freeman: *Veterinary Cytology*
Frye: *Reptiles and Amphibians 2nd Edition*
Hartmann & Levy: *Feline Infectious Diseases*
Hartmann & Sykes: *Canine Infectious Diseases*
Keeble, Meredith & Richardson: *Rabbit Medicine and Surgery 2nd Edition*
Kirby, Rudloff & Linklater: *Small Animal Emergency and Critical Care Medicine 2nd Edition*
Lewbart: *Ornamental Fishes and Aquatic Invertebrates 2nd Edition*
Lewis & Langley-Hobbs: *Small Animal Orthopedics, Rheumatology & Musculoskeletal Disorders 2nd Edition*
Mair & Divers: *Equine Internal Medicine 2nd Edition*
May & McIlwraith: *Equine Orthopaedics and Rheumatology*
Meredith & Keeble: *Wildlife Medicine and Rehabilitation*
Moriello: *Small Animal Dermatology*
Moriello & Diesel: *Small Animal Dermatology, Advanced Cases*
Pycock: *Equine Reproduction and Stud Medicine*
Samuelson & Brooks: *Small Animal Ophthalmology*
Scott: *Cattle and Sheep Medicine 2nd Edition*
Sparkes & Caney: *Feline Medicine*
Tennant: *Small Animal Abdominal and Metabolic Disorders*
Thieman-Mankin: *Small Animal Soft Tissue Surgery 2nd Edition*
Verstraete & Tsugawa: *Veterinary Dentistry 2nd Edition*
Ware: *Small Animal Cardiopulmonary Medicine*

Printed and bound by CPI Group (UK) Ltd, Croydon, CR0 4YY

23/10/2024

01777696-0005